Add **THIS** to Your Plate!

Mastering the Essentials in Cooking, Nutrition, and Fitness for the New and Seasoned Mom

Copyright © 2018 Danielle Formaro

All rights reserved. No part of this book may be used or reproduced in any manner whatsoever without prior written consent of the authors, except as provided by the United States of America copyright law.

Published by Best Seller Publishing®, Pasadena, CA
Best Seller Publishing® is a registered trademark
Printed in the United States of America.
ISBN: 978-1-946978-93-6

This publication is designed to provide accurate and authoritative information with regard to the subject matter covered. It is sold with the understanding that the publisher is not engaged in rendering legal, accounting, or other professional advice. If legal advice or other expert assistance is required, the services of a competent professional should be sought. The opinions expressed by the authors in this book are not endorsed by Best Seller Publishing® and are the sole responsibility of the author rendering the opinion.

Most Best Seller Publishing® titles are available at special quantity discounts for bulk purchases for sales promotions, premiums, fundraising, and educational use. Special versions or book excerpts can also be created to fit specific needs.

For more information, please write:
Best Seller Publishing®
1346 Walnut Street, #205
Pasadena, CA 91106
or call 1(626) 765 9750
Toll Free: 1(844) 850-3500
Visit us online at: www.BestSellerPublishing.org

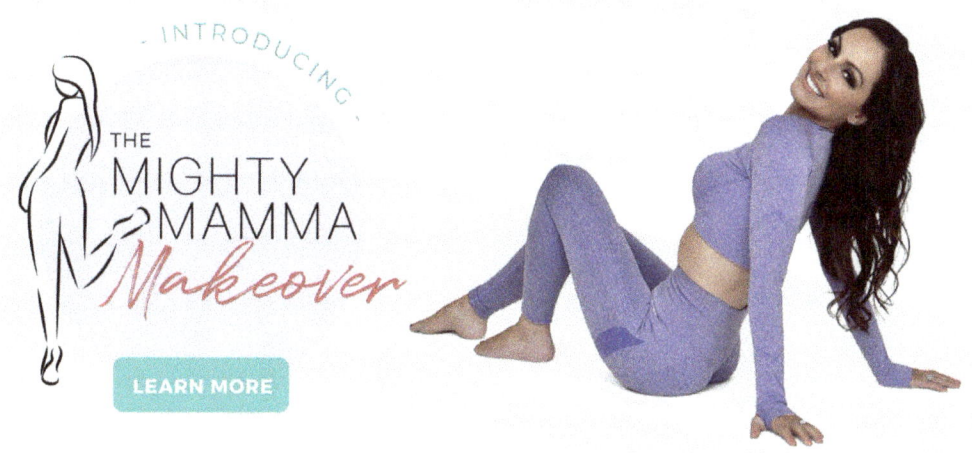

Get the results you've always wanted and keep them **forever**!

My Gift To You!

Transform your wellness routine with a special 20% discount on my Mighty Mamma Makeover Program. Benefit from personalized virtual fitness & nutrition training, tailored just for you, and flexible scheduling to match your busy life. Book your session today and take the first step towards a new you!

As Seen On:

 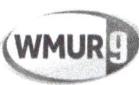 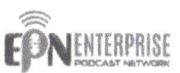 

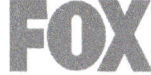 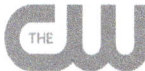 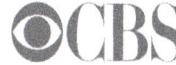

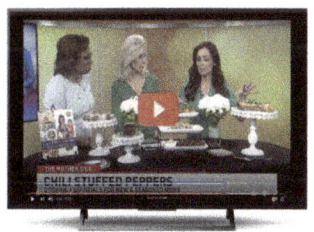 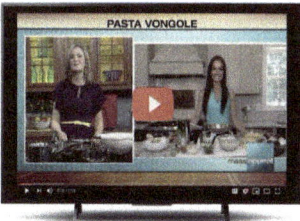 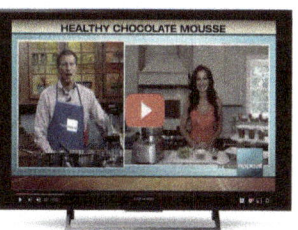

To Learn More: Go to mightymammafitness.com
Book Your Free Consultation Today!

DEDICATION

To my mom, who not only taught me how to cook, but how to put love into everything I do. From my first sauce to my first hand-rolled meatball, she was the one that started my passion for cooking. Not only did she teach me how to cook, but how to become the woman I am today. She taught me about family values, ethics, and generosity. She taught me how to gain inner strength, to be a leader, and to have the confidence to do anything I wanted in life. She made me believe if I tried hard enough, I was capable of anything. Thank you, mom, for always believing in me. You are my rock, my second set of eyes and the glue that kept our family bond so strong all these years.

To my dad, one of my biggest supporters and also one of my favorite meal partners. Not only did my dad's passion for food get passed down to me, but also his impressive work ethic. My father was and still is one of the hardest working people I know. I want to thank him for being such a great role model for me, always putting 200% into everything thing he did. My father is such a go-getter, growing up he really set the bar for what discipline and dedication looked like. Thank you, dad, for all your love and support and thank you for setting such an incredible example for our family.

To my pretty nana, who, like my mom, taught me how to cook and entertain. She had a love for hosting parties for friends and family, and it's no wonder I do too! She was a firecracker, her laugh was contagious, and all that knew her, loved her. She is greatly missed, but every time I cook, I feel her next to me in spirit. She was my biggest fan, and this book would have made her so proud.

To my son, Giorgio, who was the best baby food critic I could have asked for. I couldn't have written this book without you, as you were my inspiration from the very start. From the moment you were born you filled my plate, and will always and forever fill my heart.

To my husband, Steve, my soul mate, for all your love and support throughout this entire process. You make my heart smile, and my soul complete. I look forward to sharing many more plates together and creating many more memorable years to come.

To all the moms in the world that are ready to kick some major ass being the rock stars that they are.

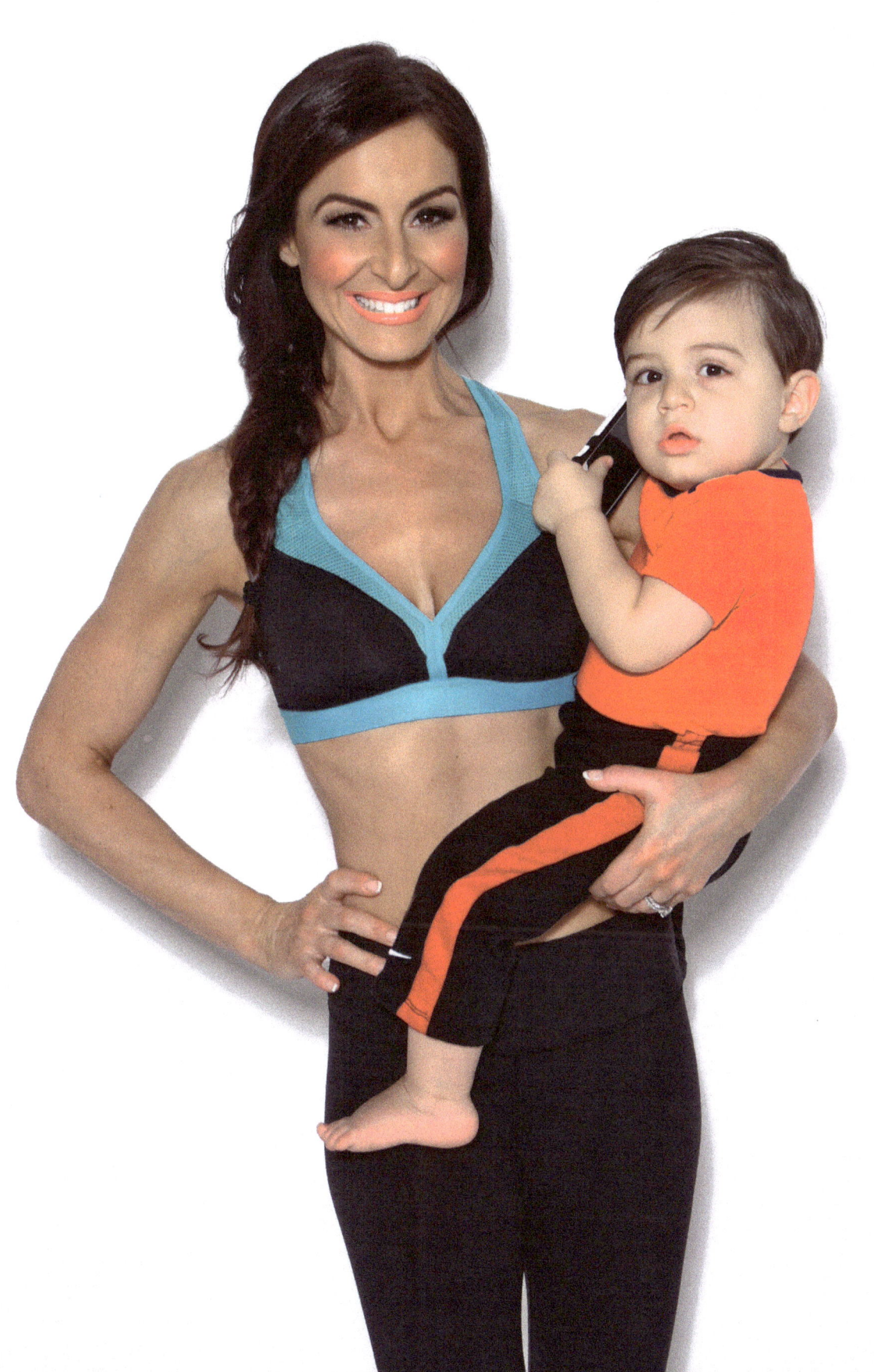

ABOUT THE AUTHOR

DANIELLE F ORMARO is an international best-selling author, a proud army wife, mother of two boys, and a fitness & nutrition professional with credentials from the prestigious Athletics and Fitness Association of America & the National Academy of Sports Medicine.

Danielle is dedicated to empowering moms through her multi-faceted approach to wellness. Her offerings include online weight loss programs, postnatal healing, wellness coaching, and live group fitness via her on-demand streaming service.

With over 20 years of experience in the food and restaurant industry, Danielle's expertise extends far beyond fitness. Not only has she opened her own nutrition supplement line, but as a former restaurateur, she blends her passions for health and cuisine by hosting online cooking classes and collaborating with major TV networks like NBC, FOX, CBS, and ABC. Through monthly demonstrations, she provides expert advice on nutrition, healthy cooking, and fitness, reaching diverse audiences nationwide.

In addition to her fitness and nutrition work, Danielle is a versatile author, offering children's books, cookbooks, and literature on motherhood. Her vision and leadership have touched lives across the globe through her "Strong as a Mother" movement, which now inspires and supports hundreds of thousands of women worldwide.

CONTENTS

Introduction 1

Creating Effective Time Management 7

Welcoming the Kitchen to the Family 11

Getting to Know Your Kitchen Tools & Appliances 13

Getting to Know Your Pots & Pans 19

Culinary Jargon Explained 25

Holy Smokes! The Truth About Oils 31
    The Skinny on Fat and Nutrition 20-21 34

Let's Get to the Meat of It 21-22 35
    Give it a Rest 36
    Playing it Safe 36

Playing it Safe In The Kitchen For Baby 39
    Foods to Hold Off On For Baby 39
    Important Notes While Preparing Food 40
    Preparation After Cooking 40
    Freezing Foods 41
    Thawing or Reheating Foods 41
    Avoiding Spreading Bacteria to other Foods 41
    Allergies and Intolerances 42
    So What's The Big Stink 43
    Preventing Choking 44

When to Add These Foods to Your Baby's Plate 45

Just You and Your Bundle of Love 49

Adding Solids to Your Baby's Plate 51

    Signs Your Baby is Ready 51

    Signs You Should Wait 51

    Recipes: Baby's First Cereals 53

    Recipes: Baby's First Purees 57

    Recipes: Favorite Puree Combos: Let's Mix it Up 65

    Recipes: Pureed Meats 76

    Creating New and Exciting Plates 77

The Family Plate 103

    Recipes: What's For Breakfast 103

    Recipes: Soups, Salads, Sandwiches 121

    Leaving a Legacy At The Dinner Table 141

    Recipes: Dinner 142

    Recipes: On The Side 195

    Recipes: The Sweet Tooth 213

Getting Back In The Saddle 233

    #momproblems 233

    Training the Mind Through Personal Development 234

    Once and For All, The Truth About Weight Loss and Carbs 235

    Portion Control 237

    Meal Prepping and Planning Ahead 239

    Finding a Fitness Program That Works For You 243

    Stop Looking At The Scale 244

    Fat Vs Muscle 245

    Finding a Success Partner 247

    Saving the Best Recipe for Last 248

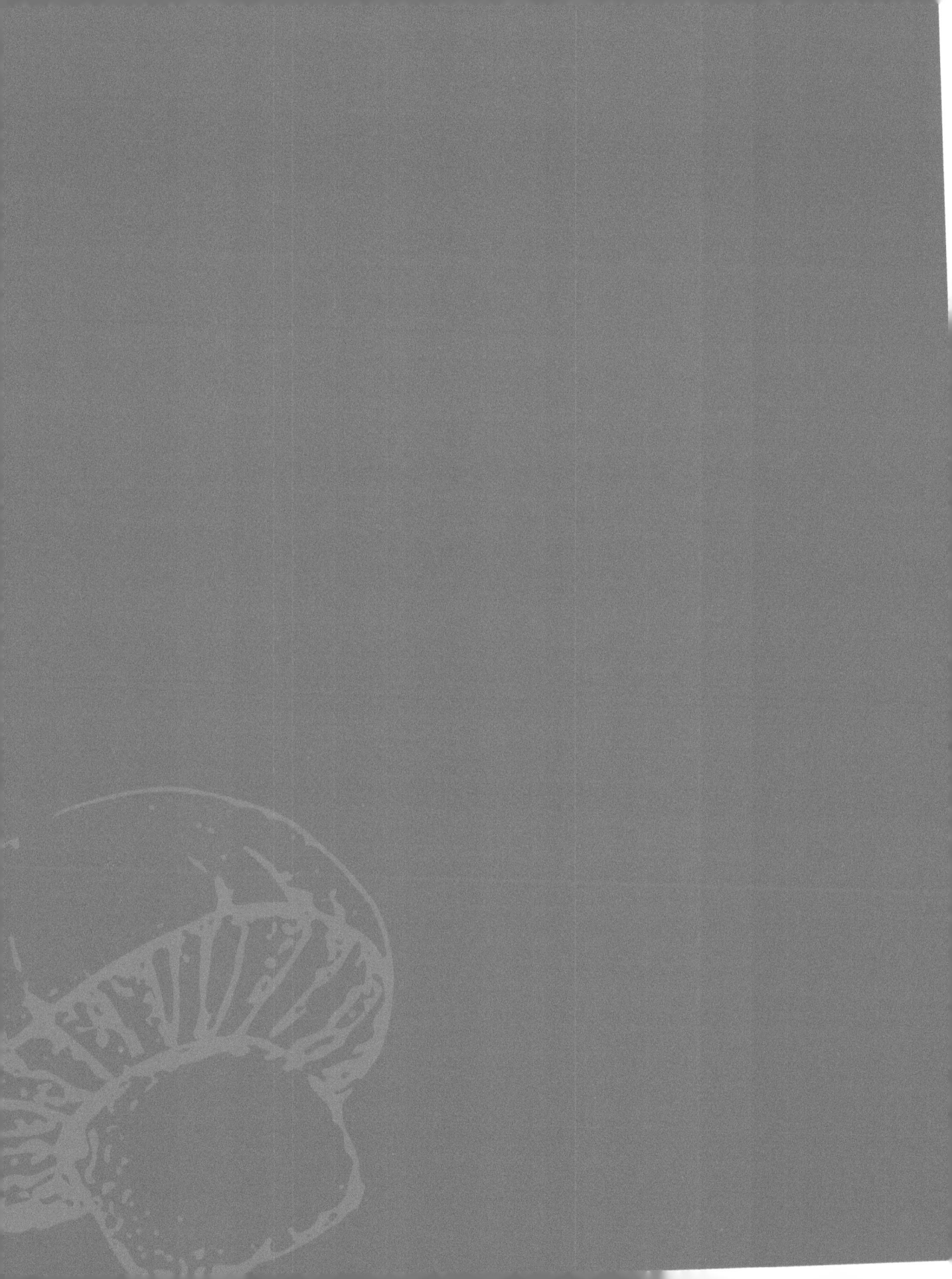

Introduction

The Woman With Eight Great Arms, Covered On The Underside By Tiny Sucker Charms...

(Quote inspired by my son's favorite children's book, "The Pout Pout Fish")

We women constantly pile new things onto our plates; if not in our minds, then literally, on our plates—hence, the dreaded mommy weight-gain! As our to-do lists continue to grow, we always (somehow) find a way to add even MORE to our smorgasbord of STUFF. It just never ends. Once upon a time, it was enough that women ran the household and raised the children. Now we've added so much more to our plates. We now have more roles than a French bakery!

Today's woman is expected to be everywhere and to be everyone ALL AT THE SAME TIME. Women are corporate executives, wives, moms, chefs, personal assistants, teachers, chauffeurs, therapists, party hosts, sex goddesses, housekeepers, janitors, magicians, and even handymen... oh, excuse me... "handy-women." We do it all, and we do it in stride. Our closets are filled to the brim with the number of hats we wear on a daily basis.

To make matters even more difficult, moms feel the added pressure of wearing multiple hats while still rocking a pre-child wardrobe. We grow miracles in our bodies, and upon delivery of our new angels from above, we are expected to go right back to our pre-baby bodies in just a few weeks! Piece of cake, right? I think we would all rather enjoy a piece of cake (with a side of hot fudge).

But seriously, am I right or am I right? The answer is YES...and that is because we ARE ALL CRAZY and bite off WAY MORE THAN WE CAN CHEW! We are superheroes, remember? We are mighty mammas! I know, I know, you may not feel like one at times, but give yourself some credit. You are stronger than you realize and you will survive. Let's just take this one step at a time, shall we?

When I first got married, I remember friends asking me how I did it all. They wanted to know how I worked full time, stayed fit and managed to find time to cook a homemade meal every night. I am not talking mac 'n' cheese my friends; I mean restaurant-style spreads like beef tenderloin and garlic mash, whole roast chicken with fingerling potatoes, or perhaps lollipop lamb chops with rice pilaf and grilled Mediterranean vegetables. Sounds good, right? (Have no fear, the recipes are listed later in this book.) I am not going to tell you it was easy, because it wasn't. I made the time. I mustered up every last bit of energy. I had it together.

When I had my firstborn, all hell broke loose with my girlfriends. "Danielle, how the hell did you do it?" You had a baby, lost all your baby weight in record time (under 5 months), you still work full-time, AND you cook dinner every night? WHAT?" Again, let me just reiterate, it was not a walk in the park. I was determined; it was my mindset.

A little about my personal plate at the time. Besides being a mom and a wife, I was a restaurant owner, an event manager for eight additional restaurants, a ballroom dancer, a group fitness instructor, a personal trainer, an online fitness-and-lifestyle coach, an author, and a master iron chef of my own kitchen (at least I like to call myself that, we can all pretend, right?). Out of all the items on my overcrowded plate, there were only two items my friends really wanted the recipe for—they wanted all my cooking recipes and along with the recipes, how I managed it all.

The one thing I love about my cooking is that it is delicious, but still healthy. I believe in moderation and making small nutritional changes that will have a large impact on your body. I will sometimes recommend organic options in some recipes, but that is because I find the quality better in some products, that's all, don't over think it. I like to call this "The Healthy Realistic Diet." Did I just coin a new phrase? I like it! Wouldn't you totally rather do a diet called "Healthy Realistic Eating" than "Starve Yourself for Months and Regain it back a Week Later Diet?" LOL I know, I am just playing around...but honestly, staying fit and healthy is all about following a permanent lifestyle, not a trend. Depriving yourself of treats, bread, and pastas for life is not realistic for most. You should be able to indulge in your favorite foods from time to time without panicking you will gain 50 pounds...that is more realistic. But self-control and portions are the key; we will dive into that later ;)

It's one thing to put a frozen dinner on the dining room table, but it's another thing to truly know how to cook from scratch and avoid prepackaged items as best we can. I know everyone is looking for quick fixes and super-quick meals, and if that is what you are looking for, this is not the book for you. The point of this book is to teach you how to REALLY cook, not just how to mix pre-cooked packages loaded with MSG into your meals. The only quick fix I will recommend is buying pre-chopped foods to speed up your cooking time.

I want you to learn how to cook from scratch. It's healthier and much more flavorful. Once you start to learn how to work with flavors, you will see how talented you really are, and you will learn to love to cook, and you will cook much faster than you did when you started. As soon as we get good at something we crave to do it more. I am no trained gourmet chef, but I must say I have mastered traditional family favorites while lightening them up to be enjoyed in a less guilty manner. Moderation...Moderation...Moderation.

One thing I have noticed over the years is how many women in America do not know how to cook. Could be the reason that a lot of women work full-time jobs? Perhaps it is a cultural thing?

Maybe it is a combination of both. Growing up in an Armenian/Italian family, I was just expected to know how to cook. The kitchen and meal times are what brought the family together, and cooking was just part of what we did together. Cooking, in my family, was how we showed our love. It was how both the men and women in my family nurtured and took care of each other. I do have to admit there was nothing better than coming home from school and having my home smell like chicken cutlets and a homemade sauce. These days, I much prefer to stay in and have dinner than go out. I can't imagine having to order out every night, or the weight gain and expense that would come out of it.

When a woman can put on a show in the kitchen, company will always be impressed, and the appreciation will never get old. Nothing feels better than when someone says, "Wow, this is so delicious, did you make these?" and you actually have the pleasure of responding, "I sure did!"

People always associate food with weight gain, and that is just an injustice. We need food! In fact, if you are trying to lose weight, you actually have to eat more often in order to speed up your metabolism. The choice in food, of course, needs to be healthy and low in saturated fats.

Food becomes the enemy of most people for two reasons: 1.) the association of food with obesity and 2.) the association of food with time spent cooking, which for the masses in America, seems like mission impossible or just downright exhausting. I think if more people were educated on how to eat healthier, they could all enjoy the wonderful flavors without the guilt. If you're thinking, "I can't even boil an egg!" have no fear—you are a mighty mamma, remember?

You created human life, and I promise you can cook a healthy meal. Now hear me out: this book is not meant to be a "clean eating, non-fat cookbook." BUT it is all of our favorite recipes we grew up loving "lightened up" so that they are healthier for us. You will hear me say this a few times: I do not believe in depriving our bodies of anything, and I do not believe in crazy fad diets. All I believe in (and it seems to work fine for me and my family) is to eat a balanced diet and be mindful of portion control. There is a science to being fit and healthy and that science is also called *balance*.

Juggling it all can be tough, but if you have the right recipe for success, you will be able to juggle it all, even in the kitchen. The trick to weight loss is not dieting; it is creating a healthy lifestyle filled with healthy choices, including your meals, and of course a decent amount of exercise.

My entire outlook on nutrition changed when I was pregnant. I remember the instructions about changing from white bread to whole grains, and how to be careful of sugars and sodas, for example. Being aware of my glycemic index was crucial! It posed a serious question to me. If we are supposed to be this careful and aware of our nutrition while creating a baby, why not continue taking care of ourselves in this manner after the baby is born? Good nutrition and avoiding junk should be just as important all the time, not just during pregnancy. This is how we stay fit for life.

In this book, you will see a lot of small changes in ingredient choices that make a big impact on your nutrition when practiced on a regular basis. You will notice, for the most part, white grains are replaced with whole grains, and processed sugars are replaced with natural sugars.

Is being a new mom going to be easy? Hell, no! But neither is anything new we have to learn. I can promise you it will be the most amazing experience of your life and will be worth every sleepless night. So what is my recipe for success? I find this one recipe to be the most sacred of all. In fact, if you can't get my cooking recipes right, at least practice perfecting this one.

THE NEW MOM RECIPE FOR SUCCESS

Ingredients

- Love
- Patience
- Practice
- Clear communication with your partner

****Note: You will need an unlimited supply of all of the above!!!****

Directions

- Combine all ingredients. Practice and repeat this step... forever.

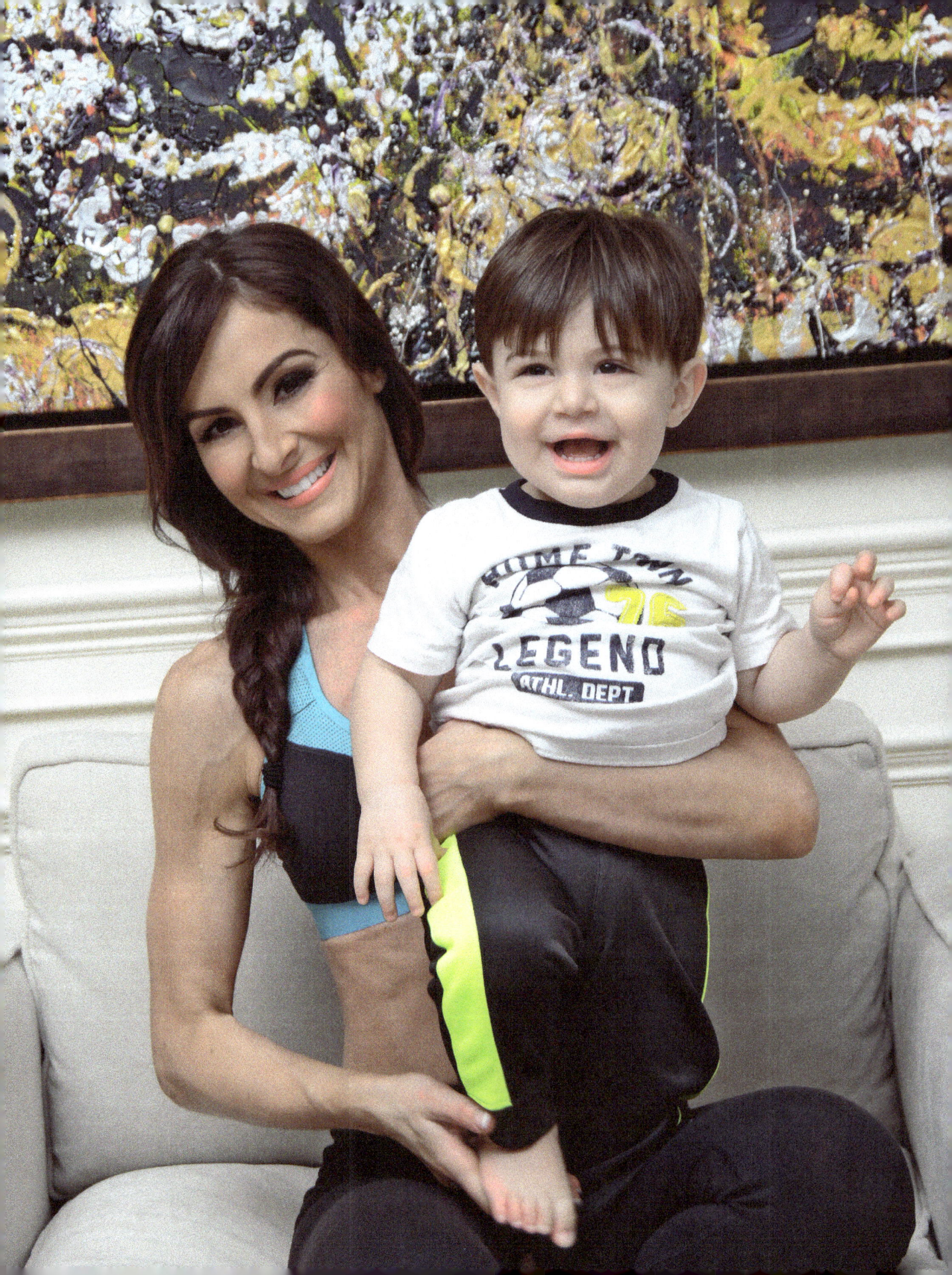

Add THIS to Your Plate!

Creating Effective Time Management

If I can give you just one piece of advice as a new mom, it is that time management is important. You will be pulled in many directions. You will want to sleep at any free moment… but sleeping won't even seem possible with the number of things piled on your plate. I remember the older generation in my family telling me to sleep when the baby sleeps. Really?! I sure wish they had shared the contact number for the fairy who would take on my responsibilities during my nap. Wouldn't it be nice if there were a boatload of magical creatures who cleaned and cooked while I was slumbering? It'd be even nicer if one of those fairies would take on my workout while I dreamed sweet dreams.

If I had slept EVERY time the baby slept, I would have accomplished ZERO. I mean the bitter truth is that you cannot do it all (especially during a nap) but with some prioritizing along with acknowledging and accepting help, you can certainly make a dent. Start by doing this:

1. Make a list of all the things you need to do each week. This includes time spent with your baby, sleep, personal goals, work, meal planning, household chores, date night with your partner and your fitness routine (yes, I said fitness routine) and anything else that you need to do that I did not mention.

2. Grab yourself a calendar that has hours on it, so you can see each hour of the day. (I am a notepad and pen type of gal, but phone or computer is great too since it has a reminder alert on it.)

3. Once you sit down in front of a calendar with the hours of the day on it, you will realize you have plenty of hours in the day to get these things done. Next, start scheduling all of the items on your checklist according to importance and how much time is needed. Then be sure to **MAKE AN ALERT ON YOUR CELL PHONE** to remind you when to start each task on the chosen day of the week. This will remind you when to start the next task and stop doing whatever else you should not be doing. This will prevent things from not getting done. We tend to procrastinate on important things by focusing on the less important things, so this alert will be like saying, "Stop washing the dishes, you need to go work out now before you miss your opportunity when baby wakes!"

4. Based on this, figure out where you may be able to outsource some of the work. For example, perhaps you have a sitter who comes for 4 hours every Saturday while you have date night with your partner and while you are gone she/he can do all your laundry for you? Check! That is two things off the list for the week! Or perhaps you hire a cleaner who can come do the heavy-duty cleaning for you every 3-4 weeks. How much of a time saver would that be? Or what about having your mom or another relative or friend come over for a few hours a week while you cook and meal prep for the upcoming week? Let's not forget your partner in all of this; unless you are a single parent, you have another parent here to help as well! Be clear with the expectations of each person's roles and at what time each day. Sit down and go over this schedule with your partner, so you both know what you expect from one another. This can avoid a lot of arguments. Believe me; communication is key!

5. One last thing I want to mention is being realistic with your major goals and the time you need to get them done. For example, if your goal is to write a book, don't schedule this entire task to get done in one day. I know you would not do that, but you know what I mean, right? So if this was a goal, perhaps you schedule 15 minutes a day to work on the first step of moving closer to that goal. Large goals will need a list of their own, broken down into steps to reach that goal. Each day you will need to schedule a part of each step into your calendar. But be sure that step's time is allocated appropriately. I like to write out my goals for the week, then I break them down day by day, hour by hour. You can even take this a step further and write your tasks out for the month and then break it down week by week and then day by day! TRUST me this works...it may seem tedious, but you will get SO much more done in the long run. On the next page, I have listed an example of what a typical day would look like for me :)

Daily Schedule Sample

5:30am: Rise, Espresso, Check Emails (30 minutes)
6:00am: Giorgio wakes, make Giorgio breakfast (30 minutes)
6:30am-7:30am: Workout, post- workout meal (60 minutes)
7:30am-8:30am: Shower, Drive Giorgio to school (60 minutes)
9:00am-11:00am: Coaching w/Scheduled Clients (2 hour block, client calls)
11:15am: Pick up Giorgio, post office run (30 minutes)
12:00pm: Lunch with Giorgio, put Giorgio Down for Nap (60 minutes)
1:00pm-3:00pm: Work Block
- Social Media Marketing (30 minutes)
- Follow-Up Calls (30 minutes)
- Check Social Media Ads (30 minutes)
- Online Challenge Group Check-Ins) (30 minutes)
3:00pm-4:30pm: Food Shopping (1.5 hours)
5:00pm-6:00p Prepare Dinner (1 hour)
6:00pm: Dinner with Family
7:30pm-8:00pm: Bedtime Routine with Giorgio
8:00pm-10:00pm: Alone time with my love
10:00pm: Bed

Again, when you are making your list, you will need to figure out how long it takes for each task to be completed and when you do schedule this in, be realistic with the amount of time you block off so you have an effective schedule that works. Doing this changed my life. Even if you do not finish each task, that is ok; doing a little at a time is better than not doing it at all. If you really want to step up your game, write out your yearly goals, then break them down month by month with a timeline, then week by week, and then day by day. That is pretty balls to the wall I know, but I bet you would be one successful mighty mamma! Now that is pretty sexy if you ask me!

One more thing I will point out again is: do not be afraid to ask for help. This has always been a personal struggle for me, but the more you ask, the easier it will get. If you question if you need help doing certain things like laundry and cleaning, ask yourself, "Is this the best way to use my time to achieve my goals?" If it is not, then you need to outsource that "stuff."

Got me? Good!

Add THIS to Your Plate!

Welcoming the Kitchen to the Family

Whether you realize it or not, your kitchen is part of the family. Did you know that according to numerous studies, the kitchen is the most used room in the house? Yes, even for those that do not cook! It is a place of gathering, eating, drinking, gossiping, and lounging.

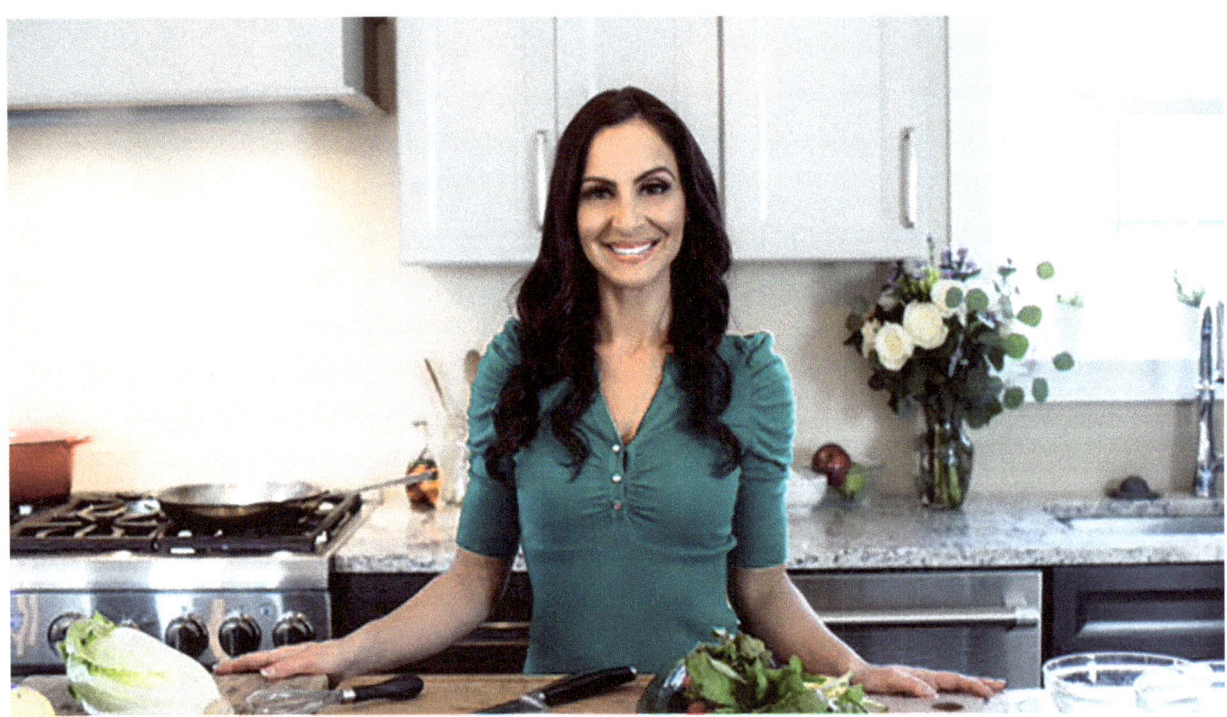

In fact, your kitchen knows every little thing about all of you! She has a big job and should be treated with respect. As you start to get comfortable with your new family member (as in *your kitchen*), you will become best friends with her. Be sure to keep this space clean and organized as it will make your life so much easier. If you are going to take the time to decorate a room in your house, start with your kitchen. The more love you put into her, the better your bond with her will be.

When you are preparing meals, there is nothing more stressful than to be surrounded by clutter—a million utensils, small kitchen appliances, pots & pans, and ingredients to deal with. Take the time to arrange things in a way that is convenient for you. For example, place the most-used items within reach of your food prep area and place items that you do not use often on the top shelves.

So what are all these items we are referring to? In the next few sections, I will go over your basic kitchen tools, small appliances, and pots and pans and why they are needed. Although in today's world the list never ends, these are the staples to start off with. You can start to collect more culinary pieces as you become more advanced in your skills.

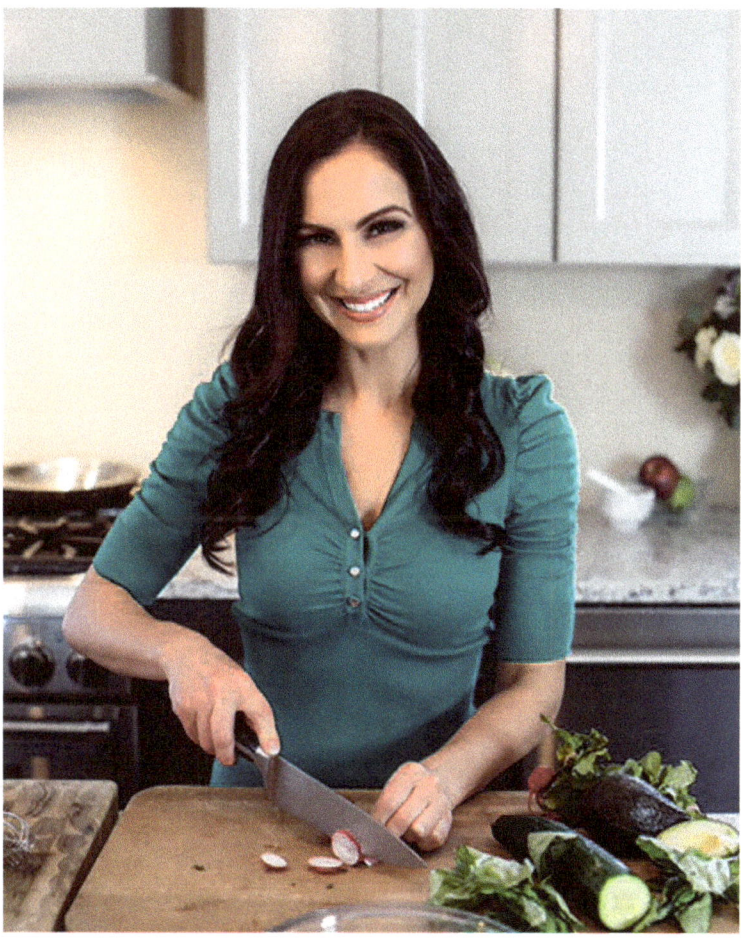

Add THIS to Your Plate!

Getting to Know Your Kitchen Tools & Appliances

Before we begin our journey together, we need to get prepared by making sure we have our essential tools and small kitchen appliances. There are so many voices telling us what we need, and so many options in our stores. How do you know who to listen to and what to purchase?

In this section, I break it down to what you really need to get started. If you want to get all fancy with new-and-improved specialty items, you go, girl… but for now, I just want you to get familiar with what I consider the MVPs of kitchen appliances.

Food processors were pretty intimidating to me in my younger years. I do not think I even knew what one was until I started working in the restaurant business. But why would I have? I really didn't make anything other than your typical beginner meals such as chicken stir-fry, and I don't mean from scratch; I mean the one you buy that is already prepackaged and frozen in the supermarket. You know which one I am talking about—the one where your only requirement was is to add chicken. Yup! That one!

As I became more skilled in the kitchen, I started getting into more advanced recipes, which resulted in me using a wider array of kitchen tools. Although there are thousands of kitchen tools these days, including 19 different types of vegetable peelers, for the sake of this book, let's just start with the essentials.

Essential Kitchen Tools

Measuring Spoons

Get something lightweight. Although the metal ones are nice to look at, I find them very heavy; a light metal or even plastic is best.

Measuring Cups

You will need a set each for liquid ingredients and solid ingredients. As with the measuring spoons, I would recommend something lightweight.

Mixing Bowls

I know you may be tempted to buy the fifteen-piece, clear measuring-bowl set, but honestly, unless you are going to be on a cooking show measuring out every little ingredient, they will just take up space in your already-crowded kitchen. Just get yourself a three-piece, plastic mixing-bowl set that comes in three different sizes and can be stored one inside the other. The bottoms should have rubber on them so they do not slip. Of the hundreds of recipes I have made, non required more than these bowls and they are light weight. The lighter you stay with your tools, the easier it is to move around your kitchen.

Cutting Boards

Invest in at least three boards. The type you choose will be all about your preference. I prefer hardwood and also love using wood when I am serving something on it, such as cheese. But again, use what is right for you. Just choose something sturdy that will not slide when you are cutting your food.

Whisks

I like to have at least two sizes: one large and one small, simply for smaller mixes and larger mixes. Be sure to get whisks with thin wires rather than thick wires, so they are well balanced when you whip eggs or creams. A solid handle is also preferred over a wired one to prevent food from getting inside.

Ladle

A deep scooping spoon is great for soups and sauces. I prefer metal with this tool.

Slotted Spoon

Pick a sturdy spoon with a stainless-steel handle that won't get too hot.

Wooden Spoons

Call me old-fashioned, but nothing gives love to your homemade sauce like stirring it with a wooden spoon. They are strong, sturdy, and will never scratch the bottom of your pan. Some chefs even like to use them for risotto since they do not transfer heat as much as metal spoons. (cool fact right?) This can prevent rapid overcooking with certain dishes. I like to have smaller and larger-sized spoons for different occasions.

Locking Tongs

Select a style with non-slip handles and scalloped tips for a firm grip. Use it for turning meats and tossing vegetables. I used them for everything these days!

Spatulas

Choose a few; one with a thin blade, one that is smaller for getting under delicate items like cookies and pancakes, and then a longer one for larger foods that may need to be flipped. I prefer a metal one for a high flame and a plastic one for more delicate items with a lower flame, such as eggs.

Knives

There are three core essentials:

- Chef's knife: eight or ten-inch
- Paring knife: three or four-inch
- Bread knife: as long as possible, twelve inches or more

In my opinion, I feel a nice knife set from a good reputable brand is the way to go. This is one thing you should not go cheap on. You will use them every day so the investment will be worth every penny, trust me! It makes chopping and prepping so much easier when you have a nice blade that cuts like silk. A nice set will last forever.

Plus, a set will normally have a nice set of kitchen shears and some added extras like a set of steak knives. Just be careful with block sets on the counter with kids! Yikes! I recommend storing all your knives in a drawer with a safety lock.

Colander/Strainer

It is nice to have a larger one with bigger holes for draining heavier liquids such as draining water from a pasta pan. At the other end of the spectrum, you will want a colander/strainer of a netted type for skimming broths or using as a quick sifter for flour when baking.

Grater

A box grater is the most versatile, with six different grate options to shred, shave, dust, and zest. Choose one with a sturdy handle that will not skid. Remember your skin can shred the same way if you slip so be careful. Sorry, that is the mom in me coming out! Plus....I have totally done this to myself!

Microplane Grater

For small tasks that require a fine grater—zesting lemons and grating Parmesan, garlic, and nutmeg. Be sure to get a nice, sharp, steel one.

Lemon/Lime Press

Don't bother with the ones that have a lemon on one side and a lime on the other; it really does not make it easier in my opinion. The best models are big enough for both a lime and a lemon and have ridges to grip fruit better.

Y-Shaped Vegetable Peeler

This will give you a better grip than a traditional swivel model for hard-to-peel foods like mangos, pears, potatoes, and butternut squash. A good peeler can be your best friend.

Potato Masher

A curved head will let you get into corners of bowls and pots.

Can Opener

A safe-cut or smooth-edge model cuts around the outside of the can, rather than the lid, produces smooth edges, and will never lower the lid into your food. Gross! I hate when that happens. Don't waste your time with electric; they don't work well and break easily. If you have an old one that is hard to turn, ditch it for a nice, easy, smooth-turning one. Again, small things like this make your time in the kitchen more enjoyable. Who wants to play test-of-strength when you just need an open can of tomato sauce?

Corkscrew

A standard waiter's corkscrew will open both beer and wine and take up much less space than a two-armed model. Plus, the fancier you go, the more likely it is they will just break. Keep it simple. If you do not know how to open a bottle, ask someone to show you; it's not as hard as you may think. Like riding a bike, once you've got it, you've got it.

Instant-Read Thermometer

Find one that is easy to read and shatterproof. Having to guess the temp with an old-fashioned, red back-and-forth arrow is just annoying. Why play guessing games when we have today's technology? This will really come in handy when you want perfectly cooked meats. It takes the guessing game out of it. The worst no-no of all time is cutting into the meat before it sets to see the temp… DON'T DO IT. We will get into this later.

Peppermill

There is nothing better than freshly ground pepper. The coarseness can really make a big difference in your dish. An easily adjustable grind setting will let you go from coarse to fine. A large hole allows easy refilling of the peppercorns.

Salad Spinner

Yes, life will go on if you don't have one, but nothing is worse than soggy lettuce, especially before the dressing is even added. You can use one with a solid bowl for both swishing greens clean and serving them. In addition, if you want to prep some salad for the next day, it will be nice and dry and won't get soggy. I am a big fan of these.

Timer

This is not something I would say you NEED, especially with cell phones, microwaves, and a stove timer, but some digital models allow for multiple time-keepings, so you can track a roast in the oven, potatoes on the stovetop, and dough in the refrigerator—all at the same time, which is just pretty damn cool.

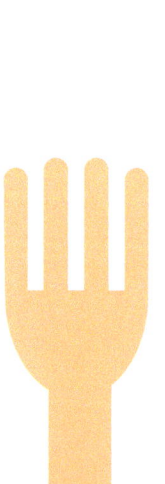

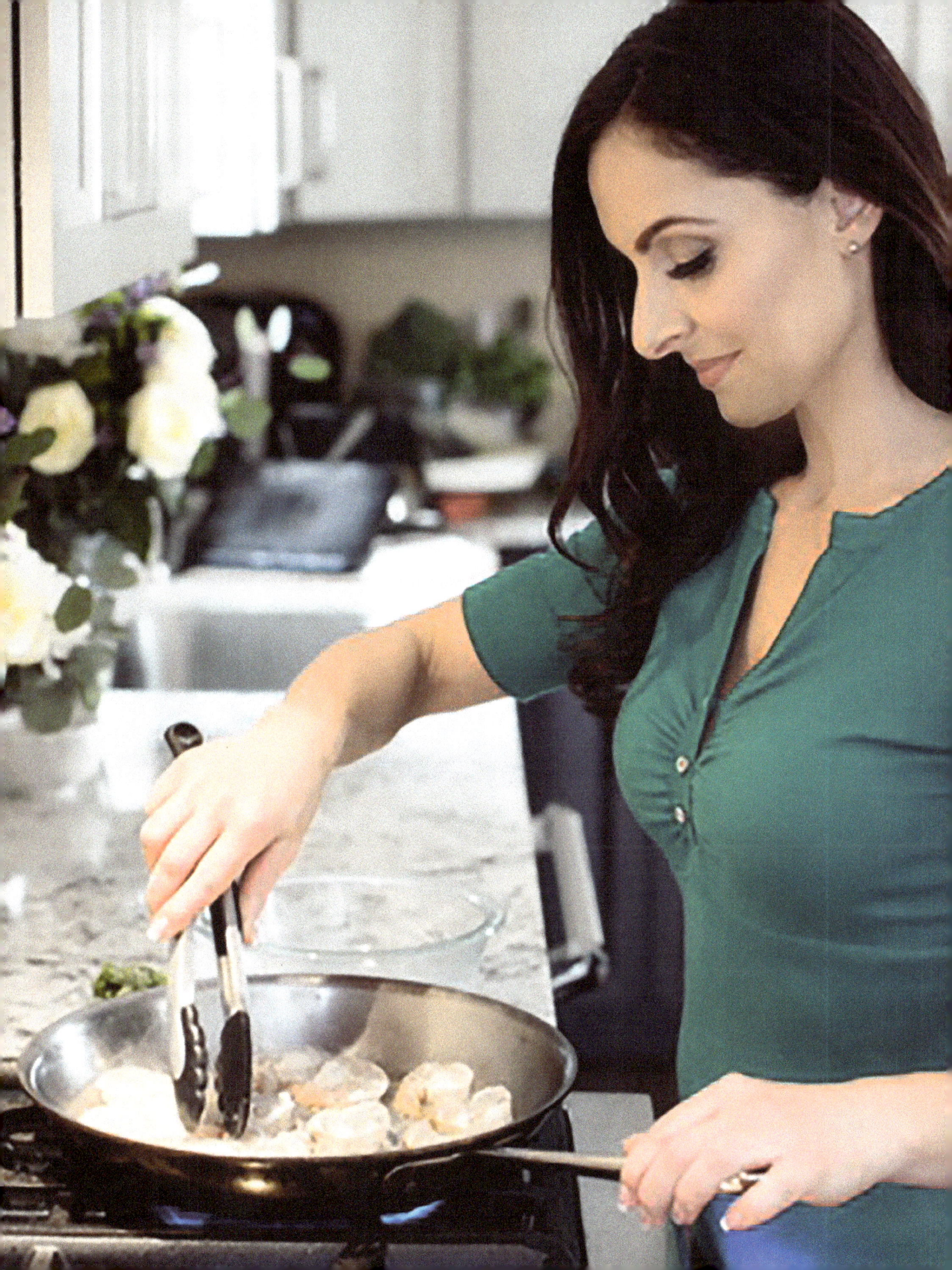

Add THIS to Your Plate!

Getting to Know Your Pots & Pans

I used to think I could use a non-stick pan for everything. Turns out, you'll never get the crust you desire if you cook everything the same way. (Who knew?) If you're a one-pan kinda gal, this section is for you.

FRY PAN

A flat-bottomed pan with a long stick handle and low sides that flare out at an angle to encourage air circulation and allows for easy flipping or turning of food.

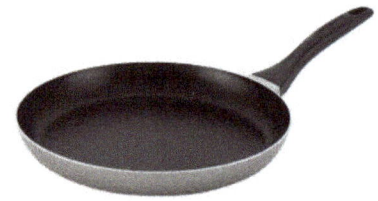

PURPOSE

Fast cooking: frying, searing, browning.

ADD THIS TO YOUR NOTES

Eight-, ten-, and twelve-inch-diameter pans are the most useful. It's a good idea to have at least one fry pan with a non-stick surface for making eggs **and one with a regular surface for higher-temperature cooking**, which is what will give you that nice seared or browned technique you find in restaurants. The biggest mistake home cookers make is they use a non-stick for everything. If you are trying to get a nice top crust on seared scallops or a nice browned chicken, it is better to use a regular frying pan. The non-stick is better for your eggs and foods that will adhere easily and burn on a regular surface.

SAUCEPAN

A heavy pan with a flat base: tall, vertical sides that are roughly the same measurement as the pan's diameter, and a long stick handle. Larger sizes should have a "helper handle" on the far side of the pan.

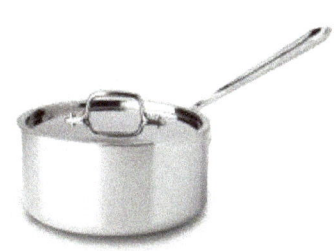

PURPOSE

Cooking with a fair amount of liquid: simmering, boiling, cooking grains, poaching eggs and making sauces.

ADD THIS TO YOUR NOTES

These are the most useful sizes: 1–1.5 quart; 2–2.5 quart; 3 quart; and 4 quart. But if you have to choose just one, select a 3 or 4 quart.

SAUTÉ PAN

A pan with a wide, flat bottom; vertical, moderate sides; and a long stick handle. Larger sizes should have a "helper handle" opposite the stick handle.

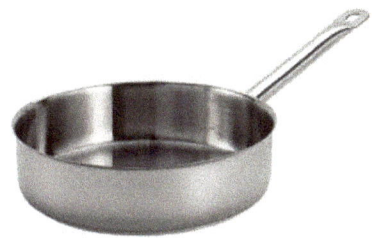

PURPOSE

Fast cooking while shaking, tossing, or stirring food: sautéing.

ADD THIS TO YOUR NOTES

A four-quart pan is the most versatile. It's a good idea to select a sauté pan with a cooking surface other than non-stick so that you can achieve the best browning and caramelization, as with the regular-surface frying pan. This pan is nice since the higher sides prevent food from falling off the sides. This is more secure than your frying pan, which is meant for smaller volumes.

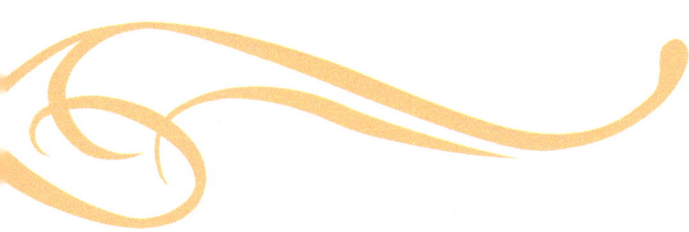

DUTCH OVEN

A large pot with vertical sides slightly shorter than the pot's diameter, two sturdy loop handles, and a heavy, tight-fitting lid (a.k.a. French oven or cocotte).

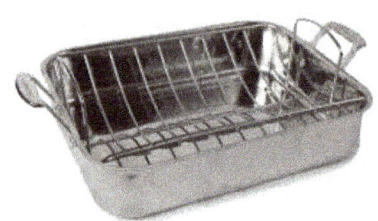

PURPOSE

Long, slow cooking, often with some liquid that's allowed to circulate inside the vessel: stews, braises, roasts, and casseroles.

ADD THIS TO YOUR NOTES

These are the most popular and useful sizes: 5 quart and 7 quart. For a quick calculation, count one quart of capacity for each serving.

ROASTER

A large, rectangular pan with low sides to allow the oven's heat to reach as much of the food as possible. It's often used in conjunction with a roasting rack, which elevates food above the cooking surface.

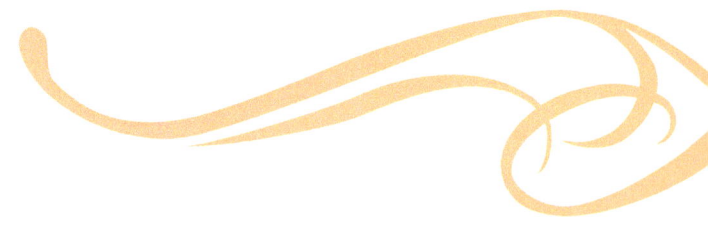

PURPOSE

Cooking in the dry heat of the oven at relatively high temperatures.

ADD THIS TO YOUR NOTES

While roasters with a non-stick finish make for easy cleanup, a roaster with a regular cooking surface has been said to create a better gravy.

GRIDDLE

A broad, flat pan often with a non-stick or stick-resistant finish that sits flat on a stovetop over one or two burners.

PURPOSE

Fast-cooking foods that benefit from a large, smooth cooking surface: pancakes, thin steaks, grilled cheese, bacon, eggs. Although you can use a non-stick frying pan, the reason I love a griddle is because you can fit more on it at one time. For example, with pancakes, it takes a fraction of the time to be able to make 8 pancakes at once versus 2 at a time in a frying pan. There are some nice electric griddles you can buy as well as the ones that go right on top of your stove.

ADD THIS TO YOUR NOTES

If you plan on cooking meat or anything else that will have juice or liquids on your griddle, look for a pan with a depression around the rim to catch grease.

GRILL PAN/ SANDWICH PRESS

A pan with a ridged cooking surface designed to resemble the grates of an outdoor grill, and low sides for increased air circulation.

PURPOSE

Higher-temperature cooking: grilling, searing, or as a sandwich press. If you live in an apartment or an environment where you may not want to grill outside when it's cold, this is a great indoor option. Although in my opinion, nothing beats the smoky flavor of a real grill, this is the next best thing.

ADD THIS TO YOUR NOTES

To attain the best grill marks on your food, select a cast-iron or enameled, cast-iron grill pan. Getting a grill pan that has a sandwich press is key so that you don't feel like you have to buy a panini maker. It works just as well, in my opinion, and now you have a two-in-one pan.

MULTIPOT

A tall pot similar to a soup or stockpot with a large perforated insert for cooking food in water and a smaller perforated insert for steaming food above water. I say *optional* with this because you can steam simply by adding a steam basket into a saucepan, adding a few inches of water and covering. I find this to be unnecessary, but if you have the room and added this to your wedding registry, why not?

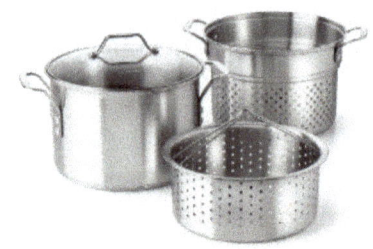

PURPOSE

Use the large insert for boiling and easy straining of large quantities of foods like pasta or corn. Use the smaller insert for steaming vegetables and other foods.

ADD THIS TO YOUR NOTES

Multipots are available in these sizes: 6 quart, 8 quart, and 12 quart. They can be used to make small batches of stock, soup, or stew.

BAKEWARE

When you first start out, just grab yourself a basic bakeware set for your favorite baked good recipes such as cookies, muffins, cakes, and perhaps a loaf. As you get more advanced, you can venture into more creative tools.

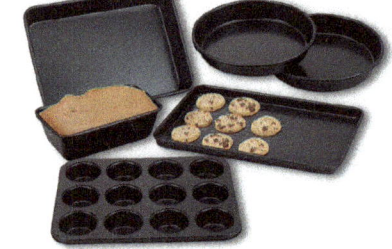

PURPOSE

You will need bakeware that will be safe in the oven and also help create the specified mold for your baked goods, such as cupcakes.

ADD THIS TO YOUR NOTES

To start, two round cake pans, a couple of cookie sheets, a muffin pan, and a loaf pan will do.

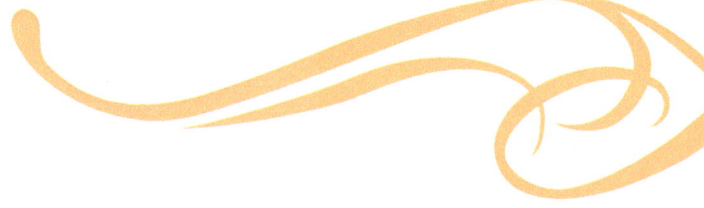

Add **THIS** to Your Plate!

Culinary Jargon Explained

Now that you have your essential tools and small appliances, and your pots and pans, you are almost ready to dive into all those amazing recipes you have been waiting to master. But before you begin, there is culinary jargon you should know. Do you know how many times I had to stop mid-recipe and google what a word or instruction meant?

Plenty of times!

Sometimes recipes can sound so intimidating because of the preparation instructions when really, it's not as difficult as it may seem. Here is a quick guide to common terms you will often see in recipes and what they mean. You're welcome!

Al dente: Pasta cooked until just firm. From the Italian "to the tooth."

Bake: To cook food in an oven, surrounded with dry heat; called roasting when applied to meat or poultry.

Baking powder: A combination of baking soda, an acid such as cream of tartar, and a starch or flour (moisture absorber). Most common type is double-acting baking powder, which acts when mixed with liquid and again when heated.

Baking soda: Baking soda is a dry chemical leavening agent, a mixture of a carbonate or bicarbonate and a weak acid and is used for increasing the volume and lightening the texture of baked goods. Always mix with other dry ingredients before adding any liquid, since leavening begins as soon as soda comes in contact with the liquid.

Barbecue: To cook foods on a rack or a spit over coals.

Baste: To moisten food for added flavor and to prevent drying out while cooking.

Batter: An uncooked pourable mixture usually made up of flour, a liquid, and other ingredients.

Beat: To stir rapidly to make a mixture smooth, using a whisk, spoon, or mixer.

Blanch: To cook briefly in boiling water to seal in flavor and color; usually used for vegetables or fruit, to prepare for freezing, and to ease skin removal.

Blend: To thoroughly combine 2 or more ingredients, either by hand with a whisk or spoon, or with a mixer.

Boil: To cook in bubbling water that has reached 212°F.

Bone: To remove bones from poultry, meat, or fish.

Bouquet garni: A tied bundle of herbs, usually parsley, thyme, and bay leaves, that is added to flavor soups, stews, and sauces but removed before serving.

Braise: To cook first by browning, then gently simmering in a small amount of liquid over low heat in a covered pan until tender.

Bread: To coat with crumbs or cornmeal before cooking.

Broil: To cook on a rack or spit under or over direct heat, usually in an oven.

Brown: To cook over high heat, usually on top of the stove, to brown food.

Caramelize: To heat sugar until it liquefies and becomes a syrup ranging in color from golden to dark brown.

Core: To remove the seeds or tough woody centers from fruits and vegetables.

Cream: The butterfat portion of milk. Also, to beat ingredients, usually sugar and a fat, until smooth and fluffy.

Cube: To cut food into small (about ½-inch) cubes.

Cut in: To distribute a solid fat in flour using a cutting motion, with 2 knives used scissors-fashion or a pastry blender, until divided evenly into tiny pieces. Usually refers to making pastry.

Deep-fry: To cook by completely immersing food in hot fat.

Deglaze: To loosen brown bits from a pan by adding a liquid, then heating while stirring and scraping the pan.

Dice: To cut food into very small (⅛- to ¼-inch) cubes.

Dollop: A spoonful of soft food such as whipped cream or mashed potatoes.

Dot: To scatter butter in bits over food.

Dredge: To cover or coat uncooked food, usually with a flour or cornmeal mixture or breadcrumbs.

Dress: To coat foods such as salad with a sauce. Also, to clean fish, poultry, or game for cooking.

Drippings: Juices and fats rendered by meat or poultry during cooking.

Drizzle: To pour melted butter, oil, syrup, melted chocolate, or other liquid back and forth over food in a fine stream.

Dust: To coat lightly with confectioners' sugar or cocoa (cakes and pastries) or another powdery ingredient.

Fillet: A flat piece of boneless meat, poultry, or fish. "Filet" means to cut the bones from a piece of meat, poultry, or fish.

Fines herbes: A mixture of herbs, traditionally parsley, chervil, chives, and tarragon, used to flavor fish, chicken, and eggs.

Flambé: To drizzle liquor over a food while it is cooking, then when the alcohol has warmed, ignite the food just before serving.

Flute: To make decorative grooves. Usually refers to pastry making.

Fold: To combine light ingredients such as whipped cream or beaten egg whites with a heavier mixture, using a gentle over-and-under motion, usually with a rubber spatula.

Glaze: To coat foods with glossy mixtures such as jellies or sauces.

Grate: To rub foods against a serrated surface to produce shredded or fine bits.

Grease: To rub the interior surface of a cooking dish or pan with shortening, oil, or butter to prevent food from sticking to it.

Grill: To cook food on a rack under or over direct heat, as on a barbecue or in a broiler.

Grind: To reduce food to tiny particles using a grinder or a food processor.

Julienne: To cut into long, thin strips, matchstick-like in shape.

Knead: To blend dough together with hands or in a mixer to form a pliable mass.

Macerate: To soak in a flavored liquid; usually refers to fruit.

Marinate: To soak in a flavored liquid; usually refers to meat, poultry, or fish.

Mince: To cut into tiny pieces, usually with a knife.

Parboil: To partially cook by boiling. Usually done to prepare food for final cooking by another method.

Poach: To cook gently over very low heat in barely simmering liquid just to cover.

Prep Time: The time it takes to prepare food before you actually start cooking it on the stove or in the oven.

Purée: To mash or grind food until completely smooth, usually in a food processor, blender, sieve, or food mill.

Reduce: To thicken a liquid and concentrate its flavor by boiling.

Render: To cook fatty meat or poultry—such as bacon or goose—over low heat to obtain drippings.

Roast: To cook a large piece of meat or poultry uncovered with dry heat in an oven.

Sauté or panfry: To cook food in a small amount of fat over relatively high heat.

Scald: To heat liquid almost to a boil until bubbles begin to form around the edge.

Sear: To brown the surface of meat by quick-cooking over high heat in order to seal in the meat's juices.

Shred: To cut food into narrow strips with a knife or a grater.

Simmer: To cook in liquid just below the boiling point; bubbles form but do not burst on the surface of the liquid.

Skim: To remove surface foam or fat from a liquid.

Steam: To cook food on a rack or in a steamer set over boiling or simmering water in a covered pan.

Steep: To soak in a liquid just under the boiling point to extract the essence—e.g., tea.

Stew: To cook covered over low heat in a liquid.

Stir-fry: To quickly cook small pieces of food over high heat, stirring constantly.

Total Time: How long it will take to make the recipe from start to finish, including prep time.

Truss: To tie whole poultry with string or skewers so it will hold its shape during cooking.

Whip: To beat food with a whisk or mixer to incorporate air and produce volume.

Whisk: To beat ingredients (such as heavy or whipping cream, eggs, salad dressings, or sauces) with a fork or whisk to mix, blend, or incorporate air.

Zest: The outer, colored part of the peel of citrus fruit.

Add **THIS** to Your Plate!

Conversion Measurements in Cooking

One of the things that still confuses me to this day is the measurement conversions. There are so many ways of explaining things in recipes, and everyone writes down something different. So in order for you to not have to Google how many cups are in a fluid ounce, I thought I would help you out with a cheat sheet chart. So when you get stuck, remember you have this page to check back into. You're welcome!

Unit of Measurement:	Equals:
Pinch or dash	less than ⅛ teaspoon
3 teaspoons	1 tablespoon
2 tablespoons	1 fluid ounce
1 jigger	1½ fluid ounces
4 tablespoons	¼ cup
5 tablespoons plus 1 teaspoon	⅓ cup
12 tablespoons	¾ cup
16 tablespoons	1 cup
1 cup	8 fluid ounces
2 cups	1 pint or 16 fluid ounces
2 pints	1 quart or 32 fluid ounces
4 quarts	1 gallon

Add THIS to Your Plate!

Holy Smokes! The Truth About Oils

When it comes to cooking healthy, the most common mistake is the misuse of oils.

Wait. What?

We all know oil provides a lot of nutritional value, but we also know fried food is so bad for us. Without getting all scientific on you, oils (especially extra-virgin oils in the purest forms) are very healthy by providing omega-3's, omega-6 fatty acids, antioxidants, and vitamins. Great, right?

Well, here's where it gets interesting. Most people don't know that each oil has a *smoke point*, meaning the heat point at which the negative side effects cancel out the nutritional value. Once the oil is heated past its smoke point, the oil begins to smoke, producing toxic fumes and harmful free radicals.

This is why fried food is so frowned upon. The high heat damages the oil, which is soaking into the food being prepared. It is the same with sautéing. You may think that by sautéing on the stove with extra-virgin olive oil is healthier than frying, but if the sauté flame goes above the oil's smoke point, you've still potentially turned a healthy meal into an unhealthy one with the large increase in saturated fat.

Horrible, right? A simple step to avoid this common mistake is to simply use an oil with a higher smoke point (such as avocado oil, which can stand heat up to 520°F!) and save that extra-virgin olive oil for your salad.

BASIC RULE: For high-temperature cooking, select cooking oils with a high smoke point. For low temperature cooking, or adding to dishes and salad dressings, chose oils with a higher omega-3 fatty acids since they promote healthy cells and decrease stroke and heart attack risk. Easy enough? Ok great, now that we have that OFF OUR PLATE, here is a short list you can refer to when in doubt.

Add THIS to Your Plate!

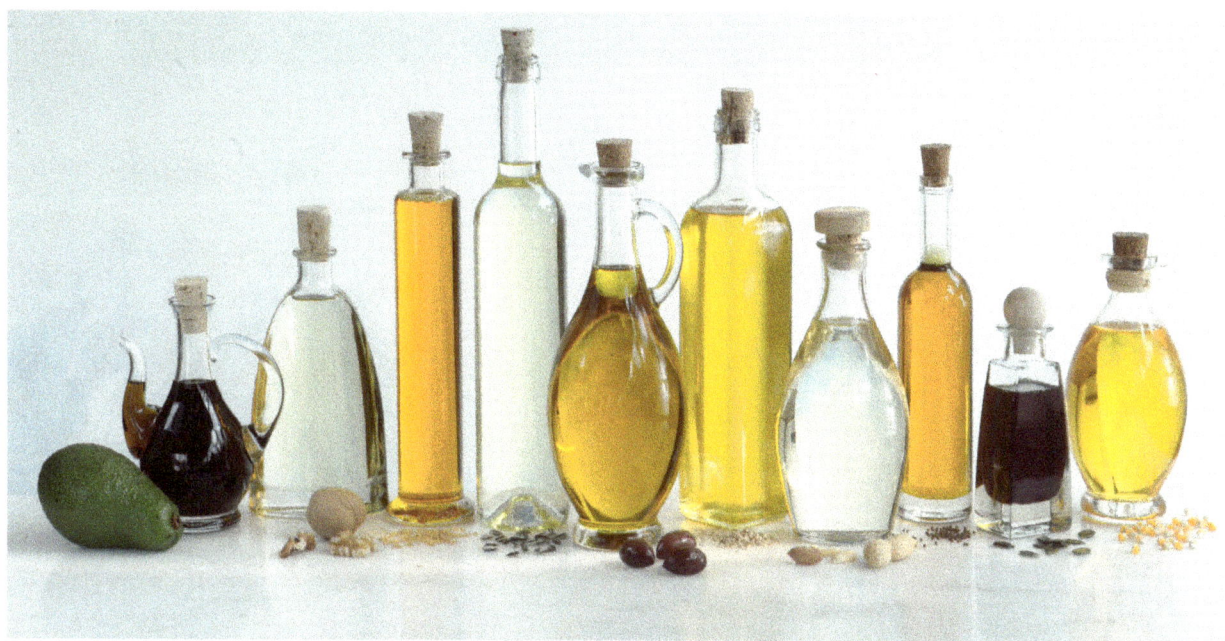

Cooking Oils	Smoke Point C	Smoke Point F
Unrefined Flaxseed Oil	107	225
Unrefined Safflower Oil	107	225
Unrefined Sunflower Oil	107	225
Unrefined Corn Oil	160	320
Extra-Virgin Olive Oil	160	320
Unrefined Peanut Oil	160	320
Semi-refined Safflower Oil	160	320
Unrefined Soy Oil	160	320
Unrefined Walnut Oil	160	320
Hemp Seed Oil	165	330
Butter	177	350
Semi-refined Canola Oil	177	350
Unrefined Soy Oil	177	350

Cooking Oils	Smoke Point C	Smoke Point F
Unrefined Sesame Oil	177	350
Coconut Oil	171	350
Vegetable Shortening	182	360
Lard	182	370
Macadamia Nut Oil	199	390
Canola Oil (Expeller Pressed)	200	400
Refined Canola Oil	204	400
Semi-refined Walnut Oil	204	400
High-quality (low acidity) Extra-Virgin Olive Oil	207	405
Sesame Oil	210	410
Cottonseed Oil	216	420
Grapeseed Oil	216	420
Virgin Olive Oil	216	420
Almond Oil	216	420
Hazelnut Oil	221	430
Peanut Oil	227	440
Sunflower Oil	227	440
Refined Corn Oil	232	450
Palm Oil	232	450
Refined Peanut Oil	232	450
Semi-refined Sesame Oil	232	450
Refined Soy Oil	232	450
Semi-refined Sunflower Oil	232	450
Extra Light Olive Oil	242	468
Rice Bran Oil	254	490
Refined Safflower Oil	266	510
Avocado Oil	271	520

The Skinny on Fat and Nutrition

Saturated Fat: Primarily from animal sources including butter, dairy products, and meats. Healthy adults should follow a diet of less than 10% of daily calories from saturated fats.

Monounsaturated Fat: Has been shown to reduce LDL cholesterol (bad cholesterol) without effecting HDL (good cholesterol). A preferred form of fat. Good sources from olive oil, canola oil, peanut oil, and avocado oil.

Polyunsaturated: Divided into omega-6 vegetable oils and omega-3 fish oils. Omega-3 fatty acids have been known to suppress atherosclerosis by decreasing platelets, and by reducing blood pressure, cholesterol, triglycerides, and blood clotting. Good sources come from vegetable oils such as sunflower oil, soybean oil, and sesame oil. Omega-3's come from fish, especially mackerel, halibut, salmon, albacore tuna, and whitefish.

Add THIS to Your Plate!
==

Let's Get to the Meat of It

The fastest way to reveal yourself as an amateur cook is to remove meat from the oven and immediately cut into the center to check the temperature. FOR THE LOVE OF MEAT, DON'T DO THAT! Let your meat rest before you prematurely cut it. Don't release all that juicy goodness! Real pros aren't afraid to use a meat thermometer.

Safe Internal Temperatures

Ground Beef & Meat Mixtures
Ground Beef, Pork, Veal, Lamb	160 °F
Ground Turkey, Chicken	165 °F

Whole Cuts
Beef, Veal, Lamb, Pork
Medium Rare	145 °F
Medium	160 °F
Well Done	170 °F

Poultry (all cuts)	165 °F
Seafood	145 °F
(or until opaque and flakes with a fork)	

Give It a Rest!

Excuse my tone, but please listen: let that beautiful piece of meat rest once you take it out. By doing so, you are ensuring the meat retains its juices, making it one succulent dish! The time taken to rest will depend on its size; a roast is best rested for **ten to twenty minutes** before carving. Steaks or chops should stand for **five minutes** (but no less than 3) before serving. A rule of thumb used by some chefs is **one-minute** resting time for every quarter pound of meat.

Playing It Safe

Remember when you are cooking for your family—especially your baby—please play it safe with your meats. Although you may like your steak medium rare, this is not the safest for your child. Please refer to the information below from the USDA safety guidelines. Remember there is always a risk of bacteria with meat, poultry, and fish. The guidelines will help reduce, but not eliminate, risk.

USDA Safe Minimum Internal Temperature Chart

Safe steps in food handling, cooking, and storage are essential in preventing foodborne illness. You can't see, smell, or taste harmful bacteria that may cause illness. In every step of food preparation, follow the four guidelines to keep food safe:

- **Clean**—Wash hands and surfaces often.
- **Separate**—Separate raw meat from other foods.
- **Cook**—Cook to the right temperature.
- **Chill**—Refrigerate food promptly.

Product	Minimum Internal Temperature & Best Time
Beef, Pork, Veal & Lamb	
Steaks, Chops, Roast	145°F (62.8°C) and allow to rest for at least 3 minutes
Ground Meats	160°F (71.1°C)
Ham, fresh or smoked (uncooked)	145°F (62.8°C) and allow to rest for at least 3 minutes
Fully cooked Ham (to reheat)	Reheat cooked hams packaged in the USDA-inspected plants to 140°F (60°C) and all others to 165°F (73.9°C)
All Poultry (breasts, whole bird, legs, thighs, wings, ground poultry, and stuffing)	165°F (73.9°C)
Eggs	160°F (71.1°C)
Fish and Shellfish	145°F (62.8°C)
Leflovers	165°F (73.9°C)
Caseroles	165°F (73.9°C)

Add THIS to Your Plate!

Playing it Safe in the Kitchen for Baby

Although we are all told preparing food ourselves is preferred over using store-bought food, there are certainly still rules to follow in the home kitchen to make sure we play it safe, especially when preparing home-cooked meals for baby. When we prepare food at home, we must be sure food handling and storage are safe, the texture is appropriate, and the methods of cooking used are those that conserve nutrients in a manner that will last, as prepared, without adding unnecessary ingredients.

Foods to Delay with Baby

- Non-USDA-approved foods
- Non-pasteurized milks or dairy products as they may contain harmful bacteria that can cause serious illness
- Shellfish
- Foods that pose a choking hazard
- Low-fat dairy products: baby needs the fat for her developing brain
- Sugar
- Salt
- Cow's milk until after baby's 1st birthday
- Honey and corn syrup (which have been known to cause botulism)

Important Notes While Preparing Food

Below you will find a simple checklist for playing it safe in the kitchen.

- Begin with good-quality food. Avoid using leftover food, and use fresh food from the start.
- Cook foods until soft and tender.
- After pureeing food, liquid (water, breast milk, or formula) can be added to thin out textures. You can change the textures as your baby gets older.
- No need to add sugar, lots of salt, seasonings, sauces, lard, or fat drippings to your infant's meals.
- NEVER add honey to baby's foods because it can cause botulism.
- Be careful with home-canned foods (if stored improperly they can have harmful bacteria); outdated cans; food from dented, rusted, bulging, or leaking cans or jars; or food from jars without labels.
- Never serve infants partially cooked or raw meat, poultry, eggs, or fish, as it can contain harmful bacteria, parasites, or viruses that could cause serious food poisoning.

Food Storage Tips

- Immediately after buying meats, poultry, fish, and dairy, store them in the refrigerator (not in the door section) and remove right before use.
- Wrap securely, so no juices drip and cross-contaminate other foods.
- Do not allow them to sit at room temperature.
- Store in the coldest part of the refrigerator, such as a bottom shelf or drawer and prepare the within 1-2 days of purchase.

Meat Preparation After Cooking

- After cooking, separate any remaining bone, skin, and visible fat. Cut food into pieces and puree to desired texture.
- Warm meat done in smaller batches is easier to puree than cold meat.
- As baby's feeding skills mature, foods can start to be served ground or finely chopped instead of pureed.

Freezing Foods

- Keep freezer clean and sanitary.
- There are many freezer-friendly storage containers you can buy in the stores, or you can simply use an ice cube tray with a cover of aluminum foil or plastic wrap. When ready to use, just remove the number of cubes in tray with clean hands and thoroughly reheat them.
- Label and date the containers and use within a month.

Thawing or Reheating Foods

- Thoroughly reheat refrigerated or frozen foods to 165°F before feeding to baby. Reheating kills bacteria which can grow slowly while food is in the refrigerator thawing. Stir the food and test the temperature before serving to baby.
- Defrost foods in the refrigerator, under cold running water, or as part of the reheating process. NEVER defrost baby foods by leaving at room temperature such as leaving on a kitchen counter or in standing water, such as a pan or bowl.
- Do not refreeze baby food that has already been thawed. Use thawed food within forty-eight hours from the time it was removed from the freezer. Meats, poultry, or fish should be thrown out if stored longer than twenty-four hours.
- If thawed in a microwave, cook immediately since parts will be warm.

Avoiding Spreading Bacteria to Other Foods

- Do not allow partially cooked meats to touch other foods or surfaces, serving plates, or utensils used to serve other foods. For example, don't use a fork to test the temperature of a piece of meat and then use it to stir your food together.
- Use separate utensils and cutting boards for meats, fish, and non-animal foods. Do not use boards with crevices and cuts as bacteria can get stored in them.
- Be sure to store meats, poultry, below-cooked, or ready-to-eat foods in a storage container to avoid them dripping on other foods in the refrigerator and contaminating other foods.
- After cooking, remove tough parts and visible fat.

Allergies and Intolerances

One of the scariest things we hear about is food allergies and intolerances. Although we cannot prevent them, we can take safer measures and have the best awareness possible. Here is a list that should be pretty helpful.

- Introduce new foods one at a time and perhaps stick with that one food for about 3-5 days. By doing so, if your baby should have a reaction or even stomach discomfort, it will be easier to target which food was the cause. Once you have done this with multiple foods with success, you can start mixing flavors.
- Introduce small amounts at first (as in 1-2 teaspoons) so your baby can get used to the flavor and texture. You will be able to see which ones she likes and dislikes by her facial expression!
- Use single-ingredient foods first. For example, if you are making applesauce, hold off on the cinnamon until you have confirmed the apples were tolerated. Then add a dash of cinnamon for flavor the following week.
- After your baby has eaten, observe closely after for a reaction.
- Common foods that cause an allergy are milk, wheat, fish, tree nuts, eggs, soy, shellfish, and peanuts.

Common Allergy Symptoms

- Diarrhea
- Vomiting
- Coughing and wheezing
- Extreme irritability
- Congestion or stiffness
- Ear infection
- Stomach pain
- Hives
- Skin rash (especially diaper rash)

Severe Allergy Symptoms

- Shock or difficulty breathing (in this case dial 911 right away or contact your nearest medical emergency service)

So What's the Big Stink?

It's tough to determine whether your baby has an allergy or just a lot of gas. My recommendation is that if your baby is gassy more than once from a certain type of food, hold off on it until she gets a little older and her tummy can handle it better. I remember green beans always did it for my son; he would get irritable and cranky every time he had them, so I just avoided them for a year. Why force it when there are so many green veggies to eat? Here is a list of some that can cause quite a stink for baby (no pun intended).

- Fruit Juice
- Dairy
- Wheat
- Beans
- Cauliflower
- Broccoli
- Garlic
- Onions

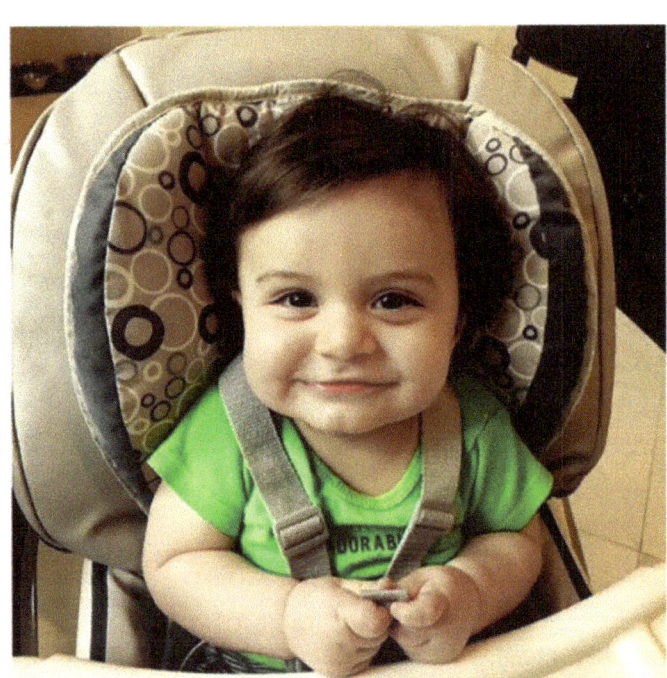

Preventing Choking

Choking is still my biggest fear today. Before we get into a short list of ways you can prevent choking accidents, first get certified in CPR so that you are prepared to handle a choking infant, toddler, or child.

Okay, so now that we have that out of the way, let's chat about a few quick and easy steps that you can take to help avoid this from ever happening.

- Never leave your baby alone while eating! Rule numero uno! Do not take this moment to clean your house or go take a shower. It takes seconds for your baby to choke. But on another note, meals should be eaten together. You should really start to introduce the importance of family time, which in my upbringing was always around the dinner table.
- When your child is ready for finger foods, cut them into very small pieces (¼-inch thick).
- Only put a few pieces on her plate at a time to avoid her wanting to put them all in her mouth at once; they tend to do this for quite a while.
- Teach him to take small bites, I used to take one first and then say, "Now you do!" Babies like to imitate, so you can set the example.

Choking Hazard Foods

- Raw vegetables (including green peas, string beans, celery, carrots)
- Cooked or raw corn kernels
- Whole pieces of canned fruit
- Whole priced of raw fruit such as apple, pear, or melon
- Whole grapes, berries, melon balls, cherries, cherry tomato (cut into quarters and remove pits)
- Uncooked dried fruit (including raisins)
- Peanut butter or soft, sticky foods can get stuck easily in the throat.

Add THIS to Your Plate!

When to Add These Foods to Your Baby's Plate

There are a lot of different opinions about when you should start adding solids to your baby's diet. Consult your pediatrician. I started solids for my son at 4 months, but some start at 6 months.

I remember referring to my pediatrician's pamphlets and favorite cookbooks regarding the age at which I could introduce certain foods. It would have been super helpful for me if I'd had a cheat sheet I could have referred to, so that is just what I did for you. Although children's needs and allergies vary, on the next page you can refer to while taking this wonderful culinary journey with your baby.

Add THIS to Your Plate!

4-6 MONTHS	6-8 MONTHS	8-10 MONTHS	10-12 MONTHS
FRUITS	**FRUITS**	**FRUITS**	**FRUITS**
Apple	Apricot	Blueberry	Citrus
Avocado	Mango	Melon	Strawberries
Banana	Peach	Cherries	**VEGETABLES**
Pear	Plum	Citrus	Beans
VEGETABLES	Prune	Coconut	Lentils
Beans (Green)	Pumpkin	Cranberries	Corn
Sweet Potato	**VEGETABLES**	Fig	Spinach
Squash	Carrot	Grapes	Tomatoes
Butternut	Parsnip	Kiwi	**MEAT**
GRAINS	Peas	Papaya	Fish (wild)
Barley	Squash-Zucchini	Persimmons	**DAIRY**
Oatmeal	**MEAT**	**VEGETABLES**	Cow Milk
Rice	Chicken	Asparagus	
	Tofu	Broccoli	
	Turkey	Beets	
		Cauliflower	
		Cucumber	
		Eggplant	
		Leeks	
		Onions	
		Peppers	
		Potato-White	
		Turnip	
		GRAINS	
		Buckwheat/Kasha	
		Flax	
		Kamut	
		Millet	
		Pasta	
		Quinoa	
		MEAT	
		Beef	
		Eggs	
		Pork	
		DAIRY	
		Cheese	
		Cottage Cheese	
		Cream Cheese	
		Yogurt	

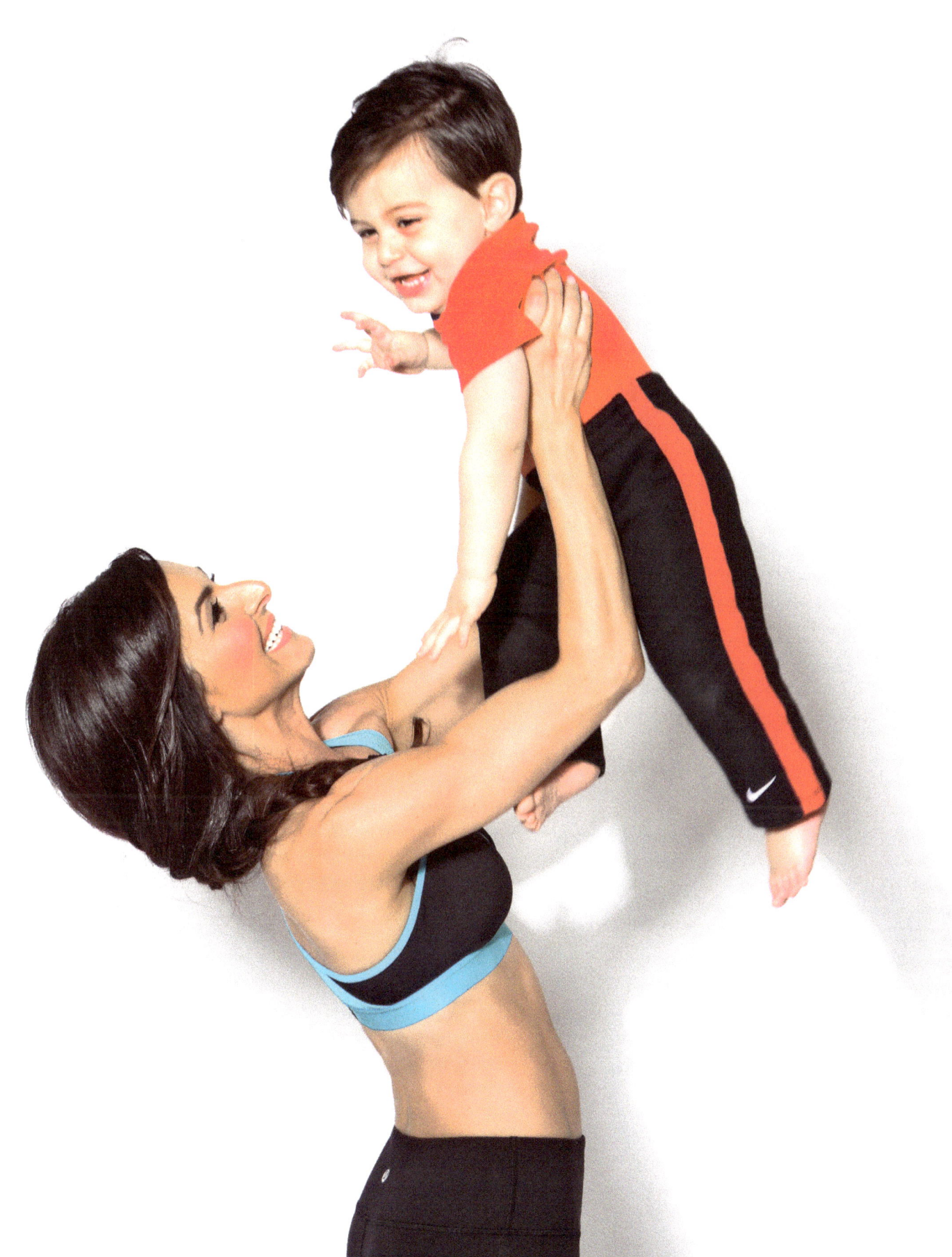

Add THIS to Your Plate!

Just You and Your Bundle of Love

The moment you hold him/her you will fall in love. Your breath will be taken away, and your heart will pound harder than ever before. Never in your wildest dreams did you feel this type of love, other than the moment you realize you are a mother. You will have the gift of falling deep in love all over again every day, for the rest of your life. You are each other's world.

Nights will be sleepless, and circles will form under those eyes, but every sleepless hour will be worth the memories that will last a lifetime. The first year was the hardest for me. My son did not sleep through the night until he was 12 months old and even then it was not consistent. As someone who used to get 8 hours of sleep a night and was a 10am riser, I found waking 2-3 times a night for the first 12 months one of the hardest things I have ever done—besides giving birth, that is. If you took the "no-sleep factor" out of the equation, it would be a piece of cake! Ok, I am exaggerating, but it would be a LOT easier.

As a multi-business owner, let's just say maternity leave was sort of comical. Although I technically took 30 days off, I was still online, doing emails, and taking phone calls... just not as much. But now I had an entirely new business to attend to, something we call "motherhood."

It is the hardest job in the world, but the most rewarding and valued by far. Let's talk about all the concerns we have before delivery. Will I be a good mom? Will I know what to do? Will I be a good provider? Will I give good advice? "OMG... I am going to be responsible for another human being FOREVER!" Sound familiar? I know, it is scary! But we all seem to manage, now don't we?

The way I was raised was that the most important thing you can give your child is love, love, and more love. With this said, a way of displaying your love in my family was to provide wonderful home-cooked meals. I associate cooking with nurturing. I never realized it until one day someone pointed it out to me. They said, "I think you love cooking so much because you just love to take care of people." And you know what? They were right!! It was my way of showing love to the people I cared about.

I think the other reason I love cooking for my family is that I love when the house smells like food; it is what makes a house a home. I love the expressions on their faces when they take their first bite.

Cooking also gives me a feeling of accomplishment. I am proud of my creations. It's an art form, hence the term *culinary arts*. To be a chef in your own kitchen, you do not have to be a trained gourmet chef; you just need a wooden spoon and a lot of love. I know it is not that easy and can be intimidating for some, but honestly cooking is one of those things that once you get the hang of it, you want to do it more and more.

I have a dirty little secret. Although I love to cook I have to admit, it took me longer than I thought to start making my infant's baby food. In fact, for the first couple of months, all I bought was organic jarred baby food. I cooked zip! Want to know why? I was tired as hell. The thought of making my own purees sounded like WAY more work than my tired mind could handle. The real reason I was not cooking is because I was not even sure where to start. I had never had a baby before, and I was scared I would do something wrong with the texture or food. It just seemed intimidating until I realized how simple it actually was.

If you are short on time, the trick is to just pick one day out of the week where someone can watch your little one, and you can make your foods in large batches then just freeze everything until you are ready to serve it. Four steamed apples for your applesauce will go a LONG way when all your baby eats is a teaspoon with each serving.

New moms do not make their own baby food for a few reasons. They either see it as a task that will take a long time and they are too tired, or they just don't know how to make it. The recipes I am about to share will go in accordance with age, from 4-6 months, up until 12 months, so as your baby gets older, you will find the recipes will delve into more complex textures for her. It will be a fun journey for the both of you. Remember all babies are different, so always talk to your doctor before introducing solids and new foods to them. Enjoy this next section, and then we will dive into 12+ months when everyone can eat the same foods together at the dinner table, although I am not going to lie, you just may want to eat some of the baby recipes yourself!!

Add THIS to Your Plate!

Adding Solids to Baby's Plate

How do you know when your little pumpkin is ready to take their first bite of solid food? Most doctors will recommend sometime between 4-6 months. Before this time, baby only needs breast milk or formula. In fact, their swallowing and digestive systems are not developmentally ready to handle solids any earlier. Although you may think the size and weight of the baby is a good factor, more goes into it than that. Below are some guidelines that will help you decide when your little one is ready to begin. The key thing to remember is if she is ready, the ideal time is when she is well rested and happy.

Signs Your Baby Is Ready

Here are some signs your baby is ready for a first bite:

- Holds her neck steady and sits with support
- Draws in his lower lip as a spoon is removed from his mouth
- Keeps food in her mouth and swallows it, rather than pushing it back out on her chin

Signs You Should Wait

Here are some signs you may want to wait a little while longer:

- Leaning back
- Turning away

- Pushing the food out of their mouths
- Sealing lips together
- Playing with the food
- Pushing the bottle or spoon away

Ok so you got all the signs from your baby, and the doctor is on board for beginning solids, so now it's on! Let's get cooking.

In this section, you will learn how to make the essential cereals and purees, and meals that are packed with nutrition and flavor for your little one to enjoy.

Recipes

Baby's First Cereals
4-6 Months

When your pediatrician clears you to start solids for your little one, cereal and grains are recommended. Cereals are a wonderful way of getting in whole grains, which are packed with carbohydrates for energy and much-needed nutrition for rapid physical and cognitive growth. You should mix a variety of grains into your baby's diet as they all provide something a little unique. Variety means more balanced nutrition, and it protects your baby against problems that may emerge with any one ingredient.

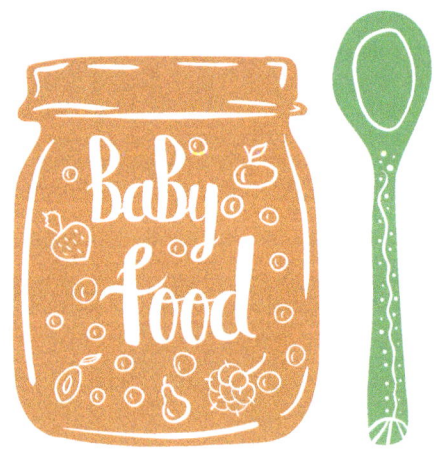

BROWN RICE CEREAL

Brown rice cereal is the perfect first food for the baby due to its dense natural nutrition and fiber. Since most store-bought rice cereals are fortified with iron, adding formula or breast milk will provide added nutrition, including iron.

 Total time: 5-6 min   **Makes** about 1½ cups

Ingredients

- ¼ cup brown rice
- 1½ cups of water, breast milk, or formula

Directions

- In a food processor or blender, add rice and process until it becomes a fine powder.
- In a small saucepan over medium heat bring 1 cup water to a light boil.
- Add the rice powder and reduce heat to low. Whisk constantly until water is absorbed and cereal is smooth and free of lumps. Add more water, formula, or breast milk as needed to desired thickness. Cook for about 5 minutes.

BARLEY CEREAL

Barley is a wonderfully versatile vitamin-rich cereal grain with a rich, nutlike flavor. Besides its amazing fiber content, it is a very good source of molybdenum, manganese, dietary fiber, and selenium, and is a good source of copper, vitamin B1, chromium, phosphorus, magnesium, and niacin.

 Total time: 12 minutes   **Makes** about 1¾ cups

Ingredients

- ¼ cup barley
- 1½ cups water

Directions

- In a food processor or blender, add barley and process until it becomes a fine powder.
- In a small saucepan over medium heat, bring 1 cup water to a light boil.
- Add the barley and simmer for 10 minutes, whisking constantly to avoid clumping.
- Mix in more water, breast milk, or formula for desired thickness. You may also add a pureed vegetable or fruit to this dish for a complete meal.

BABY'S FIRST OATMEAL

Oatmeal provides high energy for baby, is easy to digest, and improves the immune system. It is also a good source of vitamins, minerals, and antioxidants and acts as a natural laxative.

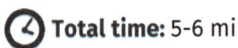 **Total time:** 5-6 min   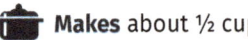 **Makes** about ½ cup

Ingredients

- ¼ cup old-fashioned rolled oats
- ¾ cup – 1 cup water

Directions

- In a food processor or blender, add oatmeal and process until it becomes a fine powder.
- In a small saucepan, bring 3/4 cup water to a light boil. Add the oatmeal powder while whisking constantly to avoid clumps.
- Simmer for 10 minutes, whisking constantly. Mix in more water, formula, or breast milk to desired thickness. You may also add any of your fruit purees as well!

MILLET CEREAL

Not only is millet known for its sweetness and nutty flavor, but it is even more well known for its important nutrients, including copper, manganese, phosphorus, and magnesium, which has been known to fight against childhood asthma.

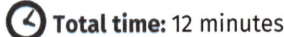 **Total time:** 12 minutes   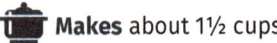 **Makes** about 1½ cups

Ingredients

- ¼ cup millet
- 1½ cups water

Directions

- In a food processor or blender, add millet and process until it becomes a fine powder.
- In a small saucepan on medium-high heat, bring 1 cup water to a light boil.
- Whisk the millet powder into the water and let sit over low heat for 10 minutes.
- Mix in more water, formula, or breast milk to desired thickness. You may also add any of your fruit purees as well!

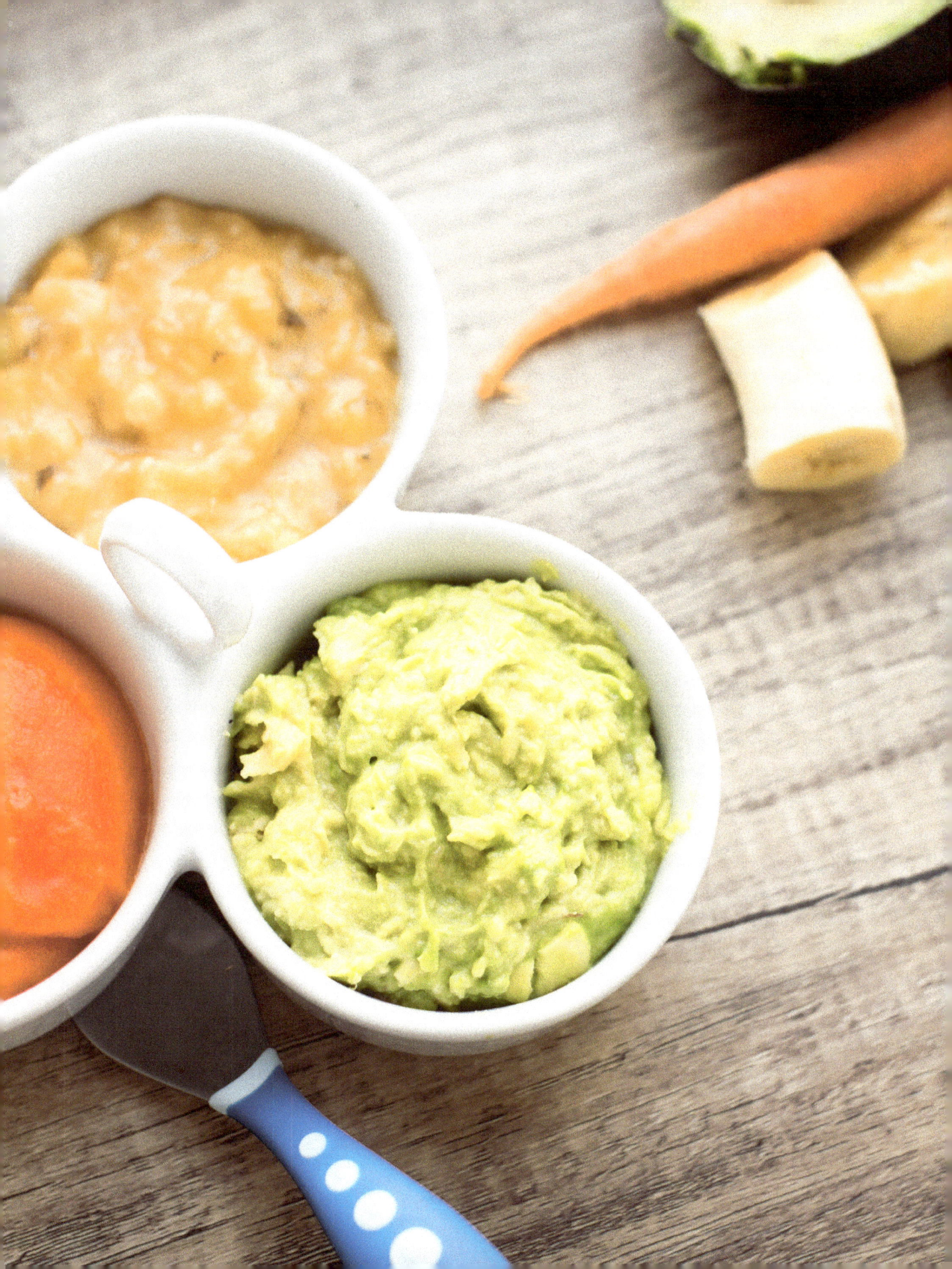

Baby's First Purees
6+ Months

Feeding my baby solids for the first time was by far one of my favorite milestones to witness. I loved watching the reaction on his face. My son has loved food from the moment I gave him his first taste of carrots. I could always tell if he liked the flavor by the rise of his two little eyebrows. It was almost as if he was saying, "Yum!" If he didn't like something, he would purse those lips together and look away. It's funny how non-verbal cues can be just as clear as saying it out loud.

Making a puree is easier than most moms think. Making baby food may seem like a time-consuming task, but if you actually take a look at the steps, it is much easier than you probably think. All we are doing for the most part is just steaming or baking the fruit or vegetable, and then just putting the cooked food right into a blender or food processor and mixing until it is nice and smooth.

Not only are purees easy to make, but they are easy to freeze for later. Whether you are a working mom or a stay-at-home mom, you will appreciate the convenience of easy frozen storage with your purees. You can simply buy freezer-friendly storage containers made specifically for freezing baby foods, or you can just use an ice cube tray with a cover and just pop the frozen cubes out and use as needed. When you start feeding your baby solids, remember to try one at a time for 3-5 days before introducing another just to be sure baby does not have an allergy or reaction. Then you can start with another type and eventually enjoy mixing all these wonderful fruits together for some new flavors. Enjoy the moments, as they will be sitting with you at the family table as a young adult before you know it!

BABY'S FIRST APPLE PIE

Remember that saying, "An apple a day keeps the doctor away?" Studies have now shown that this term is actually true! Apples seem particularly good at fending off various diseases, including cardiovascular disease and cancer. Not to mention it's a childhood favorite and will make your house smell like warm apple pie on a Fall day.

 Total time: 10 minutes   **Makes** about 1 cup

Ingredients

- 2 red apples (peeled, cored, and quartered)
- pinch of cinnamon (optional after 6+ months)

Directions

- In a large saucepan, fill about one inch of water from the bottom and place a steam basket inside the saucepan.
- Place quartered apples in the basket. On high heat, bring pan to a boil and then cover and lower the flame to medium. Steam apples for about 6-10 minutes, or until they are nice and soft and you can easily put a fork through them.
- Remove the steam basket from water and save the water on the bottom of the pan.
- Place apples in a blender or food processor and blend until nice and smooth. You may use some of the water from the bottom of the pan to make the consistency smoother if you wish. As your baby gets older and can enjoy new textures, you can mash the apples, making the consistency chunkier.

PEAR PUREE

Pears are one of my favorite purees. Because they are high in fiber, they are a great fruit to offer as a remedy to help alleviate constipation. If you have a little one with reflux, which is a common condition with infants, pears are very well tolerated. Pears are of my favorite purees to add to oatmeal, rice cereal, and even your family's pancakes. They are also great to add to not-so-liked vegetable purees as a natural sweetener.

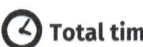 **Total time:** 10 minutes   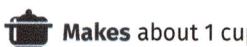 **Makes** about 1 cup

Ingredients

- 2 ripe pears (peeled and cored, quartered)
- cinnamon (optional after 6+ months)

Directions

- In a large saucepan, fill about one inch of water from the bottom and place a steam basket inside.
- Place pears in the basket. On high heat, bring pan to a boil and then cover and lower to a medium flame and steam pears for about 6-10 minutes until they are nice and soft and you can easily put a fork through them.
- Remove steam basket from water and save the water on the bottom of the pan.
- Place pears in a blender or food processor and blend until nice and smooth. You can sprinkle a little cinnamon on them for added flavor. You may use some of the water from the bottom of the pan, or formula or breast milk to make the consistency smoother if you wish. As your baby gets older and can enjoy new textures, you can mash the pears, making the consistency chunkier.

SWEET PEA PUREE

Did you know that one cup of peas contains more protein than a tablespoon of peanut butter? They also provide calcium, vitamins A and C, and iron. This is what that makes peas a wonderful first green vegetable choice for baby. They are also a wonderful first finger food when your little one is ready for that next adventure.

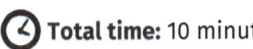 **Total time:** 10 minutes   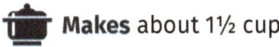 **Makes** about 1½ cups

Ingredients

- 2 cups peas (frozen or fresh)

Directions

- In a large saucepan, fill about one inch of water from the bottom and place a steam basket inside.
- Place peas in the basket. On high heat, bring pan to a boil and then lower the flame to medium and cover and steam peas for about 3-5 minutes (until they are nice and soft).
- Remove steam basket from water and save the water on the bottom of the pan.
- Place peas in a blender or food processor and blend until nice and smooth. You may use some of the water from the bottom of the pan, formula, or breast milk to make the consistency smoother if you wish. As your baby gets older and can enjoy new textures, you can mash the peas, making the consistency chunkier for him or her.

CREAMY AVOCADO

Avocado is one of my favorite vegetables for baby. This creamy delight is a wonderful source of folate, which helps promote heart health, builds new cells, and promotes growth.

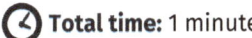 **Total time:** 1 minute   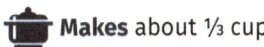 **Makes** about ⅓ cup

Ingredients

- 1 ripe avocado

Directions

- Mash avocado or add to a blender or processor and puree with a little breast milk or formula until it reaches the desired consistency.

FRESH CARROT PUREE

Carrots are an easily digestible vegetable for baby and are full of nutrients such as vitamin A, vitamin C, and calcium. Vitamin A is wonderful to promote healthy eyes and skin and also helps in fighting infection.

Total time: 10 minutes   **Makes** about 12 servings

Ingredients

- 12 carrots (peeled and evenly chopped)

Directions

- Place a steam basket in a large pot filled with 3 inches of water. Just make sure water does not touch basket.
- Place carrots in steam basket, then bring water to a boil.
- Lower flame to medium and cover and steam until you can easily put a fork through the carrots (about 7-8 minutes once water is hot).
- Transfer carrots to a blender or food processor and process to desired thickness. You can add some formula or breast milk to make it thinner.

SWEET POTATO PUREE

Rich in antioxidants, beta-carotene, vitamins C and B complex, iron, and phosphorous, sweet potatoes prove to be excellent immunity boosters. They are also high in calories, have wonderful anti-inflammatory properties, and help aid in digestion, which makes them a wonderful first vegetable. This was always a favorite with my little one.

Total time: 25-30 minutes   **Makes** about 2 cups

Ingredients

- 2 sweet potatoes (peeled and chopped)

Directions

- In a large saucepan, fill about one inch of water from the bottom and place a steam basket inside the saucepan.
- Place chopped potatoes in the basket. Bring pan to a boil and then lower flame to medium and cover and steam until a fork can poke through them (about 20 minutes, check every 10 minutes to be safe).
- Place sweet potatoes in a blender or food processor and blend until nice and smooth. You may use some of the water from the bottom of the pan, formula, or breast milk to make the consistency smoother if you wish.

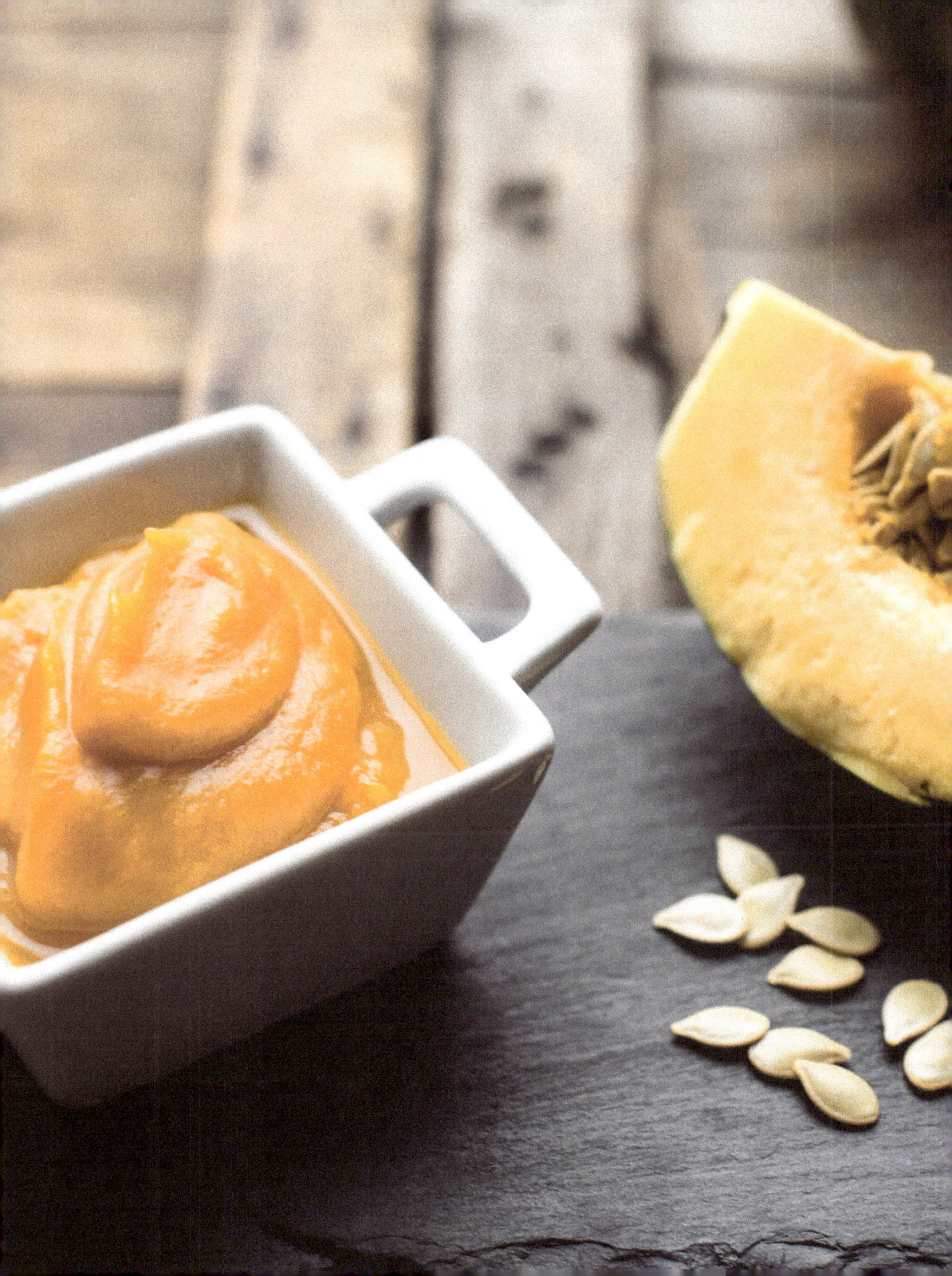

PUMPKIN, BUTTERNUT SQUASH, OR ACORN SQUASH PUREE

Pumpkin and squash have always been a favorite during the fall season. Not only do they taste yummy, but they are highly loaded with vitamin A and beta-carotene. Beta-carotene is one of the plant carotenoids that when eaten and digested, turns into vitamin A in the human body. Beta-carotene may reduce the risk of cancer as well as heart disease. These are also great sources of potassium, protein, and iron.

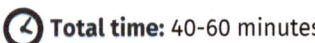 **Total time:** 40-60 minutes   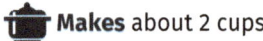 **Makes** about 2 cups

Ingredients

- 1 type of squash (such as a sugar pumpkin, butternut squash, or acorn squash) halved and seeds removed.
- water
- cinnamon and nutmeg (optional, wait until 6+ months)

Directions

- In a baking pan, place each squash/pumpkin half face down.
- Fill the baking pan with water so that it is about ¼-inch up the sides of the squash.
- Bake at 375°F for about 40-60 minutes. You will know it is done when the skin looks wrinkled and is soft when pressed.
- Scrape out the squash/pumpkin meat and place in a blender or food processor. You may add breast milk or formula to create a thinner consistency.
- **Optional:** You can add a pinch of cinnamon into the puree for added flavor. (optional after 6+ months)

TIP:

You can also buy pre-cleaned and chopped squash and just steam it. You will know it is done when you can easily stick a knife or fork through them (12 minutes or so).

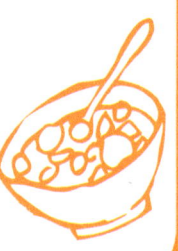

GREEN BEAN PUREE

The green bean ranks very low on the list of foods that prompt allergic reactions which is why they are a vegetable favorite. They can be known to cause some gas, so you may want to wait until your baby is at least 6 months old to try this one. They are rich in vitamin K and vitamin C, and also very high in calcium, which is wonderful for the bones.

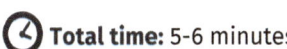 **Total time:** 5-6 minutes   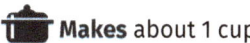 **Makes** about 1 cup

Ingredients

- 1 pound frozen green beans (frozen will be less grainy)

Directions

◎ In a large saucepan, fill about one inch of water from the bottom and place a steam basket inside the saucepan.

◎ Place green beans the basket. On high heat, bring pan to a boil and then lower flame to medium and cover and steam until they are soft (about 5 minutes).

◎ Place green beans in a blender or food processor and blend until nice and smooth. You may use some of the water from the bottom of the pan, breast milk, or formula to make the consistency smoother if you wish.

BANANA PUREE

Besides being a delicious treat for your little one, bananas also contain potassium and fiber and are also high in vitamin B6, vitamin C, and vitamin B2, which are wonderful in aiding a strong immune system. Although this may be a favorite, too much banana can cause some constipation. A little pinch of cinnamon when your baby is 6+ months is also a delicious spice to add to give a new flavor.

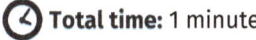 **Total time:** 1 minute   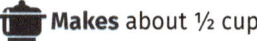 **Makes** about ½ cup

Ingredients

- 1 ripe banana

Directions

◎ Simply chop banana into 4 pieces and mash with a fork until smooth. If you wish to make it smoother, you can add breast milk or baby formula to it and blend in a blender or small food processor.

Favorite Puree Combos: Let's Mix It Up! 7+ Months

In months 4-6, we took our first big step by introducing solids to our little one and now as we move into month 7, it's time to mix things up a little. Your baby will start to eat from a spoon much more easily and will even start to eat with her hands. We learned a little bit in the previous chapter about the health benefits of our favorite fruits and vegetables, so not only will mixing these wonderful foods together be even more nutritious, but will also offer some wonderful new flavors for your baby's palate.

Although there are so many wonderful puree combos to experiment with, here are some of our favorites.

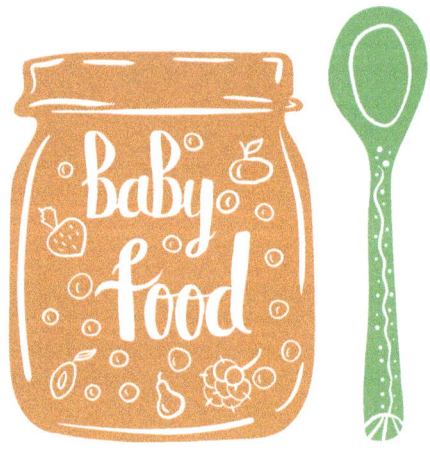

Add THIS to Your Plate!

CARROT AND SPINACH

This is a wonderful combo. As we know, carrots are wonderful for healthy eyes and skin and spinach is an amazing source of calcium. Just 1 cup of cooked spinach gives you 42 mg of calcium. Spinach also contains respectable amounts of vitamin A, iron, and selenium too.

 Total time: 10 minutes 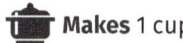 **Makes** 1 cup

Ingredients

- 2 cups carrots (peeled and evenly chopped)
- 2 cups spinach

Directions

- Place a steam basket in a large pot filled with 3 inches of water. Just make sure water does not touch basket. Then heat water on medium-high heat.
- Place carrots and spinach in a steam basket, cover, and steam until you can easily put a fork through the carrots (about 8-10 minutes once water is hot).
- Transfer carrots and spinach to a blender or food processor and process to desired thickness. You can add some water, formula, or breast milk to make thinner.

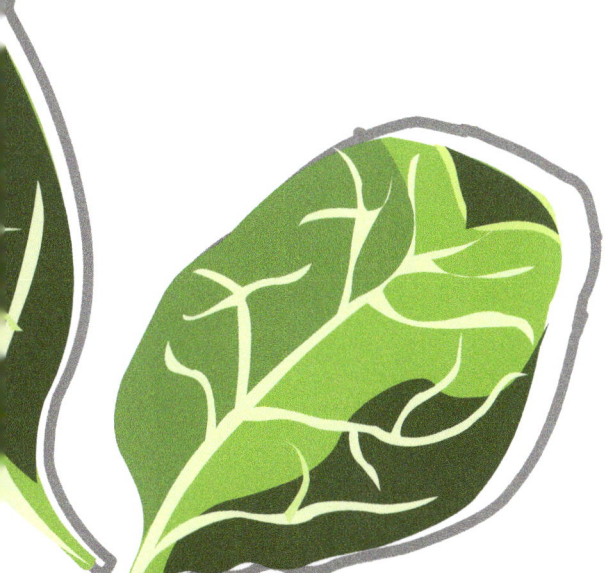

CARROT AND GREEN BEAN

This a nutrient-packed combo. The many nutrients in green beans can help you prevent a number of different conditions, including Alzheimer's, atherosclerosis, diabetic heart disease, colon cancer, asthma, arthritis, acne, ear infections, and maybe even colds and flu. Carrots help with not only vision but also cardiovascular health since they are a wonderful antioxidant.

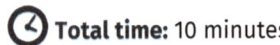 **Total time:** 10 minutes   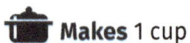 **Makes** 1 cup

Ingredients

- 2 cups carrots (peeled and evenly chopped)
- 1 lb. frozen green beans (frozen will be less grainy)

Directions

- Place a steam basket in a large pot filled with 3 inches of water. Just make sure water does not touch basket. Then heat water on medium-high heat.
- Place carrots and green beans in steam basket and cover. Steam on medium heat until you can easily put a fork through the carrots and green beans (about 7 to 8 minutes, once water is hot).
- Transfer carrots and spinach to a blender or food processor and process to desired thickness. You can add some water, formula, or breast milk to make thinner.

BANANA AND AVOCADO

Although avocado is known as one of the most amazing superfoods, I find it is more of a creamy enhancement rather than the flavor being the main attraction. By adding banana, it becomes a rich, creamy, flavorful favorite for baby.

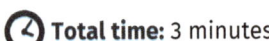 **Total time:** 3 minutes   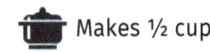 **Makes** ½ cup

Ingredients

- 1 banana
- ½ avocado

Directions

- Combine both ingredients in a blender or food processor and add breast milk or formula to achieve the desired thickness and texture.

BROCCOLI & PEAR

Broccoli, which is wonderful for heart health and growth, was always a vegetable I had to be creative with. My little one always seemed to welcome this vegetable a little bit more when I added the sweetness of pear. Your toddler will get the nutritional benefits of both while enjoying the sweet flavor of this combo.

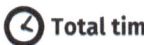 **Total time:** 10 minutes   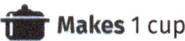 **Makes** 1 cup

Ingredients

- 1 cup broccoli (chopped)
- 2 pears (peeled, cored, and chopped)

Directions

- In a large saucepan, fill about one inch of water from the bottom and place a steam basket inside the saucepan.
- Place chopped broccoli and pear in the basket. On high heat, bring pan to a boil and then cover and steam on a medium flame until you can poke a hole through them (about 8 minutes).
- Then place cooked broccoli and pear in a blender or food processor and blend until nice and smooth. You may use some of the water from the bottom of the pan to make the consistency smoother if you wish.

BLACK BEAN AND BANANA MASH

I know this combo may seem unique at first, but it is a great mix. By adding beans to the mix, you will add protein and complex carbohydrates to the plate. They are also a great source of folate.

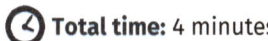 **Total time:** 4 minutes   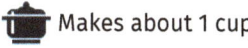 **Makes about 1 cup**

Ingredients

- 1 ripe banana
- 1 cup cooked black beans (canned or boiled fresh)

Directions

- Combine banana and beans in a bowl and mash together. You can also pulse a few times in a processor and add breast milk or formula to get a smoother texture.

BANANA & PUMPKIN

Did you know that a pumpkin is actually a fruit? Yes! Botanists consider fruits to be the portion of a plant that forms from a flower and also the part of a plant that contains seeds. Stems, leaves, roots, and even flower buds are considered to be vegetables. I love adding bananas to the mix; they were always a fruit favorite for my little one, so no matter what I added it to, he would eat it with pleasure.

Total time: 4 minutes   **Makes 1 cup**

Ingredients

- 1 large banana or 2 small bananas (mashed)
- ½ cup pumpkin puree (canned or fresh) (see pumpkin puree recipe)

Directions

- Combine bananas and pumpkin together and mix well. You may also blend and add a little breast milk or formula to make it smoother.

BANANA AND COCONUT TOFU

Tofu is a great source of iron, protein, and calcium. This exciting combo will be a new sweet tropical favor baby to try.

Total time: 5 minutes   **Makes about ¾ cup**

Ingredients

- 1 ripe banana (peeled)
- 1 cup organic tofu
- 1 tbsp. finely grated unsweetened coconut

Directions

- Combine all ingredients into a processor and blend until smooth or to desired consistency. You can add water, breast milk or formula to make it a thinner texture.

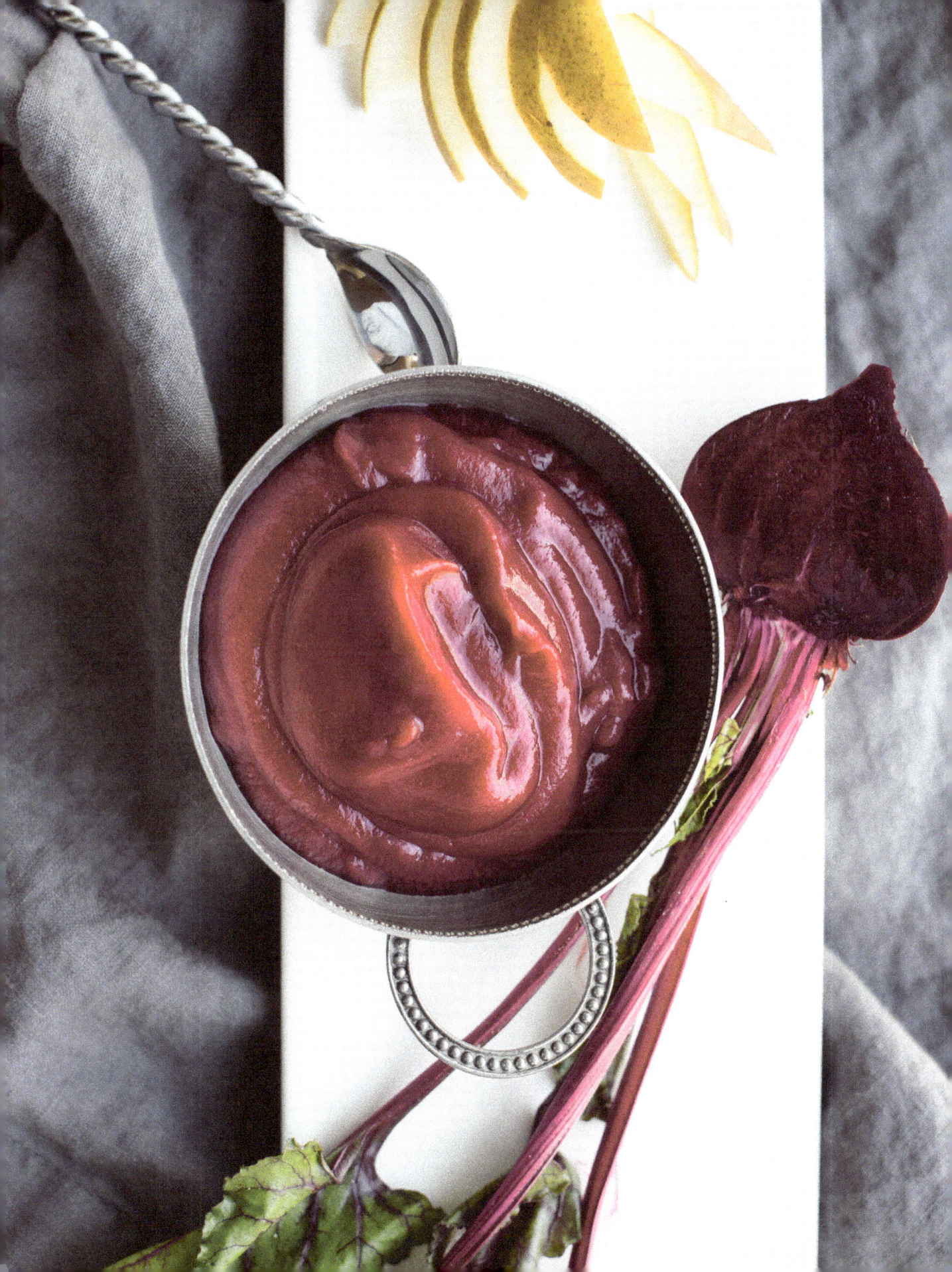

CAULIFOWER MASH WITH SWEET BEET AND PEAR

Cauliflower packs a powerful punch of vitamin C and fiber, and beets are a wonderful source of calcium, potassium, and vitamin A, which plays a large role in healthy development for your baby. I found that my little one was not a huge fan of the taste of cauliflower on its own, but when I added the sweet flavor and colorful addition of beets, he enjoyed it much more.

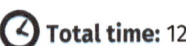 **Total time:** 12 minutes   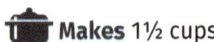 **Makes** 1½ cups

Ingredients

- 1 cup cauliflower (chopped)
- 2 beets (cleaned, greens removed, peeled, quartered)
- 1 pear (peeled, cored, and chopped)

Directions

- In a large pot, fill with about 2-3 inches of water, place a steam basket inside the pot, and then add beets, cauliflower, and pear. Cover and steam on medium-high heat until you can put a knife easily through beets (about 12 minutes, although beets may need more time).

- Combine all ingredients in a food processor or blender to create a puree of your desired consistency. You can add a little water to make a thinner consistency if needed.

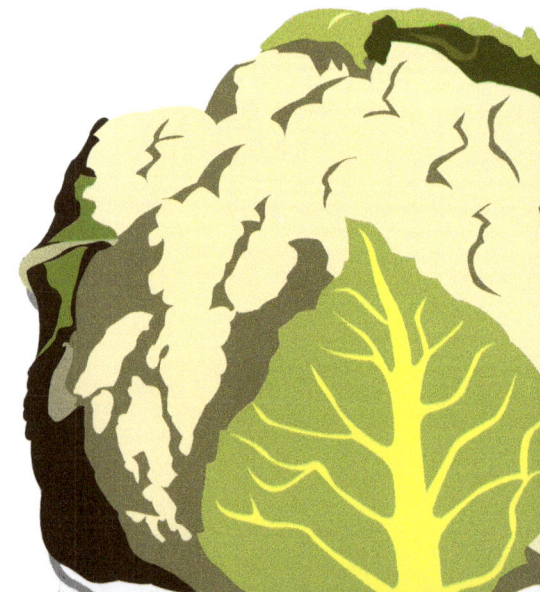

APPLE & BUTTERNUT SQUASH

This is a favorite combo of mine. I love to add a little cinnamon or nutmeg to this blend, and it has such a delicious flavor. You may need to save a few spoonfuls for yourself as well!

Total time: 10 minutes   **Makes** 1 cup

Ingredients

- 1 cup butternut squash puree (see butternut squash puree recipe, page 63)
- 2 apples (peeled, cored, and chopped)

Directions

- In a large saucepan, fill about one inch of water from the bottom and place a steam basket inside the saucepan.
- Place chopped apples in basket. On high heat, bring pan to a boil and then cover and steam until a fork can poke through them (about 8 minutes).
- Then place apples in a blender or food processor and blend until nice and smooth. You may use some of the water from the bottom of the pan to make the consistency smoother if you wish. Combine both apples and squash together in a bowl.

TIP:

You can also buy pre-cleaned and chopped butternut squash and steam with your apples. You will know it is done when you can easily stick a knife or fork through them (12 minutes or so).

BLUEBERRY, PLUM, PEACH, AND BANANA SMOOTHIE

Nothing feels more refreshing than a cold fruit delight. Now that your baby has tried so many different fruits, you can get creative by mixing your favorites together. This is one my son especially enjoyed and hopefully your baby will too!

 Total time: 10 minutes   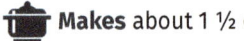 **Makes** about 1 ½ cups

Ingredients

- 1 banana (peeled)
- 1 plum (sliced in half and cored)
- 1 peach (sliced in half and cored)
- ½ cup blueberries
- water as needed

Directions

- In a blender, combine all ingredients and blend until desired consistency. Add a little water as needed.

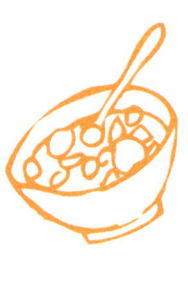

TIP:

If you wish to remove skins, you can do this by straining mixture through a fine mesh sieve set over a bowl, pushing on solids with the back of a spoon to extract as much as possible. Then discard the solids.

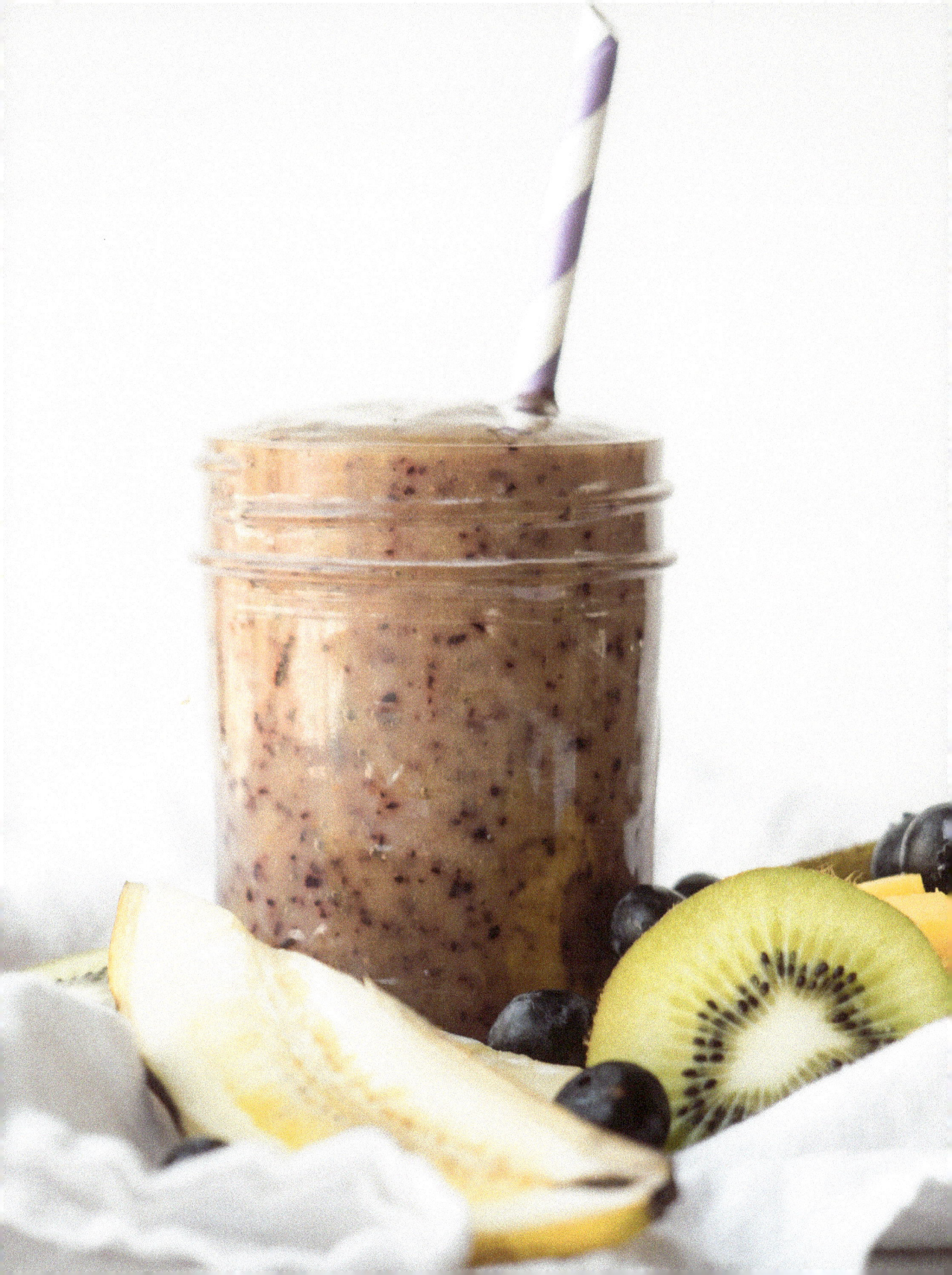

TROPICAL FRUIT SMOOTHIE

I love this blend. As I mixed these fruits together, I would get a scent of tropical vacation in the air. Although a vacation may seem like a fantasy at the moment, maybe a little sip yourself will take you to your favorite tropical island for a moment. Once your baby reaches 9 months, you can add yogurt and make this a tropical yogurt parfait. Your baby will love it!

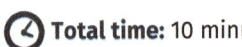 **Total time:** 10 minutes   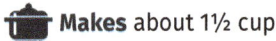 **Makes** about 1½ cups

Ingredients

- 1 banana (peeled)
- 1 mango (peeled, cored, and chopped)
- ½ cup blueberries
- ½ kiwi (skin removed)
- water if needed

Directions

- Peel and slice banana.
- Peel, core, and slice mango.
- Cut kiwi in half. Slide a teaspoon between the skin and the flesh and twist it around the edge of the fruit. Once spoon has done a complete rotation, slide under the flesh and you should be able to scoop it right out.
- In a blender, combine all fruits and blend until smooth. If you wish to decrease the thickness, you can add some water.

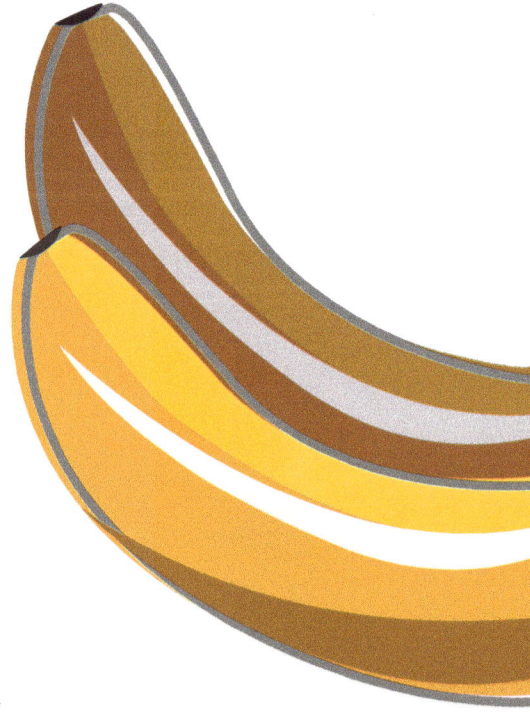

Pureed Meats
6-8 Months

Total time: About 5 minutes   **Servings:** About ½ a cup

I was surprised when my pediatrician recommended I start feeding my son meats as early as 6 months old, but again this will all vary on your pediatrician and when your baby is ready. Recent research has suggested that meat should be introduced as one of the first foods for babies, generally from 6 months of age. Why? Simply because it is high in iron. This is true for breastfed babies in particular. The iron from breast milk is very well absorbed by babies; however, when exclusively breastfed babies are introduced to solid foods, they begin to absorb less iron from their milk. This is because the iron in breast milk becomes bound by the solid food they are consuming (commonly infant rice cereal).

Thus, it becomes important to ensure that the solid food given to a previously exclusively breastfed infant is high in iron. And one of the best sources of iron is, of course, meat (beef and lamb in particular). New studies also found that that the more finely ground the meat, the more easily the body can absorb this iron. So with this said, we should get started!

Although before your baby was born you probably never prepared pureed meat, you will realize it's actually pretty easy to do. In fact, pureeing your meats is very similar to how you puree your fruits and vegetables. You simply cook your meat and then process it until smooth. The best time to puree your meat is when it is still very warm; it will just puree much more easily since it will be softer. Once you have pureed your meat, you can start to create a well-balanced meal with all food groups simply by combing your favorite vegetable purees and a choice of whole grain such as brown rice, quinoa, barley, or millet, with your meat of choice. Pretty neat, right?

Ingredients

- 1 cup cooked selected meat (preferably on the warm side) (beef, pork, chicken, veal) chopped into 1-inch chunks
- ¼ cup water or juice from when you cooked the meat

Directions

- Place chunks of meat in a food processor or blender and puree until a powdery mix is formed. Slowly add juice or water and puree until smooth or to desired consistency.
- Then add a vegetable puree and baby cereal of your choice and you will have a complete meal!

Creating New and Exciting Plates 7+ Months

BLUEBERRY & RASPBERRY CREAM OF WHEAT (7 + Months)

Cream of Wheat was one of my favorite breakfast bowls as a child, but by no means does this dish need to be served in the morning. It can be served any time of day. Berries are a wonderful antioxidant, which is great for your baby's immune system, and when served with whole grains such as Cream of Wheat, you have an added bonus because it will increase the absorption of iron from the whole grain. So not only will this be a colorful and flavorful dish, but an ingredient match, made in heaven.

Total time: 8 minutes **Makes** about 1 cup

Ingredients

- 1 cup blueberries
- 1 cup raspberries
- 1 cup breast milk or formula
- 1 cup water
- ⅓ cup cream of wheat cereal

Directions

- In a saucepan on medium heat, cook and mash blueberries and raspberries until berries have broken down to a liquid form (about 3-5 minutes).
- In a separate saucepan, bring liquids to a simmer.
- Lower heat and slowly whisk in cream of wheat cereal, stirring constantly until well blended and smooth (about 1-2 minutes)
- Then stir in berry mixture and serve.

YOGURT, CUCUMBER, AND MINT SOUP (10-12 Months)

This is what I call the perfect baby detox soup, since yogurt is a wonderful probiotic and garlic has been known to boost the immune system. Mint is known to not only clean the palate, but it also promotes digestion, soothing stomachs in cases of indigestion or inflammation.

Prep time: 10 minutes **Total time:** 15 minutes **Servings:** Makes about a cup

Ingredients

- 8 oz. plain Greek yogurt
- ½ cucumber (minced)
- ⅛ tsp. raw garlic (minced)
- 1¼ tsp. fresh mint (minced)

Directions

- In a small bowl, combine all ingredients. Serve cold.

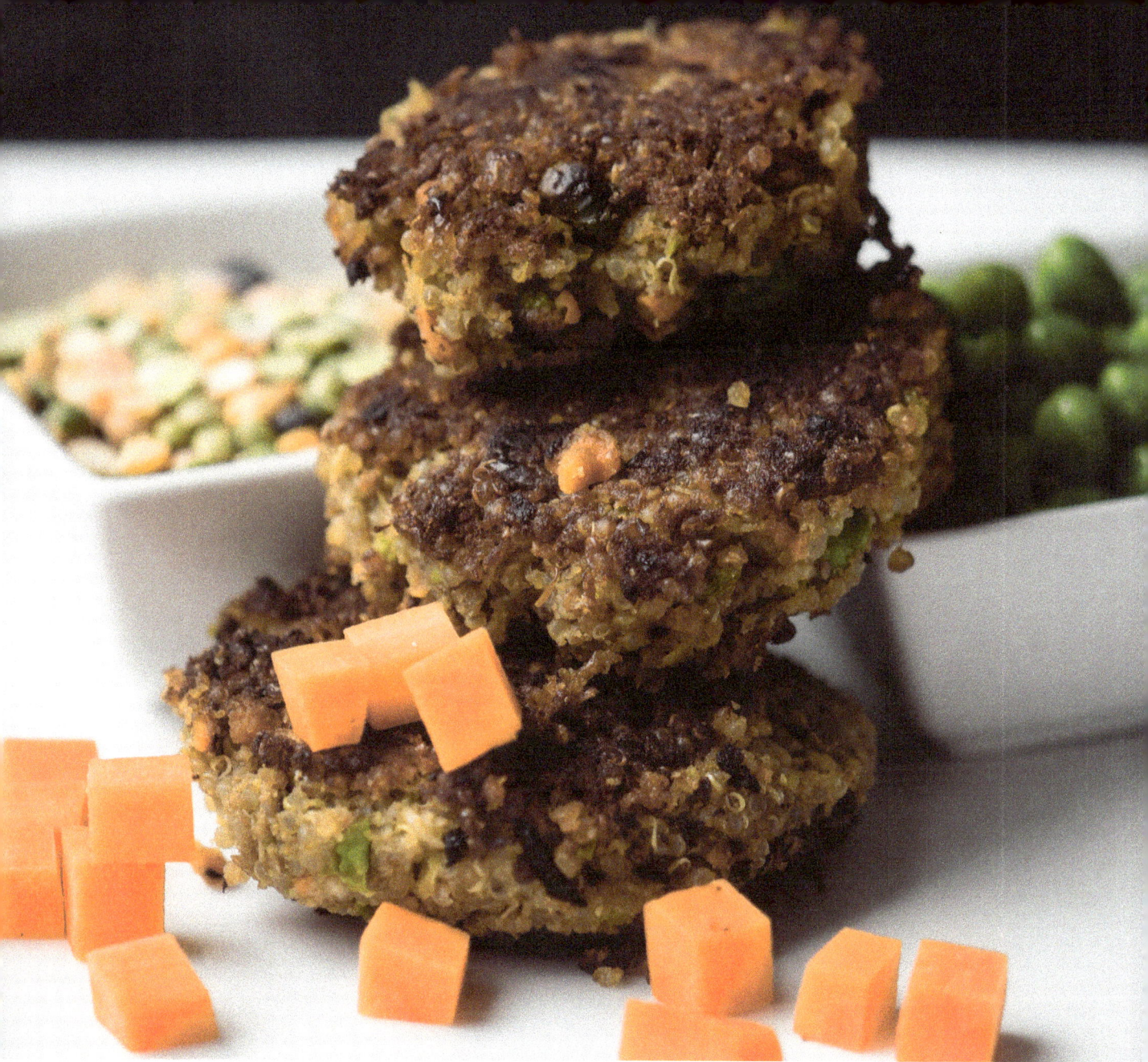

QUINOA & LENTIL MINI BURGERS (7+ Months)

This ethnic-inspired meal provides a good source or protein, vegetables, and whole grains. This is a great way to start to introduce new spices and flavors as well. I strongly believe introducing as many flavors early will help avoid picky eaters later. Children more often than not do not try certain foods due to something psychological as opposed to just the taste alone. Adding flavorful spices such as cumin and garlic will create some wonderful aromas in your kitchen and also new exciting flavors for your baby's palate.

QUINOA & LENTIL MINI BURGERS (7+ Months)

 Prep time: 15 minutes   **Total time:** 1 hour   **Makes** 14 mini burgers

Ingredients

- 1 cup cooked quinoa
- 3 tbsp. high smoke point cooking oil like avocado oil
- 2 carrots (peeled and minced)
- ½ cup onion (minced)
- 1 garlic clove (minced)
- ¾ cup whole-grain bread crumbs (about 3 slices of whole-grain bread needed)
- 1 (15 oz.) can cooked lentils (drained and rinsed if there is a lot of fluid in can)
- 1 cup peas
- ½ tsp. cumin

Directions

- Prepare quinoa by following instructions on its packaging.
- Meanwhile, in a large non-stick skillet on a medium-high flame, add oil and let heat for a minute.
- Add carrots and onions and sauté until soft (about 5 minutes).
- Add garlic and cook one minute, then turn off heat and put mixture aside.
- Prepare bread crumbs by breaking the slices of bread into pieces and placing in a blender or processor and processing until bread become a fine crumb.
- Put all the peas and half of the lentils and in a food processor or blender and process until smooth and pasty.
- In a large bowl, combine all ingredients (carrot, onion and garlic mixture, bread crumbs, peas, lentils, quinoa, and cumin).
- To prepare the patties, scoop mixture into a 1/4 measuring cup and use a spoon to press it flat. Then turn it over into your hand with a spatula to remove from cup. Then lay on a tray. Repeat this process until all of the mixture is gone.
- In a large, non-stick skillet on medium-high heat, heat about ¼ cup oil (just enough to coat the entire bottom of pan).
- Place as many mini-burgers as you can fit into the pan without crowding it. You will need room to flip them.
- Cook each side for about 1 minute or until you get a nice, golden brown crust. You may have to turn the heat to high to get a nice crisp, just be careful not to burn them. If you don't cook long enough get a crust, they are more likely to fall apart.
- Repeat until all of the burgers are cooked. You may need to add more oil each batch. Let cool a little before serving so you can break into bite-sized pieces for your baby.

RED BELL PEPPER MEDITERRANEAN HUMMUS (10 + Months)

As a daughter of an Armenian mother, hummus was a kitchen staple in my Mediterranean family. Garbanzo beans are a great source of protein and folate and also serve as a nice complex carbohydrate. This spread pairs well with vegetables, or ground chicken, lamb, or beef. You may even save some for the rest of the family as well!

Prep time: 10 minutes   **Total time:** 20 minutes   **Makes** about a 1½ cups

Ingredients

- ½ roasted bell pepper (store bought or home roasted with skin removed)
- 1 (15 oz.) can chickpeas
- 1 small garlic clove (chopped)
- ¼ tsp. cumin
- ½ cup Greek yogurt
- 3 tbsp. olive oil
- ⅛ tsp. paprika

Directions

- Set oven to broil, and place a rack at least 6-8 inches from broiler. Slice a bell pepper in half and place face down in a roasting pan. Roast for 7-8 minutes, remove from oven, wait 2-3 minutes to cool off a bit, and discard the skin. If you want a shortcut, you can buy them in the store already roasted.
- Place all ingredients in a blender or food processor, and process until smooth. Be careful all chickpeas get blended, and there are no remaining giant whole chickpeas softened.

BABY'S CREAMY PUMPKIN PIE (10+)

When I first tasted this creamy delight, I went to cloud nine. The creamy texture and flavor reminded me of pumpkin pie without the crust or guilt. My little one loves this combo. What I like even more is that since the consistency is thick and creamy, it is a nice dish to have your baby practice using a spoon on her own since the mixture sticks well to the spoon as she aims for her mouth.

Total time: 5 minutes   **Makes** almost 2 cups

Ingredients

- 7 oz. plain Greek yogurt
- 7 oz. prepared pumpkin puree (canned or homemade)
- ⅛ tsp. nutmeg

Directions

- Combine all ingredients in a medium-sized bowl. Stir well.

BAKED SWEET POTATO FRIES (7 + Months)

I contemplated placing this recipe in the "family sides" section of this book because although it is a baby favorite, it is an adult favorite too! In fact, you may want to double this recipe and save some for the entire family. This is a wonderful first finger food since you can chop the fries into small pieces and they will be soft and easy to chew. Although I used cumin in this recipe, I encourage you to try other new spices each time you make them, such as curry or a blend of nutmeg, cinnamon, and allspice. Just remember to season lightly.

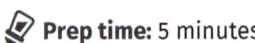 **Prep time:** 5 minutes   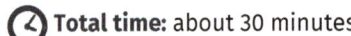 **Total time:** about 30 minutes   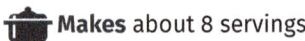 **Makes** about 8 servings

Ingredients

- 2 sweet potatoes (peeled)
- ⅓ cup high smoke point oil such as avocado oil
- ½ tsp. cumin (optional)

Directions

- Pre-heat oven to 425°F on bake.
- Slice potatoes into 4-5 slices, then cut in the other direction to create sticks.
- In a bowl, combine sweet potato sticks, oil, and cumin. Then toss to be sure potatoes are well coated.
- Then line a tray with parchment paper and lay sticks out onto the tray without any overlap.
- Cook for 20-25 minutes or until cooked fully through.

TIP:

For an even crunch I liked to flip them after the first 10 minutes.

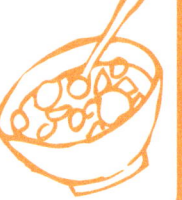

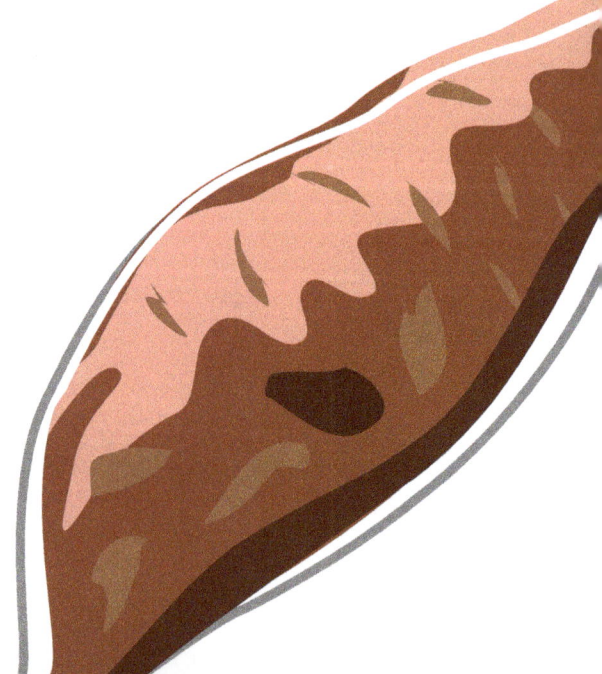

BLACK BEAN, AVOCADO & CHICKEN SALAD (7+ Months)

This dish is the perfect blend of complex carbohydrates, vegetables, and protein. Got a busy day ahead? This dish will provide a lot of energy for baby. What is so fun about combining these dishes is that most likely your baby has already tried the beans and avocado during the puree stage. By adding chicken and cumin, your baby will be familiar with the texture, yet intrigued by the new flavors.

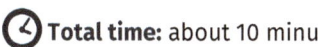 **Total time:** about 10 minutes 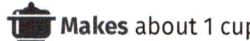 **Makes** about 1 cup

Ingredients

- ½ cup cooked chicken breast (see pureed meats recipe for desired texture for baby)
- ½ cup cooked black beans
- ½ small, ripe avocado, pitted
- pinch of cumin
- breast milk or formula

Directions

- Place beans and avocado into a food processor and pulse to desired texture. You may also use a hand masher if you prefer a chunkier texture. Add breast milk or formula for a smoother/thinner texture.
- Scoop mixture into a bowl and then add chicken. Stir together ingredients and serve!

IRISH STEEL-CUT OATS WITH PEAR AND CINNAMON (9+ Months)

As your little one matures, you will start to want to feed your little one more mature textures. A nice step up from the instant-porridge-like oatmeal will be steel-cut oats. Although no different in nutritional value, this will add a new and exciting texture for your baby to munch on. Since oatmeal can have such a plain taste, adding pear and cinnamon to the dish will perk things right up.

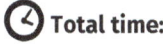 **Total time:** 35 minutes 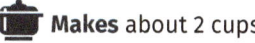 **Makes** about 2 cups

Ingredients

- 2 pears (shredded or grated)
- 1 cup Irish steel-cut oats
- 3¾ cups water, formula, or breast milk (or combo of both)

Directions

- In a saucepan, stir in oats, pears, and water, formula, or breast milk, and bring to a boil.
- Then reduce to a simmer for 30 minutes, stirring occasionally.
- Once oatmeal is tender, sprinkle with cinnamon and serve.

Danielle Formaro

CREAMY PUMPKIN RISOTTO (7 + Months)

Risotto is a favorite northern Italian rice dish cooked in a broth to a creamy consistency. Although I used pumpkin in this recipe, you can substitute any vegetable puree to create an entirely new dish for next time!

Prep time: 6 minutes **Total time:** about 36 minutes **Makes** 3 cups

Ingredients

- 2 tsp. butter
- 2 shallots (minced)
- 1 garlic clove
- 1 cup Arborio rice
- 4 cups chicken or vegetable broth
- 2 cups fresh or canned pumpkin puree
- pinch of nutmeg
- pinch of cinnamon

Directions

- Melt butter in a skillet on medium heat.
- Add shallots and cook for 2 minutes. Then add garlic and cook for one minute.
- Add and stir in rice and cook for about 1 minute to absorb flavors of garlic and shallots.
- Add one cup of broth and stir frequently until all liquid is absorbed into the rice.
- Then add another cup of the broth and repeat. Repeat this with the remainder of broth one cup at a time until rice is tender.
- Add pumpkin puree, cinnamon, and nutmeg to risotto and stir all contents together.
- You can also add more broth or add entire mixture to a blender if you feel you wish to have a smoother texture your baby can handle.

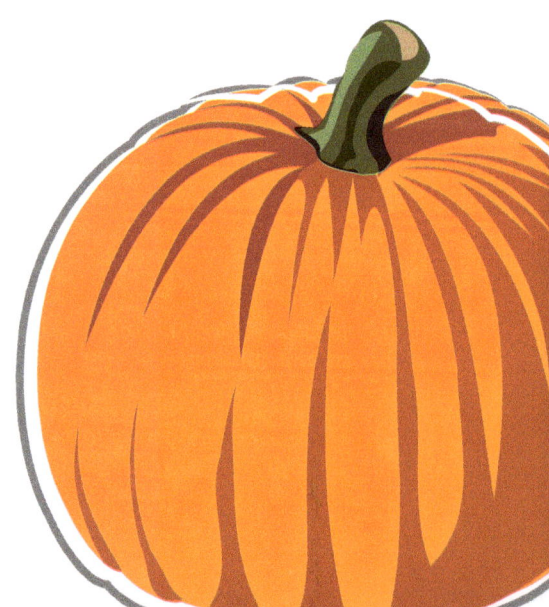

COUSCOUS WITH BROCCOLI, CAULIFLOWER, GARLIC AND OIL
(7+ Months)

Couscous is a staple of North Africa. Couscous is more than just "the food so nice they named it twice." Cute, right? Couscous is a tiny pasta made of wheat or barley; wheat couscous is the most widely available version in North America, and most of it is "instant" or quick-cooking. It also has a wide variety of health benefits, including the ability to prevent certain cancers, increase heart health, prevent bacterial and viral infections, promote normal metabolism throughout the body's systems, control fluid levels in the body, improve digestion, help weight loss efforts, heal wounds, build muscles, and boost the immune system. Now add this with some of our favorite vegetables and seasoning, and you have one healthy dish!

 Prep time: 15 minutes   **Total time:** about 35 minutes   **Makes** about 3 cups

Ingredients

- 2 cups water
- 1 cup couscous
- 1 cup broccoli (chopped)
- 1 cup cauliflower (chopped)
- ¼ cup olive oil
- 1 garlic clove (chopped)
- Parmesan cheese, for sprinkling (optional)

Directions

- In a medium saucepan, bring water to a boil. Add couscous, cover and reduce heat to low and cook for 15 minutes. Once finished, fluff with fork. Set aside.
- In a large pot, fill with about 2 inches of water, place a steam basket inside pot, and then add broccoli and cauliflower, cover and steam on medium-high heat until soft (about 6-7 minutes). Once cooked, remove from pan and finely chop vegetables and set aside.
- Meanwhile, in a small saucepan, on a low flame heat the oil, add garlic, and cook for 1 minute or until golden in color. Be careful not to burn
- In a dish, combine couscous, vegetables, oil, and garlic. Sprinkle with Parmesan cheese and serve.

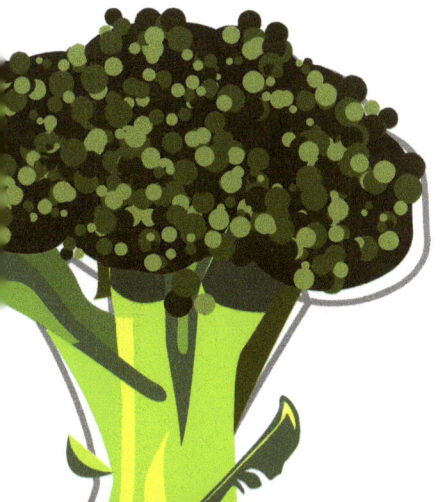

TURKEY APPLE MEATBALLS (9 + Months)

These are so juicy and flavorful you may need to hide them from the rest of the family. When I made these, I found myself popping one in my mouth around the clock. I took that as a good sign this recipe was a keeper. The secret to keeping these little balls moist was adding the apple. It not only kept them juicy but added a nice sweet surprise to each bite.

 Prep time: 25 minutes   **Total time:** about 50 minutes   **Makes** about 22 x 1-inch balls

Ingredients

- 1 red apple (peeled, cored, and grated)
- 1 lb. ground organic turkey
- 2 tbsp. yellow onion (minced)
- 1 egg (beaten)
- ½ cup whole-wheat bread crumbs (about 2 pieces of whole-wheat bread processed)
- 1 tbsp. tomato puree
- 1 garlic clove (minced)
- 1 tbsp. Parmesan cheese
- 1½ tbsp. fresh or dried flat-leaf parsley

Directions

◎ Pre-heat oven to 350°F.

◎ In a medium-size bowl, combine all ingredients with your hands until blended.

◎ Line a baking pan with parchment paper. Form into mini-balls (1 inch), and align on baking pan (about the size of a silver dollar; makes about 22 mini meatballs).

◎ Bake for about 20 minutes or until slightly golden and internal temperature reads 165°F. Allow to cool and enjoy!

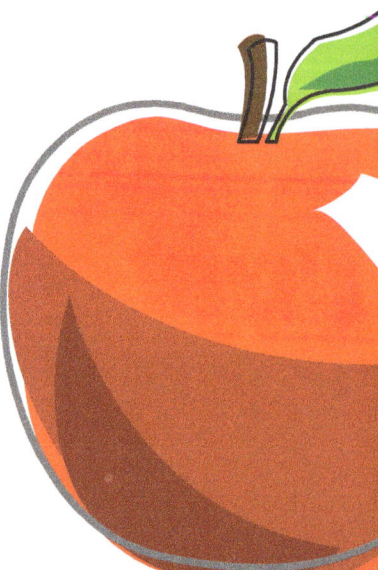

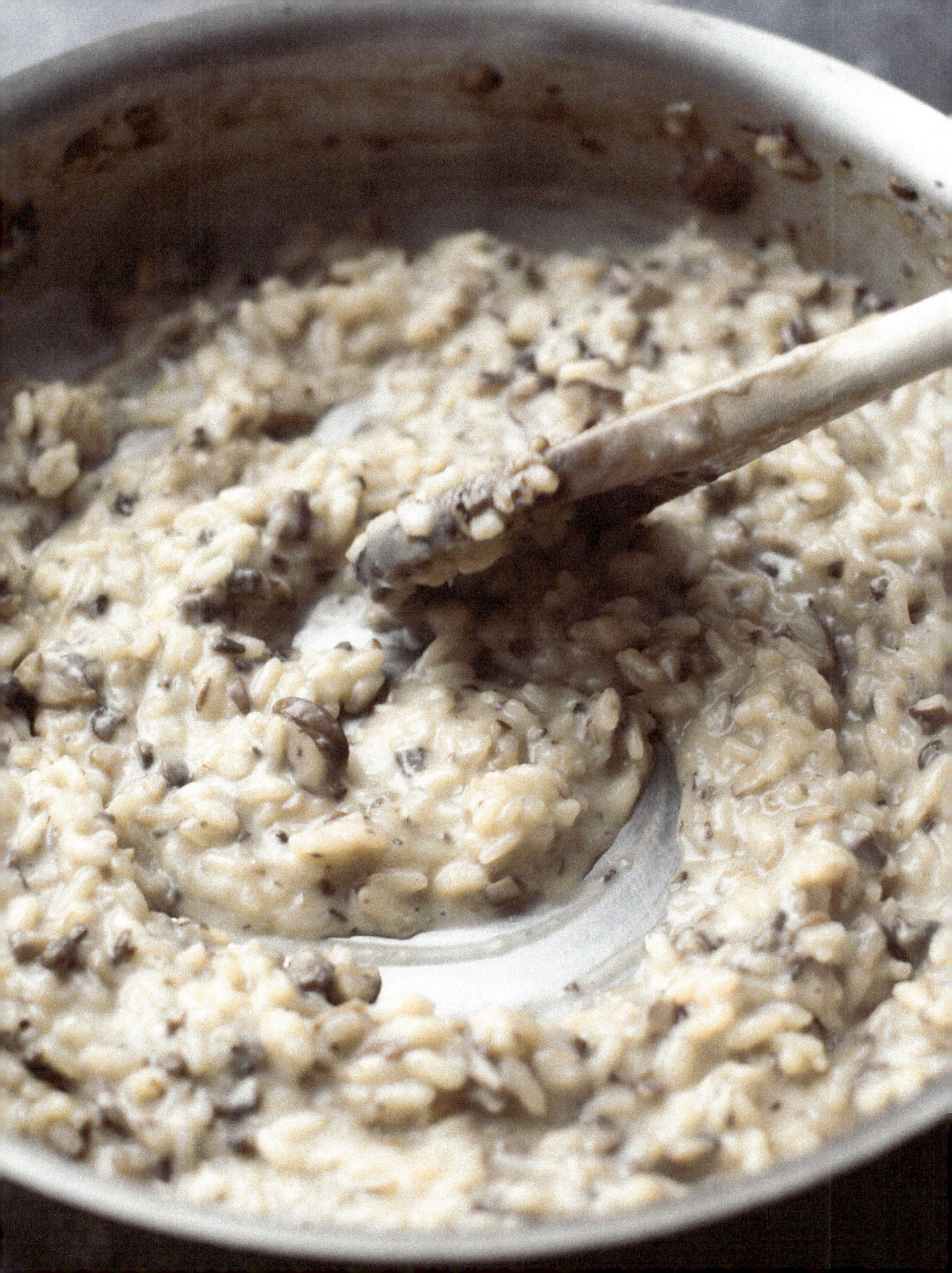

TRUFFLE MUSHROOM RISOTTO (9+ Months)

This Italian rice dish will have your mouth watering as you prepare it. You will have plenty left over, don't worry! Truffle oil became my go-to when my son did not want to eat something. All I had to do was drizzle a little truffle oil and a little Parmesan cheese, and he was as happy as a clam. Truffle oil can be easily found in most grocery stores these days or even online if need be. You will fall in love with the flavor, but be careful not to overdo it. It is a very strong, flavorful oil, and just a small amount will go a long way.

Prep time: 6 minutes   **Total time:** about 36 minutes   **Makes** 3 cups

Ingredients

- 2 tbsp. olive oil
- 4 tbsp. butter
- 2 shallots (minced)
- 16 oz. portobello mushrooms (finely chopped)
- 1 cup Arborio rice
- 3-4 cups chicken broth
- 1½ tsp. white truffle oil
- ¼ cup Parmesan cheese plus some for sprinkling

Directions

- Heat oil and melt 2 tablespoons of butter in a skillet on medium heat. Add shallots and cook for 2-5 minutes, stirring occasionally. Be sure not to burn them.
- Then add mushrooms and cook until soft.
- Add rice to pan and cook for about 1 minute to absorb flavors of shallots and mushrooms.
- Add one cup of broth and stir frequently until all liquid is absorbed into the rice.
- Add another cup of the broth and repeat. Repeat this with remainder of broth one cup at a time until rice is tender.
- Once rice is tender add last 2 tablespoons of butter and stir to melt and add a nice smooth glassy finish to risotto. Then remove from heat.
- Lastly, stir truffle oil and Parmesan cheese into the risotto.
- Serve with a sprinkle of Parmesan cheese. It will smell amazing and don't worry; there will be plenty left over for the adults!

You can also add more broth or add the entire mixture to a blender if you feel you wish to have a smoother texture your baby can handle.

LENTIL, VEGETABLE AND BROWN RICE BOWL (9+ Months)

Lentils have always been a favorite to cook for my little one. Not only does he love the flavor, but lentils are an excellent source of molybdenum and folate. They are a very good source of dietary fiber, copper, phosphorus, and manganese. Additionally, they are a good source of iron, protein, vitamin B1, pantothenic acid, zinc, potassium, and vitamin B6. This is a wonderful, well-balanced comfort food dish packed with nutrition. You can even let your little one start practicing feeding himself with a spoon with this dish.

Prep time: 15 minutes   **Total time:** 30 minutes   **Makes** about 5 cups (enough for a week!)

Ingredients

- ¼ cup olive oil
- 2 carrots (diced)
- 1 stalk of celery (diced)
- ½ onion (diced)
- 1 clove of garlic (minced)
- ¼ cup chicken broth or water
- 1 (15 oz.) can cooked lentils (drained and rinsed)
- 1 cup cooked brown rice (follow package instructions to cook rice)
- 3 tbsp. of olive oil
- Parmesan cheese (optional)

Directions

- In a large skillet, heat oil.
- Add carrots, celery, and onion and sauté until tender (about 15-20 minutes).
- Add garlic and sauté one minute.
- Pour in chicken broth or water and let cook for another minute.
- Combine rice and lentils to mixture and cook until entire mixture is heated.
- Stir in olive oil.
- Serve in small bowl and sprinkle the top with Parmesan cheese (optional).

MUSHROOM & ARTICHOKE POLENTA
(9+ Months)

Polenta was once considered peasant food in northern Italy because it was plentiful and cheap. Naturally, polenta became a diet staple in the winter months when food was scarce. Polenta is usually made from yellow cornmeal, although white cornmeal can also be used. Today, polenta is enjoyed all over the world. Because it is made from corn, polenta is also gluten-free. It is right behind wheat and rice as the most important grain in the world. In addition, it's one of the best foods to supply long-lasting energy. The wonderful part about polenta is you can switch up this dish with many other vegetables as well.

Prep time: 10 minutes   **Total time:** 25 minutes   **Makes** about 3 cups

Ingredients

- 3 tbsp. butter
- ½ cup canned artichoke hearts (drained & chopped)
- ½ cup mushrooms (diced)
- 2-2½ cups vegetable or chicken stock
- ½ cup quick-cooking polenta

Directions

- In a skillet, melt 2 tbsp. butter on medium heat.
- Add mushrooms and artichokes and then and cook on medium-high heat until softened (about 8-10 minutes).
- Transfer vegetable mixture to a blender or food processor and blend to a smooth texture.
- In a saucepan, bring 2 cups of broth to a simmer.
- Slowly add polenta and whisk until it becomes thickened and smooth (about 5 minutes), then add maining 1 tbsp. of butter. The texture of the polenta should be that of scrambled eggs: soft and creamy. If it is too thick, you may add more broth.
- In a bowl, scoop out a serving of polenta and top with a serving of the vegetable mixture and serve immediately.

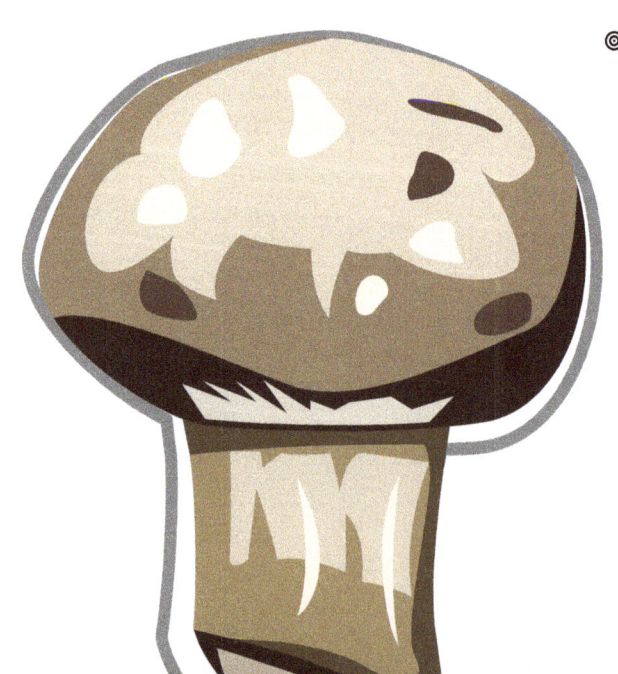

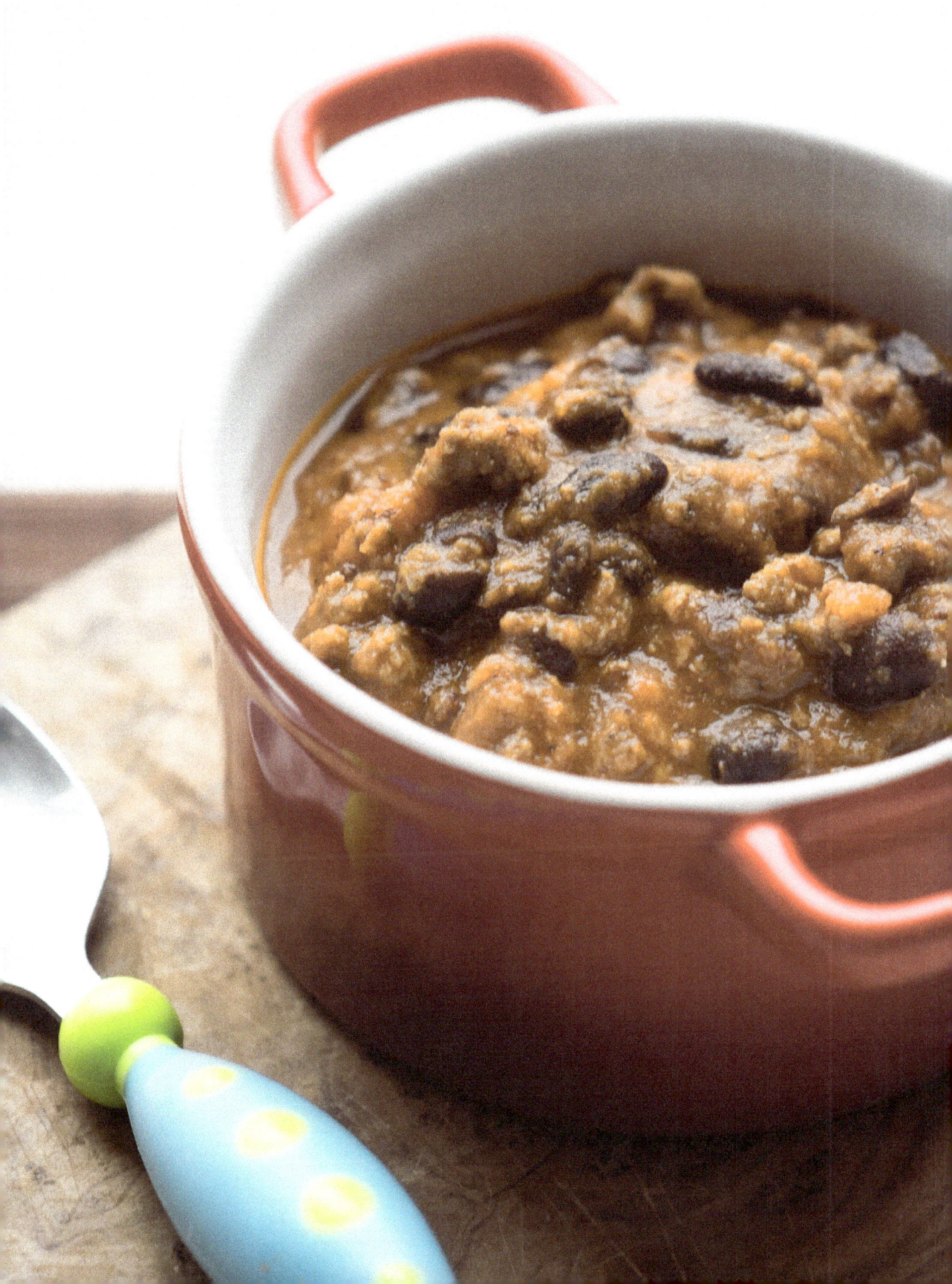

BABY'S FIRST CHILI (9 + Months)

Perfect meal for baby's first game day! This recipe is so yummy. Before you process it, you can save some for the rest of the family as well! This classic favorite is protein-rich and full of fiber. Beans are a wonderful complex carbohydrate and a top source of folate. So grab a spoon and enjoy a bite with your little one!

Prep time: 10 minutes   **Total time:** 35-40 minutes   **Makes** about 3 cups

Ingredients

- 3 tbsp. olive oil
- 3 tbsp. white onion (minced)
- 1 small garlic clove (minced)
- ½ pound lean ground organic sirloin
- 1 cup black beans
- 5 tbsp. tomato puree
- ¼ tsp. cumin
- ⅛ tsp. paprika
- pinch of chili powder
- ¾ cup chicken or vegetable broth
- 1 cup cooked brown rice

Directions

- In a large skillet with a medium flame, heat oil. Add onions and cook until softened, about 2 minutes. Then add garlic and cook another minute.
- Add ground sirloin and cook until meat is browned and cooked all the way through (about 8-10 minutes or so).
- Add black beans, tomato puree, cumin, paprika, chili powder and ⅔ cup broth to the pan. Stir well to combine ingredients. Then reduce heat to simmer, cover and let cook for 15-20 minutes, stirring occasionally. You can use more of the broth if you feel it is too thick.
- Then serve with bed of brown rice.

TIP:

You can even put mixture into a blender and pulse a few times if you want it more as a chunky puree.

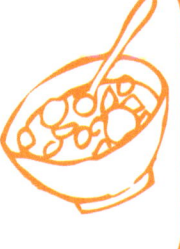

VEGGIE NUGGETS (10 + Months)

Does your little one turn her head away from vegetables such as broccoli? This will do the trick! I remember trying to find creative ways to get my son to eat some broccoli and this passed with flying colors! They cannot resist the flavors of the cheese and garlic, and you will find yourself sneaking in a taste too! Makes for a great finger food.

 Prep time: 5 minutes   **Total time:** about 30 minutes   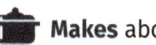 **Makes** about 8 servings

Ingredients

- 1 head broccoli (about 2 cups, chopped fine)
- 1 cup carrots (ground)
- 1 cup whole-grain bread crumbs (about 3-4 slices of any whole-grain bread)
- 1 egg
- ¼ cup scallions (chopped fine)
- ⅔ cup cheddar cheese
- 1 garlic clove (minced) (about a ½ tsp.)

Directions

- Pre-heat oven to 400°F on bake.
- Fill a medium pot with about 2-3 inches of water, place a steam basket inside pot, and then add broccoli, cover and steam on medium-high heat until soft (about 6-7 minutes). When finished, finely chop broccoli and put aside.
- Prepare whole-grain bread crumbs by breaking bread into pieces and putting in a blender or food processor until it becomes fine crumbs.
- Place carrots in a blender or processor and process until ground.
- In a large bowl, combine all ingredients (broccoli, carrots, bread crumbs, egg, scallions, cheese, garlic). The mixture will be on the wet side.
- Using a cookie scoop (1 or 2 tbsp. size), place veggie nugget scoops on a parchment-lined tray. With your two fingers, press slightly down on each so there is a flat side on each, making it easier to flip them. You can also form into small mini patties.
- Bake 16-18 minutes (flip halfway through to cook each side evenly).

Danielle Formaro

SPINACH AND MOZZARELLA TATER TOTS (10+ Months)

"Tater tots" immediately bring me back to elementary school. I can still remember the smell of hot dogs, tomato soup, and tater tots. In this recipe, we have given these kiddie favorites much more nutritional value than those old-school tots you may have been used to. These classics are a wonderful, well-balanced meal: a great blend of complex carbohydrates, dark leafy greens, and dairy.

Prep time: 25 minutes **Total time:** 55 minutes **Makes** about 30 tots

Ingredients

- 3 medium russet potatoes, peeled
- 1 tbsp. whole-wheat flour
- 2 cups loosely packed spinach (finely chopped)
- ½ tsp. onion powder
- 1 cup shredded mozzarella cheese
- avocado oil

Directions

- Pre-heat oven to 450°F.
- Place whole peeled potatoes in a large saucepan and cover with water about two inches above the potatoes. Bring to a boil and cook potatoes until parboiled, about 6-7 minutes; drain well and let cool.
- Using a box grater, finely shred potatoes. Next, try removing as much water as you can from potatoes by placing them in a dish towel or cheesecloth and squeezing water out of them.
- Transfer potatoes to a large bowl. Stir in flour, spinach, onion powder, and mozzarella. The mixture should on the dry side, but easy to form.
- Line a tray with parchment paper. Form potatoes into tots (about 1½ tsp.) and line them each of them up on the tray.
- Bake at 450°F, 15 minutes on each side.

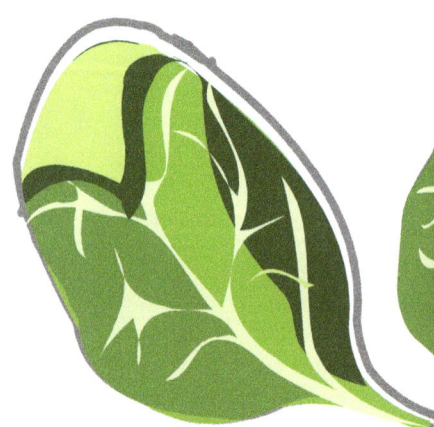

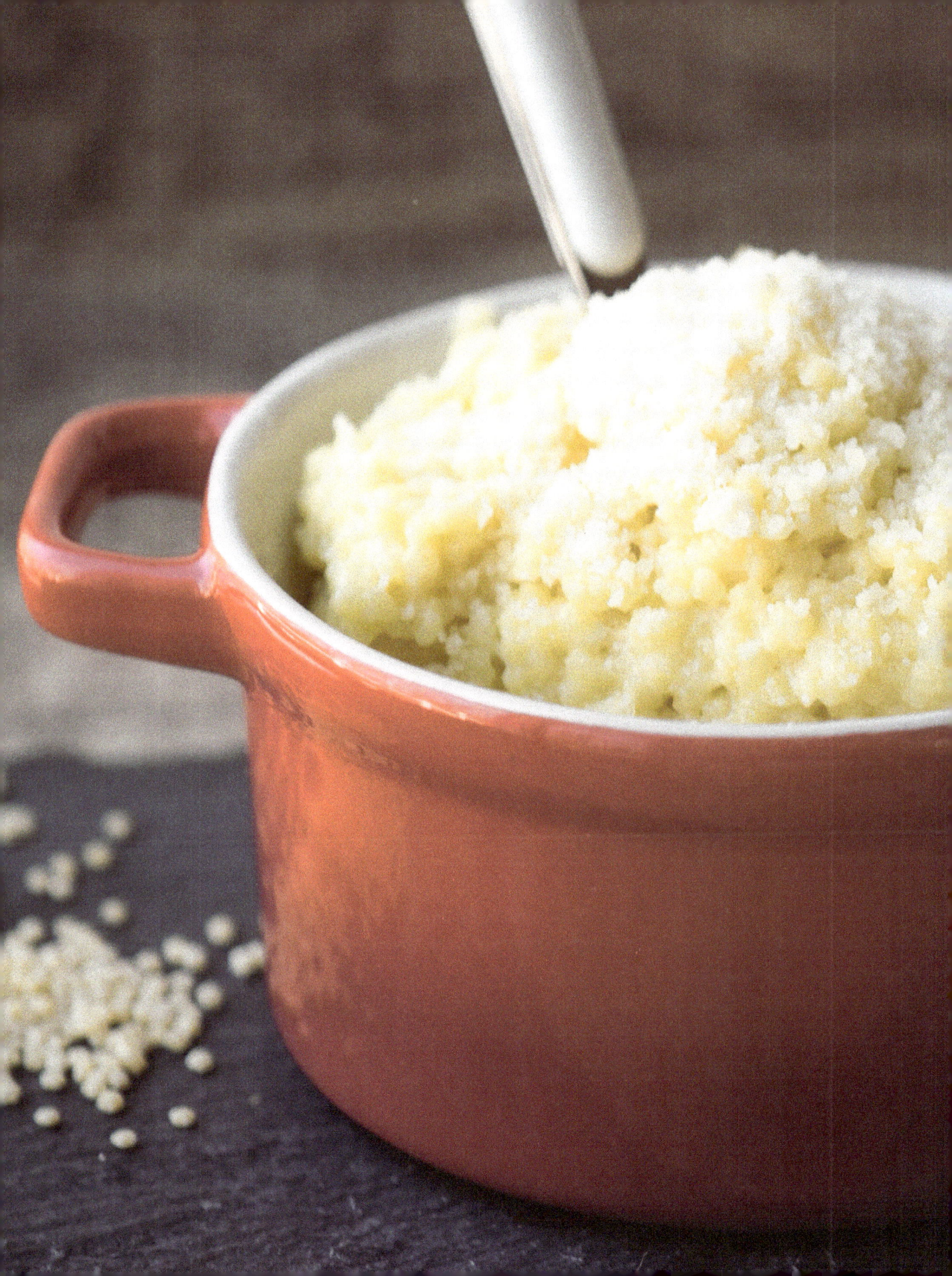

PASTINA: BABY'S SICKIE-POO COMFORT FOOD (10+ Months)

If you are Italian this meal is no stranger to you. Pastina, the smallest type of pasta produced, has been the base of one of the biggest childhood favorites for years. My mom used to make this dish for me whenever I did not feel well. It is kiddie comfort food at its best, and I will admit I still make it for myself to this very day! It is loaded with protein and cold home remedy fluids. It is also easy for the tummy to hold down on sickie-poo days. Babies all the way up to adulthood can't resist a serving of their mom's pastina! This creamy pasta, egg, and cheese dish has always, and will always be, a staple of every Italian mom's kitchen.

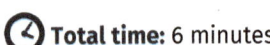 **Total time:** 6 minutes   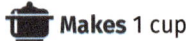 **Makes** 1 cup

Ingredients

- 1 cup water or homemade chicken stock (brewed from the bones) or canned broth if you don't have homemade
- ¼ cup pastina
- 1 egg lightly beaten
- 1 tsp. butter
- 1 tbsp. Parmesan cheese

Directions

- In a small saucepan, bring water or chicken broth to a boil.
- Lower heat to medium and add pastina, stirring frequently.
- Once water is absorbed, stir in the beaten egg and butter and then cook for another minute or two until egg is cooked (will cook very fast).
- Serve in a small bowl and sprinkle the top with a little extra love (a.k.a. Parmesan cheese).

SICKIE-POO PARENT TIP:

Every parent should have a homemade broth brewed with the chicken bones frozen and ready to go for emergencies in their freezer. Especially when you get sick! Convenience is key when illness strikes in the home. So freeze your stock or chicken soup in your freezer and prepare yourself! See page 134 how to make fresh homemade chicken soup.

CHICKEN SAUSAGE, GARLIC, TOMATO, AND BASIL WITH ORZO PASTA (11+ Months)

Now that your baby is almost a year old, her tummy should be ready to take on more citrus fruits such as tomatoes. Tomatoes are the major dietary source of the antioxidant lycopene, which has been linked to many health benefits, including reduced risk of heart disease and cancer. They are also a great source of vitamin C, potassium, folate, and vitamin K. This dish yields a lot so mommy and daddy can enjoy a few servings too!

 Prep time: 6 minutes   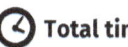 **Total time:** 25 minutes   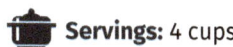 **Servings:** 4 cups

Ingredients

- 2 cups cooked wheat orzo
- 3 tbsp. olive oil
- 3 links uncooked organic non-spicy chicken sausage (casing removed)
- 2 garlic cloves (minced)
- 16 oz. can diced tomato
- Pinch of Italian seasoning
- large handful of basil (about 10 leaves chopped finely)
- Ground Pecorino Romano cheese for sprinkling

Directions

- To prepare the orzo following instructions on packaging.
- In a skillet, heat oil in pan on medium heat.
- Add chicken sausage and cook on medium-high until lightly browned on all sides (about 5-7 minutes). You can buy pre-cooked chicken sausage as well. If this is the case, remove the casing, finely chop it, and sear in a skillet for 5 minutes to brown it up a little.
- Add garlic to sausage for one minute.
- Add tomato to the pan, lower to medium heat, and cook for another 10 minutes.
- Add Italian seasoning and mix together.
- Add basil and cook 2 more minutes.
- Stir orzo pasta into skillet and combine all ingredients together.
- Serve in a bowl and sprinkle Pecorino Romano cheese.

Danielle Formaro

VEGETABLE RATATOUILLE (11 + Months)

Sometimes getting your baby to eat vegetables is not easy, but a little bit of Parmesan cheese on top always enticed my little one to dive in. This dish has so many beautiful colors, which is always a good indicator of a nutritious meal. This is also a wonderful dish to combine with a choice of meat such as chicken.

Prep time: 15 minutes   **Total time:** 35-40 minutes   **Servings:** about 2 cups

Ingredients

- ¼ cup a high smoke point oil like avocado oil
- 2 cloves of garlic (minced)
- ½ red bell pepper (diced)
- 1 cup yellow onion (diced)
- 1 zucchini (diced)
- 3 red tomatoes (diced)
- 2 cups eggplant (diced)
- A handful of basil or about 10 large leaves (chopped)
- Parmesan cheese (optional)

Directions

- In a large skillet, heat oil on medium flame.
- Add all vegetables (do not add basil yet) to the pan, raise flame to medium-high and then stir vegetables to coat with oil.
- Cook vegetables for about 20 minutes (until tender and soft) stirring occasionally.
- Add chopped basil and cook another 5 minutes.
- Serve chunky or puree in a blender or processor to an appropriate consistency for your baby.
- Serve with a sprinkle of Parmesan cheese (optional)

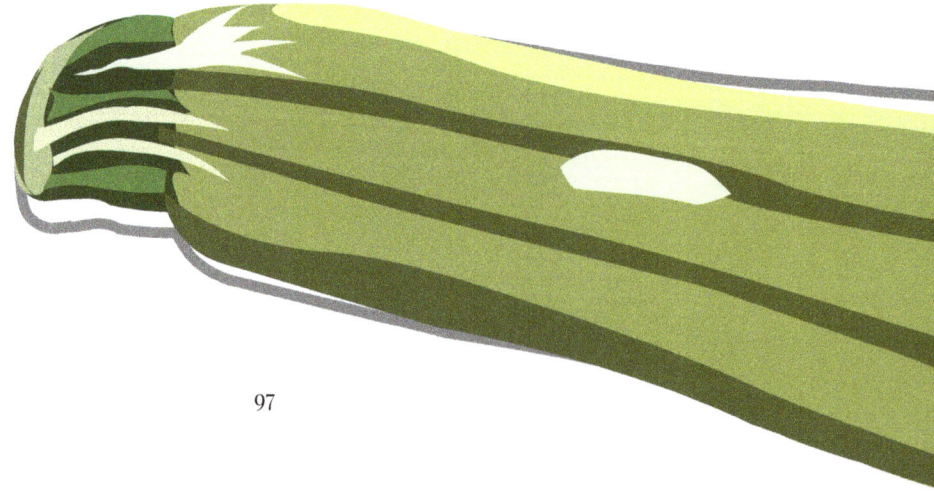

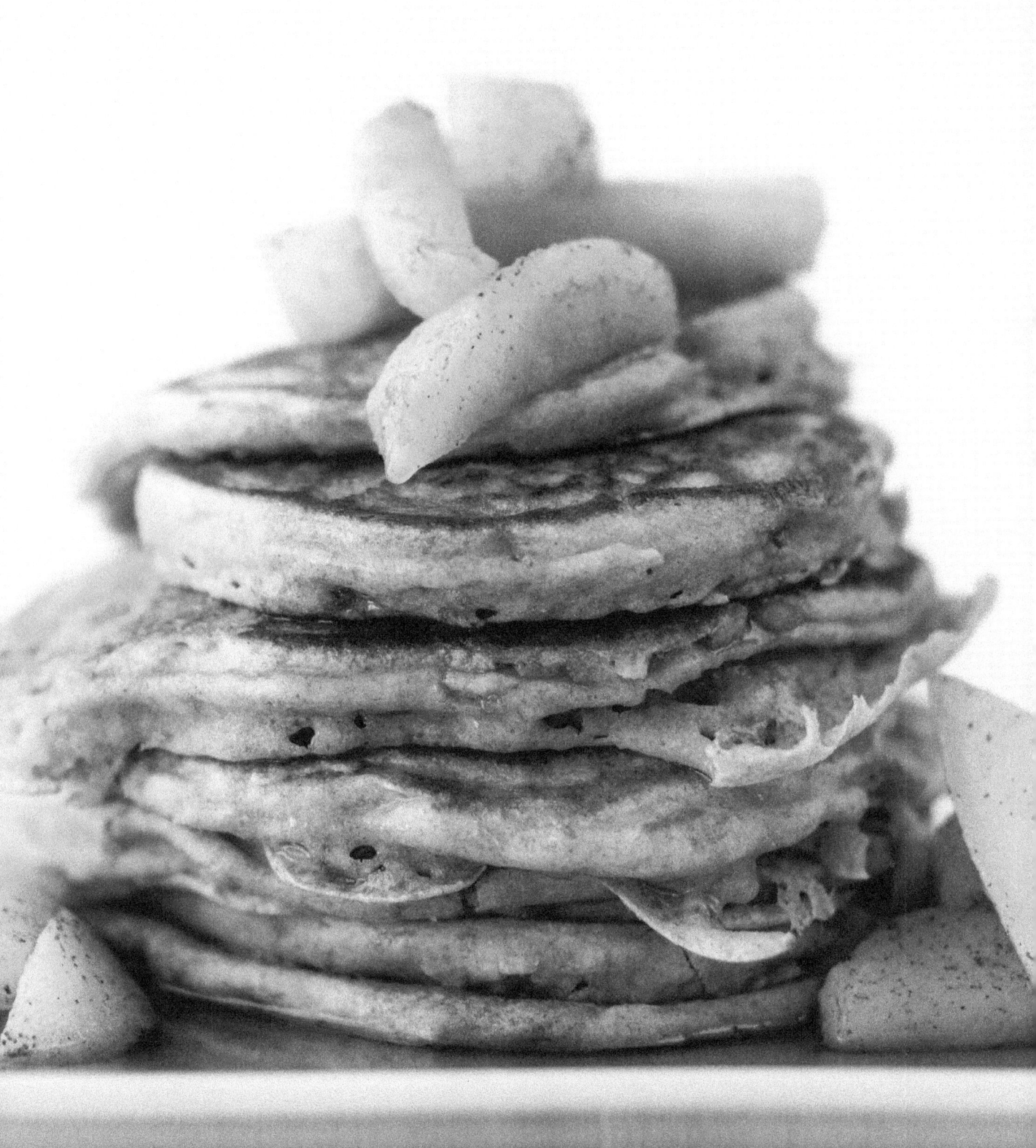

APPLE CINNAMON WHEAT PANCAKES
(10 + Months)

These whole-grain sweet apple pancakes are a favorite with my son. Wheat can taste a little bland, but when you add the apples, it becomes a sweet, mouthwatering treat. This will be a nice energy booster to start the day with the balanced blend of simple and complex carbohydrates from the wheat and apples. Milk is also a wonderful source of calcium. This meal is a wonderful representation of all the major food groups.

Prep time: 10 minutes   **Total time:** 20 minutes   **Servings:** about 12 pancakes

Ingredients

- 1½ cups organic whole-wheat flour
- 3 tsp. baking powder
- ½ tsp. ground cinnamon
- 1½ cups milk (whole milk will make them thickest)
- 1 large egg (beaten)
- 1 tsp. pure vanilla extract
- 4 tbsp. butter (melted)
- 2 favorite apples of your choice (peeled, cored, and shredded)

Directions

- Combine flour, baking powder and cinnamon in a small bowl and set aside.
- Combine milk, egg, vanilla extract, and butter in a medium bowl, and whisk together.
- Add flour mixture to wet mixture and mix together until there are no lumps.
- Add shredded apples to the batter, and mix together.
- Heat large, nonstick skillet over medium heat. Pour ¼ to ⅓ cup of batter onto the skillet and cook 2 to 3 minutes, or until sides start to bubble. Then with a spatula, flip to the other side, and cook for an additional 1 to 1½ minutes.
- Continue with remaining batter.

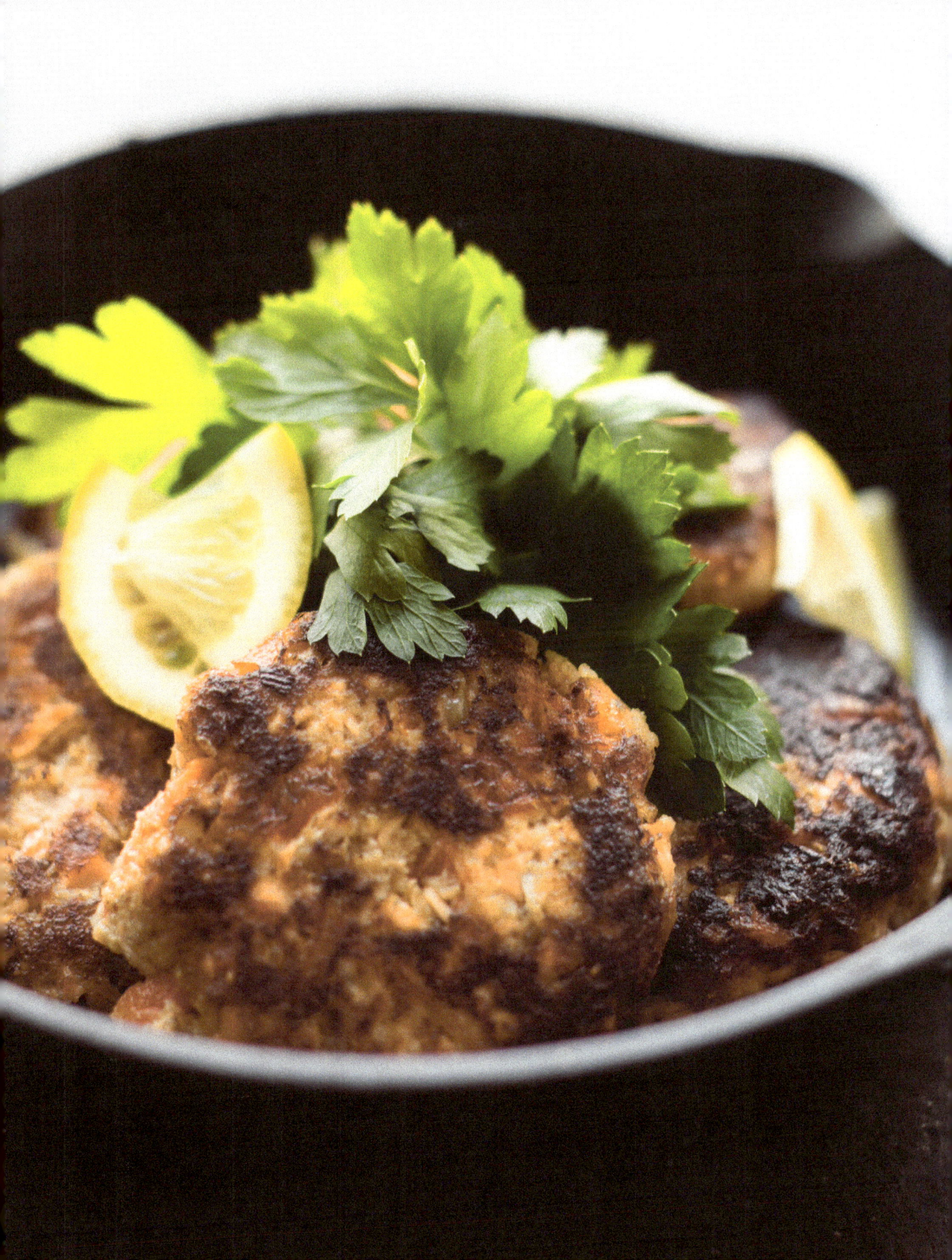

FRESH SALMON CAKES (10+ Months)

Fish are excellent sources of lean protein. Most often we see crab cakes on the menu, but the nutritional content of salmon is favored in my house. Salmon contains omega-3 fatty acids DHA and EPA, which can enhance baby's cognitive development and visual acuity. I started my little one young with these flavors to get him used to it quickly. As I mentioned before, the earlier you can have your little one try new flavors (at the appropriate age that is), the better. This gets them used to healthy options from the start.

 Prep time: 10 minutes   **Total time:** About 50 minutes   **Servings:** Makes 6 patties

Ingredients

- 1 x 8 oz. salmon fillet
- 1 tbsp. white onion (minced)
- 1 egg (beaten)
- 2 slices of whole-wheat bread
- 1 tsp. Dijon mustard
- 1 tbsp. roasted red bell pepper (minced; jarred or self-roasted)
- 3 tbsp. avocado oil

Optional Dipping Sauce

- ½ cup Greek yogurt
- 1 tsp. lemon juice
- ⅛ tsp. fresh or dry dill

OPTIONAL DIPPING SAUCE:

You can also put a nice thin layer of the yogurt dipping sauce over the salmon cake before cutting up for baby. It will be flavorful and moist.

Directions

- Pre-heat oven to 350°F.
- Place salmon in oven safe dish. Then bake for about 20-25 minutes. Remove from oven and set aside.
- If roasting your own red bell pepper, set the oven to broil. Then slice the bell pepper in half and turn it face down in the roasting pan. Roast in the oven for about 8 minutes, being careful not to burn it. Remove and let pepper cool a bit and then you can peel and discard the skin. Then mince one tbsp. and put aside.
- In a blender or processor, break wheat bread into small pieces and then process into breadcrumbs.
- In a bowl, break salmon up into fine pieces. Add onion, egg, wheat bread crumbs, Dijon mustard, and roasted red bell pepper.
- Combine all ingredients and then divide into 6 cakes/patties. Refrigerate them for about 10-15 minutes.
- In a skillet on a medium-high flame, heat oil. Add the patties to the pan and cook about 2 minutes on each side (should be a golden-brown color; be careful not to burn them). You may need to batch them if they do not all fit. If needed, you can add a little more oil to the pan, so they do not stick.
- Cut into bite size pieces for baby based on your discretion. I used to let mine break them apart on his own. Serve warm.

Add THIS to Your Plate!

CHERRY, APPLE, AND YOGURT SMOOTHIE (10+ Months)

Yogurt can contain beneficial bacteria and function as a probiotic. This can provide a variety of health benefits that go well beyond those of plain milk. Cherries are delicious and rich in antioxidants, such as anthocyanins and catechins, which fight inflammation. Together, this makes one super dense dose of nutrition.

 Prep time: 10 minutes   **Total time:** 15 minutes   **Servings:** Makes about 1 ½ cups

Ingredients

- 1 cup cherries (pitted and stems removed)
- 2 apples (peeled and cored)
- 7 oz. Greek yogurt

Directions

- Pour about 1 inch of water into a small saucepan. Put cherries and apples into steam basket and cover. Bring to a boil over high heat until fruit is tender (about 6 minutes).
- Remove from heat, and remove from basket.
- Blend or process all fruit until smooth and then stir in yogurt and mix well.

Congrats! Now that your baby is one year old, in this next section your baby can now enjoy the remaining recipes with the rest of the family!

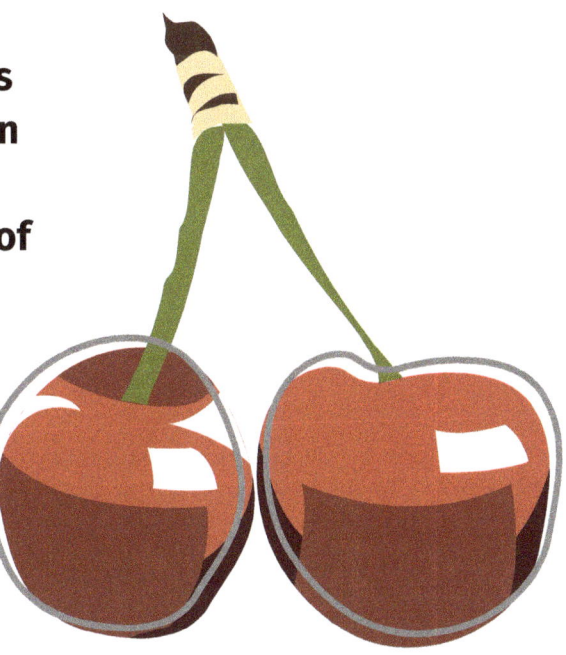

Add THIS to Your Plate!

The Family Plate Recipes

What's For Breakfast

Breakfast, the most important meal of the day. Right? Yes, it is important. However, it all depends on what you are eating! Did you know that certain foods can give you more energy while others can actually make you just want to go right back to bed?

Eating a nutritious breakfast sets the tone for the day and promotes weight maintenance and weight loss by maintaining blood glucose levels and your metabolism. To make this even more simple, while you slept your body went without food and water for, let's say, 8 hours (depending on how long you sleep, I know most of us moms may be running on 5-6 hours these days right?) and the only way to get it moving again is to fuel it! If you don't get it moving again, it will just take longer than normal to get moving at a fast pace again. This can cause weight gain due to a slow-running metabolism.

Now, I am not saying you have to eat a huge breakfast at a certain time in the morning, but you should be getting something in before your lunchtime. I personally make a late breakfast around 10:00 a.m. and my lunch is three hours later. So it's not so much about the time you first eat, but more a matter of staying regulated so that your body always has fuel to keep cranking that metabolism. Bottom line, start the day off right; eat a nice, nutritious meal that will get your blood pumping for the day.

I remember that, growing up, my brother loved Fruity Pebbles and I loved Cocoa Puffs. We were complete opposites. I loved anything chocolate (shocker ... right, ladies?) and he loved anything strawberry. Although my mom was amazing in the kitchen, breakfast was not really a huge production in my house, at least not that I can remember. Dinner was completely the opposite. I never really liked breakfast, to be honest, and if my mom was able to force anything down my throat, it was either a bite of a banana or those Cocoa Puffs.

In the '80s we didn't know or didn't care to know how much sugar was in those magical boxes with the exciting little toys at the bottom. Do they still do that? Those sugary cereals are seriously a great way to have your kid sugar-crash in school, and then have you wondering why they couldn't pay attention. Perhaps they should have had a V-8? How about, perhaps, they should have had a nice nutritious breakfast made by mom. #truth

As I got older, I started to enjoy breakfast more. I think I really started to enjoy breakfast in my college years. No surprise, right? Those were the times when a hangover was part of your weekly curriculum. Breakfast is, and will always be, a great way to help those horrible day-after headaches. That and a LOT of water!

I started enjoying eggs, potatoes, waffles, and all that delicious goodness. The older I got, the more I started to appreciate breakfast in all its art forms. I became obsessed with brunch. What a wonderful occasion to talk about the gossip from the night before. Everything became, "Let's do brunch." I think breakfast just became more fun the more I started to learn how tasty and delicious the food—and the gossip—could actually be. I think I also loved the fact that that there were no rules to breakfast. It could be big, small, casual, or a little fancy pants. Mimosa anyone?

I think the other big reason I started to enjoy breakfast was because it was that part of the day when everything and everyone had a chance to start over again, with a clean slate and a new plate. Hey! That rhymed! What's better than being the first one to wake up in the house? I love that! It is pure bliss, or the calm before the storm, as I like to call it.

The recipes below are a list of my favorite simple-yet-delicious healthy recipes that my family and I have always enjoyed. They are either recipes you may have made before or ones which you have always wanted to learn to make yourself. So enjoy, and do not be afraid to pour a mimosa while preparing them. Have a great rest of the day, as it has just begun!

BANANNA-BLUEBERRY WHEAT PANCAKES

I can't say enough about these amazing healthy and flavorful pancakes. Like my French toast, I swapped white flour for whole-wheat flour for the added nutrition and fiber boost. The banana keeps them nice and moist while the blueberries add something sweet and tart. You can also use almond milk instead of buttermilk; I just the like the fluffiness of the buttermilk. Remember to go light on your syrup; you don't want to ruin this healthy goodness by overdoing the sugar. Moderation is key!

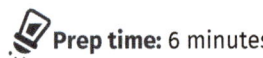 **Prep time:** 6 minutes   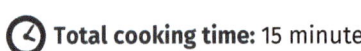 **Total cooking time:** 15 minutes   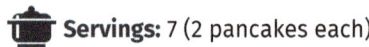 **Servings:** 7 (2 pancakes each)

Ingredients

- 1½ cups organic whole-wheat flour
- 3 tsp. baking powder
- 1 dash of salt
- 1½ cups fat-free buttermilk
- 1 large egg (beaten)
- 1 tbsp. pure grade A maple syrup
- 1 tsp. pure vanilla extract
- 5 tbsp. unsalted butter (melted)
- 2 bananas (mashed)
- ½ cup blueberries

Directions

- Combine flour, baking powder, and salt in a small bowl and set aside.
- Then whisk together buttermilk, egg, maple syrup, vanilla extract, and butter.
- Add flour mixture to wet mixture and mix together until there are no lumps.
- Stir in bananas and blueberries just until blended.
- Heat a large, non-stick skillet over medium heat. Pour ¼ to ⅓ cup batter onto the skillet and cook 2 to 3 minutes or until sides start to bubble. With a spatula, flip to the other side for an additional 1½ minutes.
- Continue with remaining batter.
- Serve with pure grade A maple syrup.

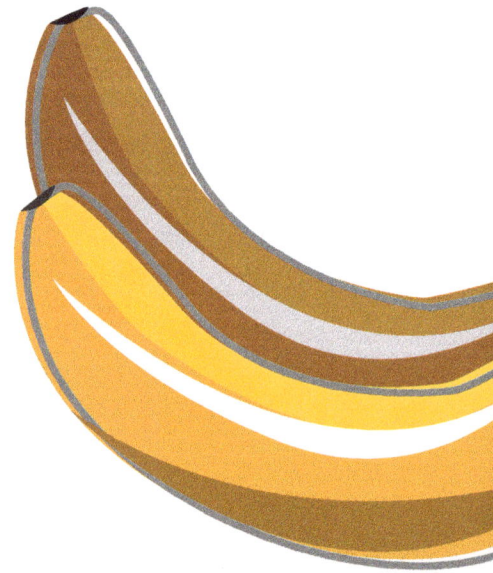

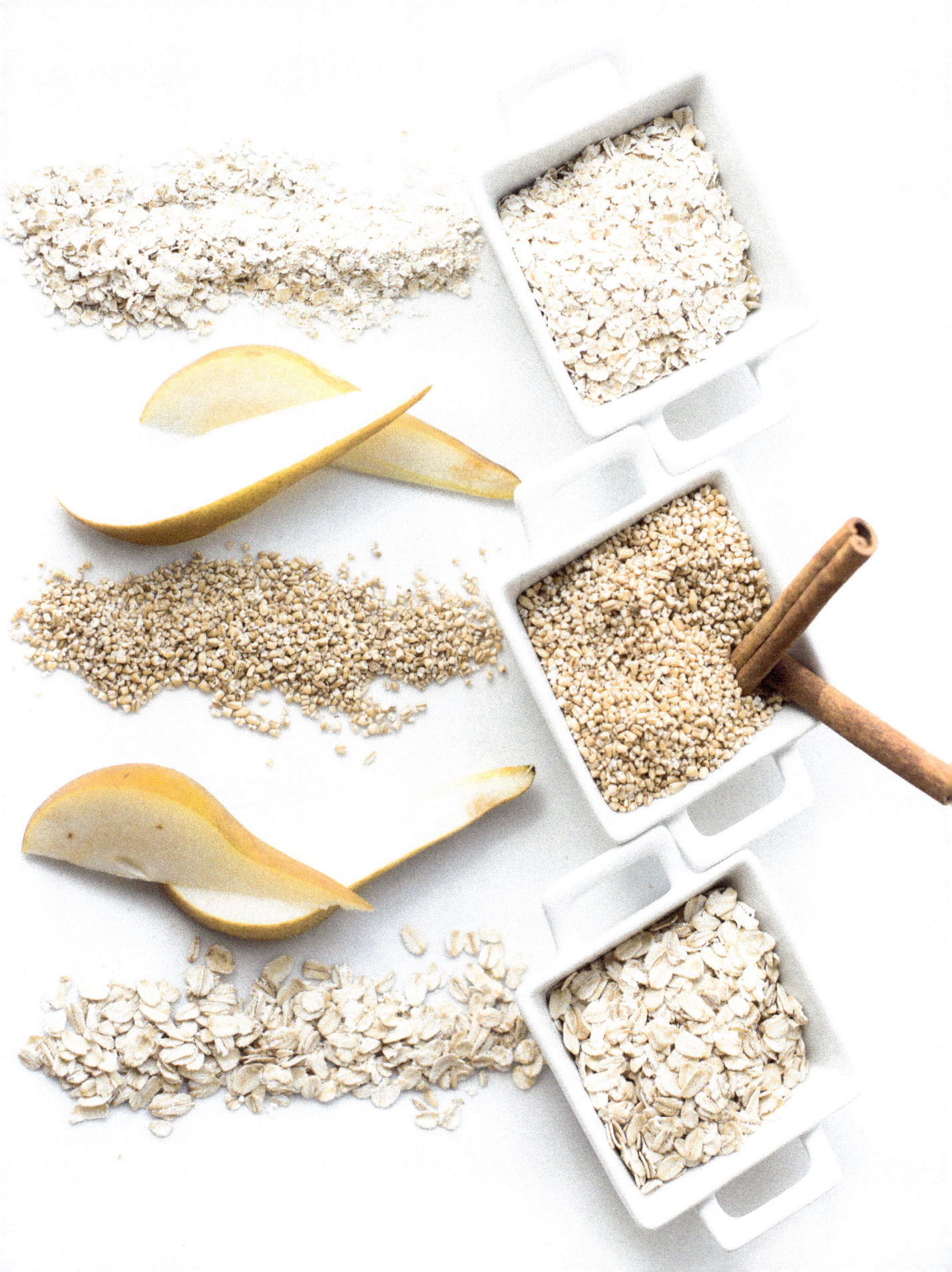

STEEL CUT OATS WITH BANANA, APPLE & CINNAMON

How do you take your oats? Would you like steel-cut or rolled? What is the difference between the two, you may ask? It is simple: steel-cut oats are relatively unprocessed, while rolled or quick oats are processed for a faster cooking time. The good news is both have the same nutritional content. Steel-cut oats and quick oats are high in vitamins E, B-1, and B-2. Eating three servings of whole grains, including steel-cut oats or quick oats, reduces the risk of having a heart attack or dying from heart disease by 30 percent, according to Harvard University's Nurses' Health Study.

For me, which type of oat I will choose all depends on what I am making. I grew up on instant oatmeal from the grocery store thinking I was eating the healthiest breakfast ever, when in fact, most store-bought, instant oatmeal packets are LOADED with sugar! Are you surprised? I know, so were most of my clients. So when it comes down to making oatmeal in the morning, if you are going to do one thing, do this: make it yourself and do not buy anything prepackaged. I know a variety of flavored oatmeal is tempting, but just don't do it.

So why steel-cut for this recipe? It is simply just a texture preference for me. I like a variety. I like to use old-fashioned rolled oats or quick oats for my baking recipes, but when I have them as a main dish, I like the slightly chewy texture, similar to brown rice, versus a traditional porridge-type dish with the rolled oats. I will warn you; they do take longer to cook. While quick oats will take a few minutes, steel-cut oats you will have to cook for at least 25-30 depending on your stove. A little trick: you can always shorten the cooking time by ten minutes just by soaking them overnight.

This is also a great recipe to have for breakfast if you are trying to lose weight because whole grains will keep you full a lot longer. The unprocessed grain will digest more slowly and will provide energy from the complex carbohydrate it contains. What a great way to start off the day!

 Total prep time: 2 minutes   **Total time:** 32 minutes   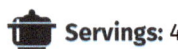 **Servings:** 4

Ingredients

- 4 cups water 1 cup steel-cut oats
- 2-3 bananas (sliced)
- homemade or store-bought organic applesauce (4 oz.)
- cinnamon

Directions

- Bring water to a boil in a medium saucepan.
- Stir in oats, reduce heat to low.
- Simmer uncovered over low heat, stirring occasionally, for 25-30 minutes or until it reaches your desired texture.
- Remove from stove, and stir in applesauce.
- Before serving, add sliced banana on top and sprinkle cinnamon on top.

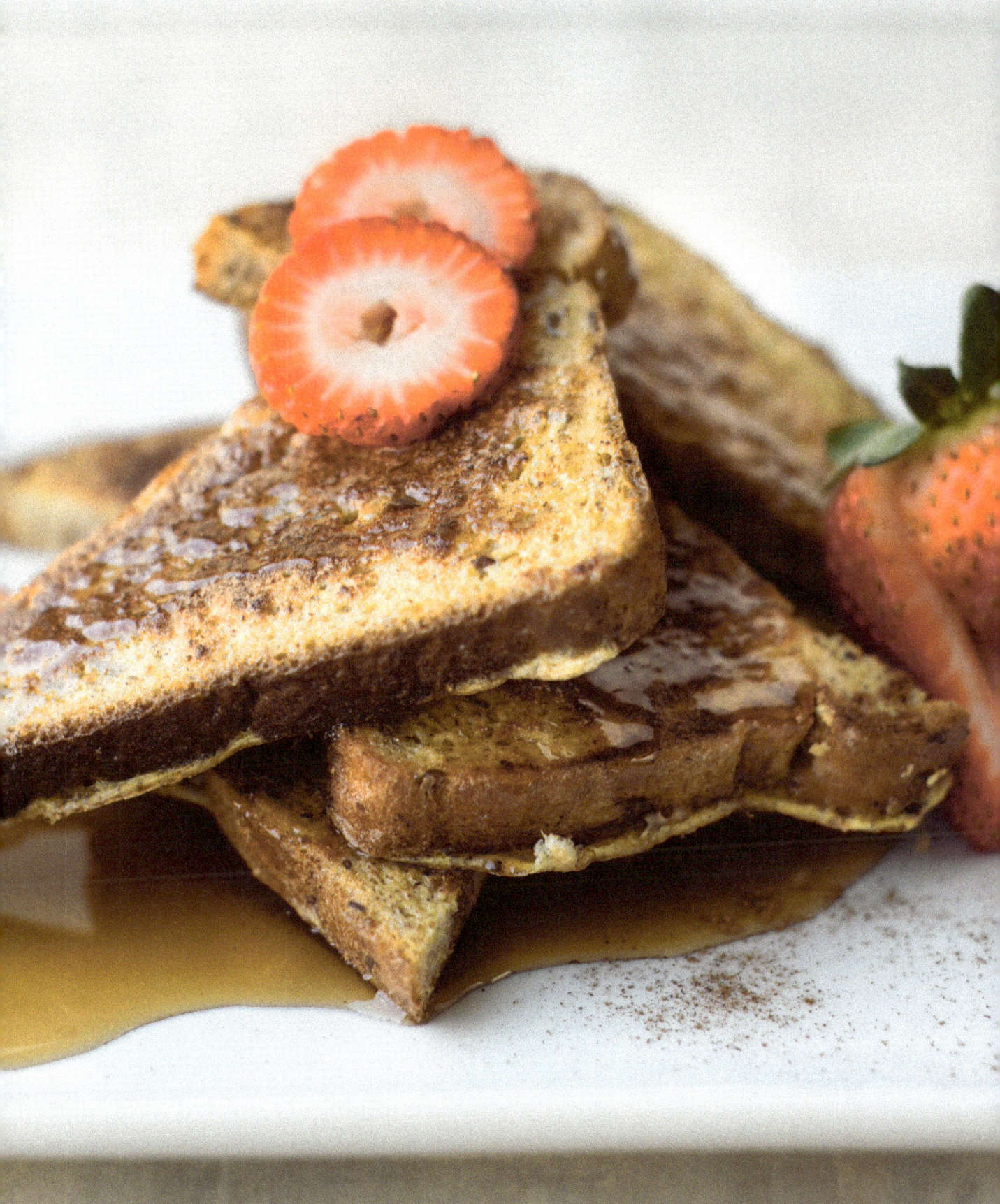

WHOLE-GRAIN FRENCH TOAST

French toast, like pancakes, are often thought to be an unhealthy option for a lot of people I have breakfast with. What gives French toast a bad name is the traditional super-thick white bread that is then drenched in maple syrup and butter. I get it! You are right. Which is why just a small change to whole-grain bread is a better choice simply because you will now add much more nutrition to the plate. Why? I will break it down to a simple explanation.

Whole-grain breads are less processed than white breads, which are highly processed and of limited nutritional value. The fact that whole grains are not highly processed is the very reason they maintain most of their nutritional value. The other major difference is the big "F-word." Fiber! The more unprocessed and higher in fiber a food is, the longer it will take the body to break it down. What does this mean? It means you most likely will feel full longer, and that typically acts as a natural aid to weight loss.

So when you think about it, this is a VERY healthy dish! You have a dish that contains eggs, which are high in protein and omega-3's, and choline, which promotes normal cell activity, liver function, and transportation of nutrients to the entire body, and you have the fiber and nutrition from your daily dose of whole grains. What more could you want for your family? Now just go easy on that maple syrup!

 Total prep time: 10 minutes   **Total time:** 20 minutes   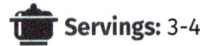 **Servings:** 3-4

Ingredients

- 6 eggs (beaten)
- ¼ cup almond milk
- ½ tsp. vanilla
- ½ tsp. cinnamon
- 6 slices of whole-grain bread of your choice (I like wheat)
- chopped fruit of your choice (strawberries, blueberries, banana)
- pure grade A maple syrup

Directions

- In a small bowl, combine eggs, almond milk, vanilla, and cinnamon.
- Take each piece of bread and dredge both sides in the egg mixture.
- On a non-stick skillet or griddle, cook each side on medium heat for about 1 minute.
- Serve topped with your favorite fruit and a light drizzle of grade A maple syrup.

HOMEMADE CRUNCHY NUT GRANOLA

I love granola. Isn't it just a staple pantry favorite? The thing I love the most about this comforting delight is that we can use it in so many different ways. Most of us associate granola with granola bars, but really, it is just a fantastic roasted blend of oats, nuts, and dried fruits. In this book, you will see granola used not only as a breakfast option but also as a dessert classic.

But what makes one granola better than another? In my opinion, it is two things: (1) The oat/nut/fruit ratio and (2) the wet-to-dry ingredient ratio, which is actually even more important than number one. If there is not a good oat/nut/fruit ratio, it may taste boring, bland, or too sweet. But if you do not have the right ratio of wet and dry ingredients, you may not get that crisp finish you so desire. I find the recipe below to be the perfect blend.

The biggest issue I saw with so many store-bought recipes is that they contain a ton of sugar. To be frank, why the heck would anyone want to add more unnecessary carbohydrates to a high-carb food? That is exactly what sugar is, a simple carbohydrate. I can't tell you that my recipe below has NO sugar, but what I can tell you is that it has a fraction of the sugar contained in most store-bought recipes. This is the reason why learning to make things from scratch at home is best.

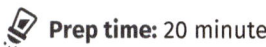 **Prep time:** 20 minutes   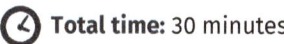 **Total time:** 30 minutes   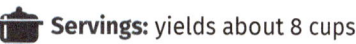 **Servings:** yields about 8 cups

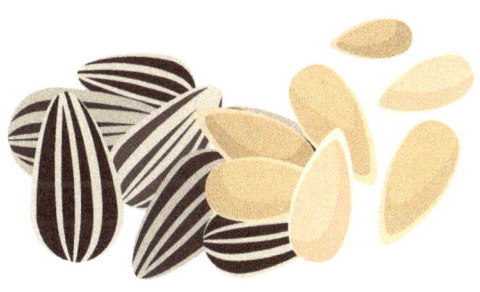

Ingredients

- ¼ cup pumpkin seeds (roasted)
- ¼ cup sunflower seeds (roasted)
- 3 cups rolled oats
- 1 cup raw dry-roasted mixed nuts (I like almonds and cashews)
- 5 tbsp. grade A maple syrup
- ½ tsp. cinnamon
- ⅓ cup agave nectar
- ¼ cup olive oil
- 1 tsp. vanilla
- ¼ cup apple juice
- ¼ tsp. salt
- ½ cup raisins
- ½ cup dried cranberries

Directions

- Pre-heat oven to 325°F on bake.
- On a baking pan, spread pumpkin and sunflower seeds and bake in oven for about 5-8 minutes for a light roast.
- In a large bowl, combine oats, pumpkin seeds, sunflower seeds, and nuts. Toss to combine.
- In a small bowl, combine maple syrup, cinnamon, agave nectar, oil, vanilla, apple juice, and salt.
- Pour the wet mixture over the dry mixture and combine.
- Spread the mixture in an even layer on the prepared baking sheet. Bake for 20 minutes and then remove from the oven and add the raisins and cranberries to mixture. With a pair of spoons, toss the granola mixture a little on the baking pan to combine the fruit.
- Be sure mixture is still in an even layer on baking sheet and then return back to oven and cook an additional 10 minutes or so or until the granola is golden brown.
- Let cool completely before storing. The granola will harden after it is cool.
- Serve over regular or frozen yogurt, fruit, or even have with milk as a cereal!

TIP:

This makes a great gift in a nice Mason jar with a cute ribbon.

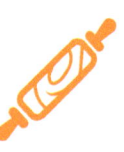

CHERRY TOMATO, MOZZARELLA & BASIL EGG-WHITE OMELETTE

Most of us are used to sautéing garlic in the evening for our dinner entrees, but as an Italian, I welcome garlic at any hour of the day, including breakfast. Your kitchen will smell like an Italian restaurant, while your omelette will taste like a margarita pizza without the crust.

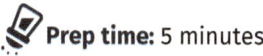 **Prep time:** 5 minutes   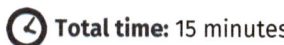 **Total time:** 15 minutes   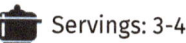 Servings: 3-4

Ingredients

- 2 tbsp. high smoke point oil such as avocado oil
- 1 garlic clove (sliced)
- ¾ cup cherry tomatoes (sliced in half)
- handful of basil (10 leaves, chopped)
- 5 egg whites (beaten) or ¾ cup liquid egg whites
- ½ cup shredded mozzarella cheese
- salt and pepper

Directions

- In a non-stick frying pan, heat oil on a medium flame.
- Add garlic to the pan and sauté until golden brown (about 1 minute).
- Add tomatoes and sauté for about 5 minutes.
- Add basil and cook for about 20 seconds.
- Pour egg whites into the pan.
- Mixture will start to set on the outer edges, then sprinkle shredded mozzarella over the top.
- With a spatula, gently push the edges toward the center of the pan to get the uncooked eggs hot on the pan's surface. Continue cooking, tilting the pan and gently moving cooked portions as needed.
- When the surface of eggs is thickened, and no visible uncooked egg remains, fold omelette in half with a spatula or utensil, and then slide omelette onto a plate.
- Season with a little salt and pepper.
- Serve immediately.

TIP:

I like to drizzle extra-virgin olive oil over the top with a sprinkle of Parmesan cheese, and red pepper for a little bite.

ROAST POTATOES WITH SAUSAGE, PEPPERS & ONIONS

This is a comfort breakfast at its best. If you are a sausage lover, you can still enjoy the flavor without the guilt. Pork sausage has 290-455 calories and 23-38 grams of fat per link. Turkey and chicken sausage have 140-160 calories and 7-10 grams of fat for the same amount. That's hundreds of calories and fat grams dodged per link. Cool, right? I got your back, moms! If you want to take the yumminess to another level, you can top an egg over easy right of the top of your serving, wow!

Enjoy this amazing recipe cuddled up in a blanket next to the fire. You may even want a little nap afterward. Wouldn't that be nice?

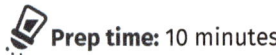 **Prep time:** 10 minutes   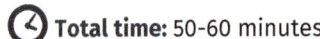 **Total time:** 50-60 minutes   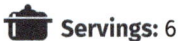 **Servings:** 6

Ingredients

- 4 russet potatoes (cut into ½-inch chunks)
- 1 red onion, chopped
- 1 lb. mini sweet peppers (assorted colors, sliced in half)
- ⅓ cup avocado oil or light cooking oil with a high smoke point
- 2 tbsp. Greek seasoning
- 1 tsp. pepper
- 1½ tsp. coarse, kosher sea salt
- ⅛ tsp. crushed red pepper
- 1 (10 oz.) package chicken sausage (Your choice;) (already cooked, no casing, sliced ¼-inch, diagonally).

TIP:

I love to make a few eggs over easy and throw them right on top of my potatoes and let the yolk run all down the potatoes. It is just yummy goodness!

Directions

- Pre-heat oven to 400°F.
- In a large bowl, combine all ingredients except the chicken sausage. Then transfer to a large baking dish. Be sure potatoes are in a single layer in order to cook well.
- Bake for 35 minutes. After 35 minutes, give potatoes a little toss with a set of utensils and cook of another 10 minutes or until soft.
- If you wish to have them a little on the crispy side, after you are finished baking, broil the potatoes for an additional 5 minutes for a more well-done potato. Keep an eye on them so they do not burn! When broiling, make sure pan is on upper shelf of oven about 6 inches from the broiler.
- Meanwhile, in the skillet on medium-high flame, heat 3 tbsp. of oil. Add sausage to the pan and cook until nice and browned or follow instructions on package. It is already cooked; this is to just give it a little sear.
- When potatoes are done, add the sausage to potatoes and toss together.

STEAK 'N' EGGS WITH PETITE HOMEFRIES

This classic is a favorite of mine for brunch. I sometimes make a nice chimichurri sauce on the side for some added pleasure. Although you can cook your eggs any style, there is something about placing the egg right on top of the steak, so when you cut right in, the running yolk just enhances the flavors of that yummy piece of meat. Although I chose rib-eye steaks in this recipe, you can use any steak you wish! I find that rib-eye is a nice option since it is nice and tender. Although skirt steak and hanger steak are also wonderful selections, you just have to really know how to cook them in order for them not to come out super tough.

The trick to a good steak sear is to cook on a very high flame. That is how you will get that nice crispy crust on your steak that you get in the restaurants. It is mouthwatering. This is a protein-packed meal at its best. In my opinion, this is the breakfast of champions and definitely a crowd pleaser.

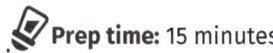 **Prep time:** 15 minutes   **Total time:** 45 minutes   Servings: 4-6

Ingredients

- 2 large Idaho potatoes (cleaned well, cut into 1-inch cubes, skin on)
- ¼ cup avocado oil or cooking oil with a high smoke point
- 1 cup white onion (diced)
- 1 tsp. fresh chopped or dried oregano
- salt & pepper to taste
- 2 x 8 oz. rib-eye steaks about ½-inch thick (cleaned and trimmed)
- 4 eggs

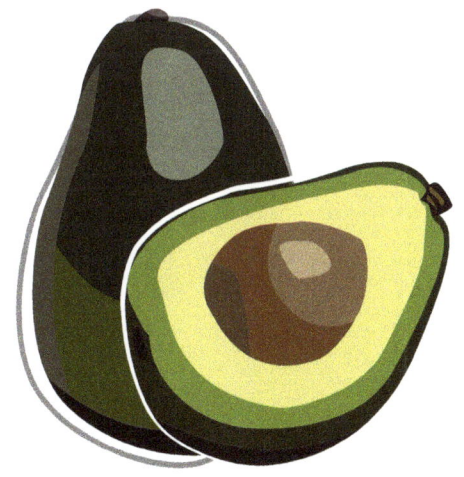

STEAK 'N' EGGS WITH PETITE HOMEFRIES

Directions

THE PETITE HOMEFRIES

- Pre-heat oven to 450°F.
- In a bowl, combine potatoes, oil, onion, oregano and season with salt and pepper (I use about a ½ to 1 tsp. of salt and ½ tsp. pepper).
- Then spread potatoes in a single layer on a baking sheet and roast for 25 minutes.
- After 25 minutes, they will be cooked, but not yet very crisp. I typically take them out, give them a toss, scraping the browned bits on the pan, and then cook another 10 minutes in the oven, so all sides are nice and crispy. You can even broil them for a few extra minutes for an even crispier finish.
- While your potatoes are cooking, you can start your steak.

THE STEAK

- Drizzle each side of steaks with a little oil and then sprinkle each side with salt and pepper.
- On grill or non-stick grill pan on high heat, cook steak about 4 minutes on each side. Pan should be nice and hot before you add steak in order to brown each side well. Center will be medium, or a nice, hot pink center. If you prefer a less pink center, you can cook to your desired temperature or doneness.
- After your steak is ready, you can start your eggs.

THE EGGS (sunny-side up)

- In a non-stick frying pan on medium heat, add a little oil. Crack eggs carefully into the pan without separating the yolk from the egg white.
- As you begin to cook, you will start to notice the egg changing color. The clear will become more of a solid white. Cook until tops of whites are set (solid white), but yolk is still runny.
- Then simply tilt the pan, and slide the egg gently onto a serving dish. You may need to prepare eggs in batches until all are cooked.

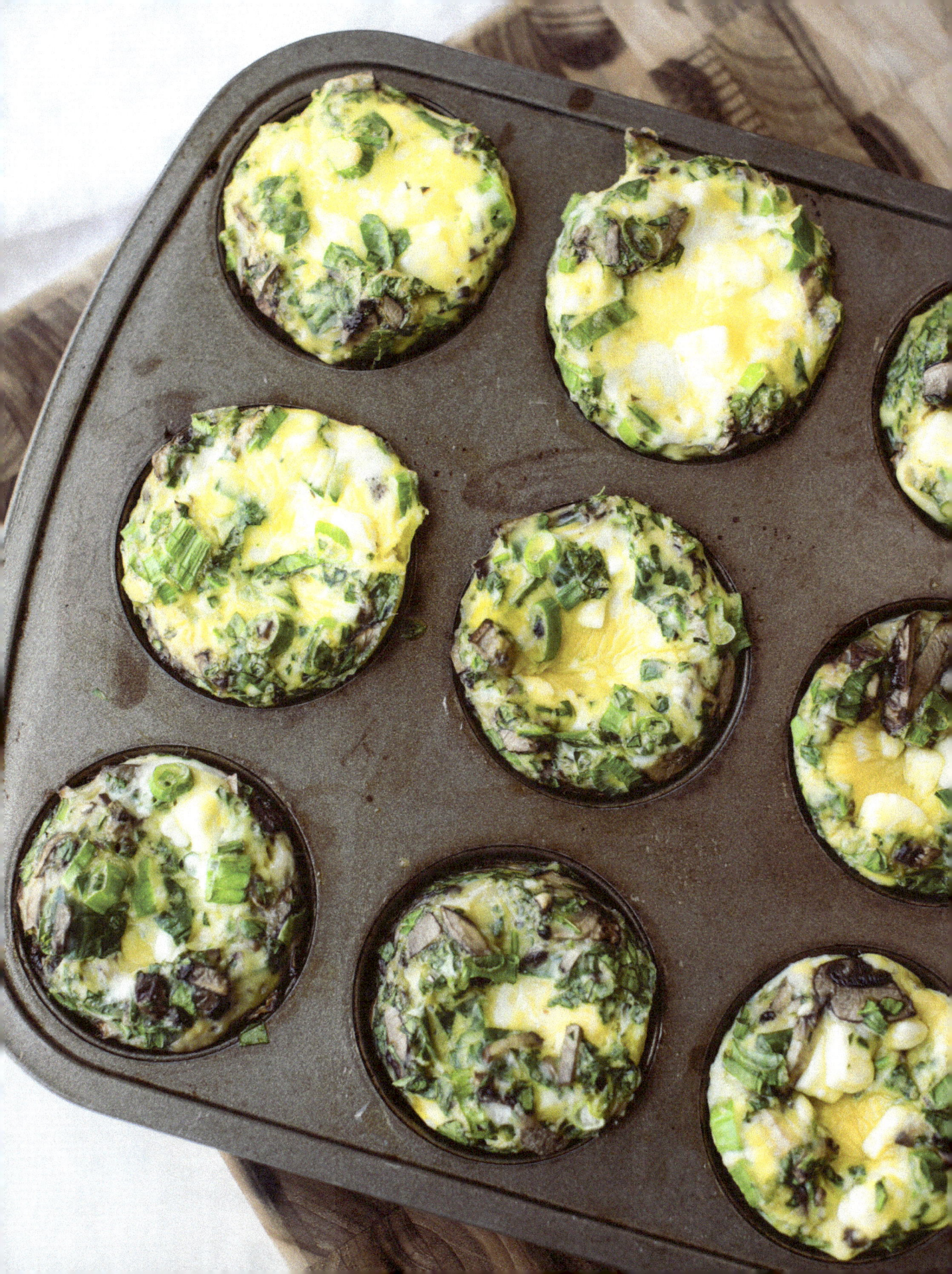

GREEK-STYLE CRUSTLESS MINI QUICHES

This is a wonderful, healthy alternative to traditional quiche since the crust is typically high in calories. If you are trying to cut back on white carbohydrates, you really will not miss the crust as these tasty little quiches are dynamite without it. You can also choose other vegetables if you wish, keeping ratios about the same. This is just my favorite combo!

If you're planning a brunch with the girls or perhaps going to a friend's house, these always bring a smile to the girls' faces. They are easy to make in bulk, and also easy to transport. If you really want to be fancy, you can serve these on a cupcake stand. How cute would that be?

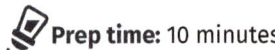 **Prep time:** 10 minutes   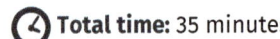 **Total time:** 35 minutes   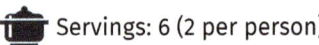 Servings: 6 (2 per person)

Ingredients

- 12 eggs (beaten)
- 4 tbsp. scallions (thinly sliced)
- 2 cups loosely packed spinach (chopped)
- ¾ cup feta cheese (crumbled)
- 1 cups white button mushrooms (diced)
- dash freshly ground pepper

Directions

- Pre-heat oven to 350°F.
- In a large bowl, beat eggs. Then add the remaining ingredients, and mix to combine.
- Spray a non-stick baking spray over a non-stick 12-hole cupcake tray. Then pour mixture evenly into the non-stick 12-hole cupcake tray.
- Bake for about 20 minutes.

CARROT-BRAN MUFFINS

Issues with irregularity? Try a bite of this! One of the most remarkable properties of wheat bran is that it is highly rich in fiber and therefore is a great way to improve constipation problems.

Similarly, wheat bran can be very recommended in diets of people with obesity, since the outer layer of the cereal increases the absorption of nutrients. Furthermore, it is a method to control appetite and increase satiety, so you feel you need to eat less. It is the perfect way to start off the day.

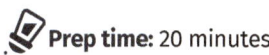 **Prep time:** 20 minutes   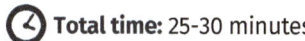 **Total time:** 25-30 minutes   **Servings:** yields about 12-13 regular-sized muffins

Ingredients

- 1 cup wheat bran
- 1¼ cups whole-wheat flour
- ¼ cup brown sugar
- 4 tsp. baking powder
- ¼ tsp. salt
- ½ tsp. baking soda
- 1 tsp. cinnamon
- 3 eggs (beaten)
- 1¼ cups buttermilk
- 1 tsp. vanilla
- ¼ cup raw honey (melted)
- ⅓ cup grade A maple syrup
- 1 cup shredded carrots
- ⅓ cup raisins
- chopped pecans (optional)

Directions

- Preheat oven to 350°F.
- In a large bowl, mix together dry ingredients—wheat bran, whole-wheat flour, brown sugar, baking powder, salt, baking soda, and cinnamon.
- In a small bowl, beat eggs, and put aside.
- In a small bowl, combine liquid mixture—buttermilk, vanilla, honey, maple syrup, and eggs.
- Slowly pour liquid mixture into dry mixture, and stir until completely combined.
- Add carrots and raisins to muffin mixture, and mix until blended.
- In a nonstick, 12-cup, regular muffin pan, pour mixture into muffin cups, and then top each serving with some chopped pecans (optional).
- Place in middle rack of oven, and bake on 350°F for 25 to 30 minutes (until toothpick comes out clean).

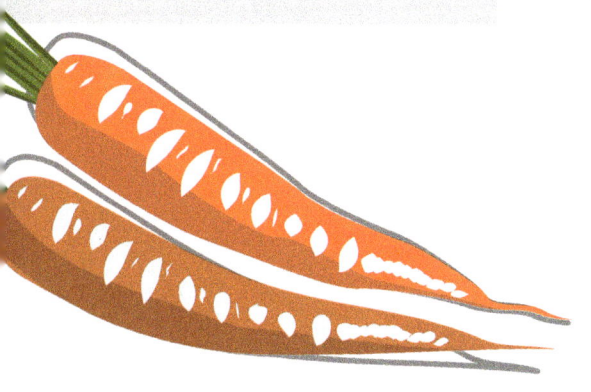

EGGS OVER EASY WITH TRUFFLE OIL AND PARMESAN

Eggs are one of the most nutritious foods on the planet. They are the perfect food; they contain a little bit of almost every nutrient we need. Although they can be high in cholesterol, they do not necessarily raise cholesterol in the blood, so don't be so scared of a little yolk. This is such a simple dish to make, but you will be surprised by the punch of flavor you get hit with. Whenever I made this for my friends I get the same response: "Danielle, I never thought to use truffle oil on my eggs!" After this recipe, you may not be able to go without it.

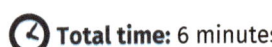 **Total time:** 6 minutes   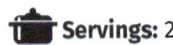 **Servings:** 2

Ingredients

- 1 tbsp. avocado oil or high smoke point cooking oil
- 4 eggs
- white truffle oil for drizzling
- Parmesan cheese

Directions

- Heat oil in non-stick skillet over medium-high heat.
- Break each egg and gently slide into the pan, one at a time keeping the yolk intact.
- Reduce heat to low-medium. Cook until whites are completely firm and yolks begin to thicken but are not too hard (about 4 minutes or so).
- Then with a spatula, gently and quickly flip each egg over and cook for one more minute.
- Tilt pan and slide into dish. Repeat for the other 2 eggs if you had to do batches.
- Drizzle lightly with some white truffle oil and sprinkle with Parmesan cheese. Serve immediately.

TIP:

Serve with a nice piece of whole-wheat toast!

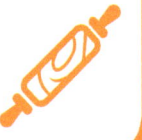

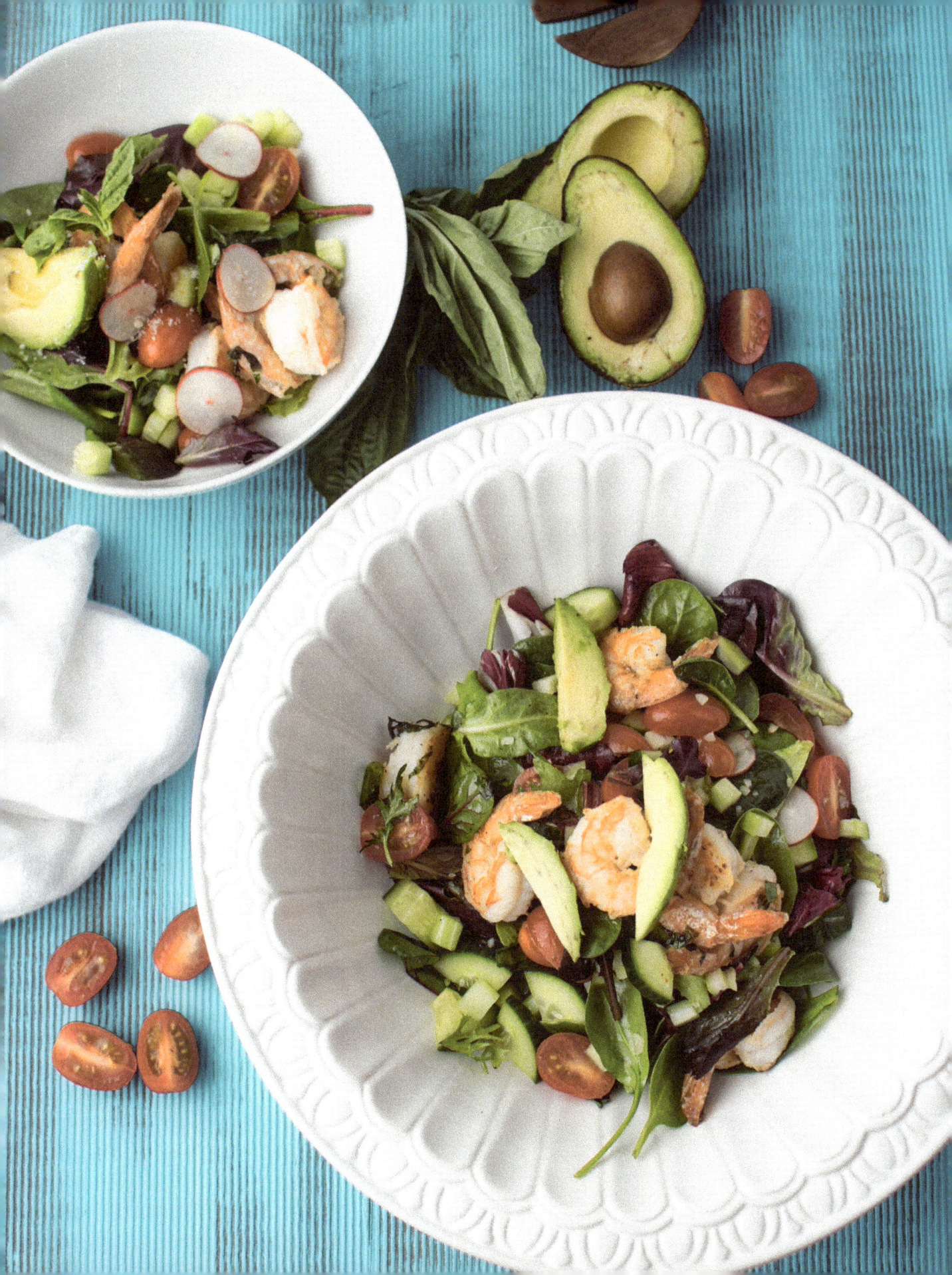

Soups, Salads, and Sandwiches

GRILLED BASIL & GARLIC SHRIMP SALAD WITH GARLIC-LIME DRESSING

What makes this a favorite salad of mine is the combination of garlic and lime juice. This will almost remind you of a pesto dish, but jazzed up with some citrus. It is the perfect salad to make for an unforgettable BBQ. So you can toss the store-bought, bagged stuff, and add this to your plate instead!

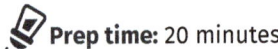 **Prep time:** 20 minutes   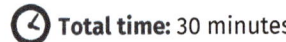 **Total time:** 30 minutes   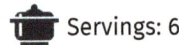 **Servings:** 6

Ingredients

The Shrimp
- 2 lbs. large raw shrimp (peeled, cleaned, tail shell removed)
- 3 cups fresh basil (chopped)
- 3 tbsp. avocado oil
- 3 tbsp. Parmesan cheese
- 2 garlic cloves (minced)
- ½ of a lime (juiced)
- salt and pepper

The Salad
- 6 cups mixed greens (chopped)
- 1 English cucumber (peeled & chopped)
- 2 stalks celery (chopped)
- 2 radishes (sliced)
- 2 avocados (chopped)
- 1 cup cherry tomatoes (halved)

Garlic-Lime Dressing
- ½ cup extra-virgin olive oil
- ¼ cup freshly squeezed lime juice
- 4 garlic cloves (minced)
- 1 tsp. freshly ground pepper
- pinch of salt

Directions

- In a bowl, combine shrimp with all ingredients, season with salt and pepper, cover, and let marinate for a minimum of 10 minutes in the refrigerator. An hour would be preferred.
- In a small bowl, prepare the dressing by combining all ingredients and whisking together. Set aside.
- In a large salad bowl, combine all salad ingredients and toss, then set aside.
- Pre-heat grill or a grill pan to medium-high.
- Grill shrimp about two minutes on each side.
- Remove from grill, add to prepared chopped salad.
- Add dressing (you may want to add half first before the rest depending on how dressed you like your salad) and toss the salad together.

MIXED GREEN GARDEN SALAD WITH LEMON, GARLIC & HERB DRESSING

The garden salad should just be named the "Safe Salad." It is that one salad you know everyone will like. Adding the chopped mint to this classic will really give it a new, refreshing taste. Guests may not really know what it is, but will compliment how tasty your salad is.

Total prep time: 15 minutes   **Servings:** 6

Ingredients

Salad
- 3 cups packaged mixed greens
- 3 cups romaine lettuce (chopped)
- 2 cups cherry tomatoes (halved)
- 1 medium onion (chopped)
- 1 cucumber (chopped)
- 1 cup fresh mint (chopped)

Garlic/Lemon Herbed Dressing
- ¾ cup extra-virgin olive oil
- ¼ cup balsamic vinegar
- 3 garlic cloves (crushed)
- 3 tbsp. fresh lemon juice
- 1 tsp. Dijon mustard
- ¼ tsp. onion powder
- 1 tsp. fresh oregano
- 2 tbsp. fresh basil (finely chopped)
- ⅛ tsp. salt
- ⅛ tsp. pepper

Directions

- Combine all salad ingredients in a large bowl and set aside.
- In a separate bowl, combine all dressing ingredients and whisk together.
- Dress salad with desired amount. Toss and serve.

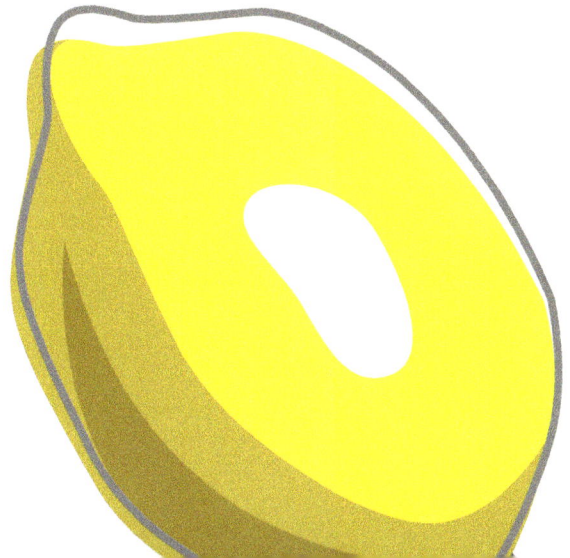

PROSCIUTTO, MOZZARELLA & FIG PRESS

There is something so pleasurable about combining something salty and sweet. Traditional panini tends to be a little on the heavy side since the bread typically needs to be thick to press. I find using a nice hearty whole-grain bread works just as well and provides a little more nutrition and fiber to the plate. The trick to making sure this does not get soggy is to layer the fig in between the meat and the cheese. Always put your wet ingredients in between a barrier from the bread, and you will never have to worry about it getting too mushy on you.

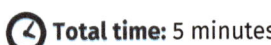 **Total time:** 5 minutes   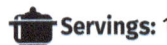 **Servings:** 1

Ingredients

- 2 pieces thick, whole-grain bread
- 3-4 slices prosciutto
- 2 slices fresh buffalo mozzarella
- 1½ tsp. fig spread
- coconut oil spray

Directions

- Warm a sandwich griddle or panini maker on medium-high heat.
- Spray each side of bread with coconut oil spray.
- Prepare sandwich by layering first with prosciutto, then spread the fig on the prosciutto (not the bread, so it does not get soggy), then lastly layer with the mozzarella, and then place an other slice of bread on top.
- Place sandwich on sandwich press or panini maker (sprayed with non-stick spray) and then press to cook. If you are using a sandwich press, cook on medium heat and be sure to flip the sandwich over after one minute and cook the other side for another minute. Total cooking time should not exceed a few minutes or when cheese is melted, and bread is toasted.

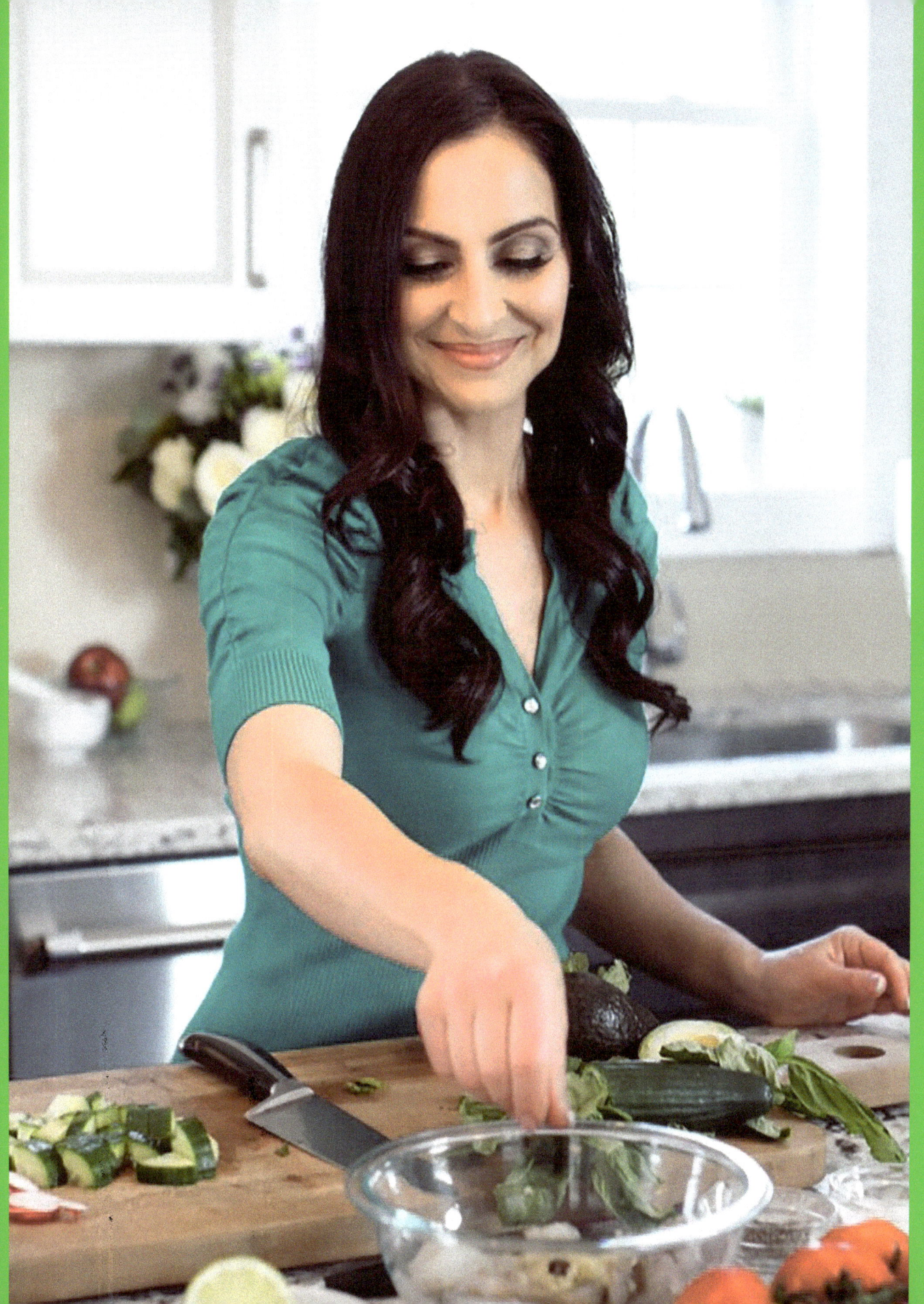

TOMATO, MOZZARELLA, AND BASIL SALAD (Mozzarella Caprese)

This is probably the easiest salad to put together yet one of the most enjoyed. The first time I had this salad was in Italy at a very young age. The dressing was nothing but vinegar and olive oil with a little salt and pepper. The one thing Italians nailed was using simple ingredients and creating extraordinary dishes. This is food simplicity at its best. If you want to jazz it up, it pairs well with the garlic lemon herbed dressing in the garden salad recipe in this book on page 122.

Total prep time: 8 minutes   **Servings:** 6

Ingredients

- 3 large beefsteak tomatoes (pits removed & sliced)
- 8 oz. fresh buffalo mozzarella cheese (sliced)
- bunch fresh basil (10-12 leaves)
- balsamic vinegar
- extra-virgin olive oil
- salt
- pepper

Directions

- On a platter, layer in a sideways fashion the tomato, mozzarella, and basil and keep alternating this layer until finished. Then drizzle the top with vinegar, oil and salt and pepper to taste.

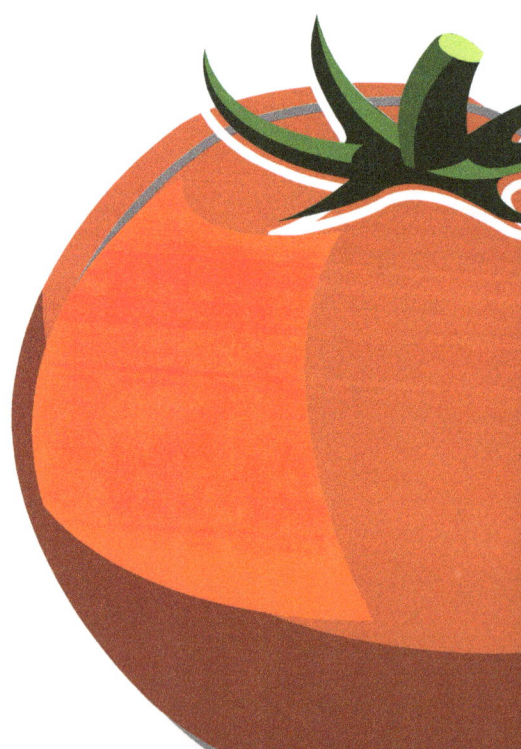

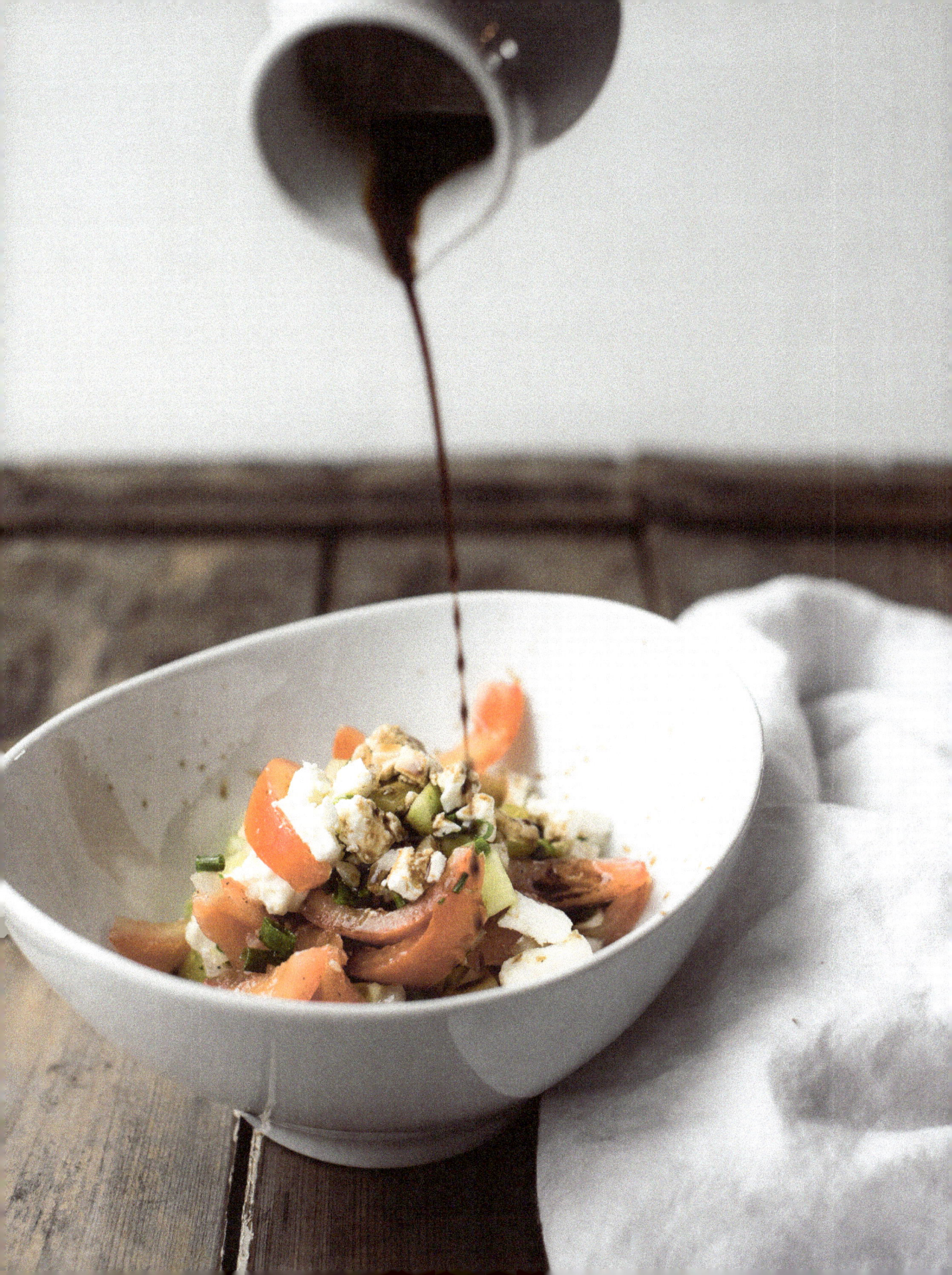

FRESH VINE-RIPE TOMATO, CUCUMBER & FETA GREEK-STYLE SALAD

This is a traditional salad you will see served at most Greek restaurants and it is just so fresh and delicious. This salad is to the Greeks as tomato Caprese salad is to the Italians. You will not really need much salt, if any, since the feta cheese contains enough salt to season this salad, but you can be the judge.

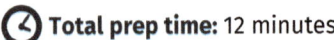 **Total prep time:** 12 minutes 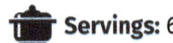 **Servings:** 6

Ingredients

- 6 vine ripe tomatoes (pitted & chopped)
- 1½ cups fresh feta cheese (if you can get it from a Mediterranean specialty store it will be nice & fresh)
- 4 scallions (chopped)
- ¾ cups sweet Vidalia onion (chopped)
- 1 large seedless cucumber (chopped)
- ⅓ cup extra-virgin olive oil
- ¼ cup balsamic vinaigrette
- salt and pepper to taste

Directions

- Combine all ingredients in a bowl and toss a few times with a pair of utensils, and serve.

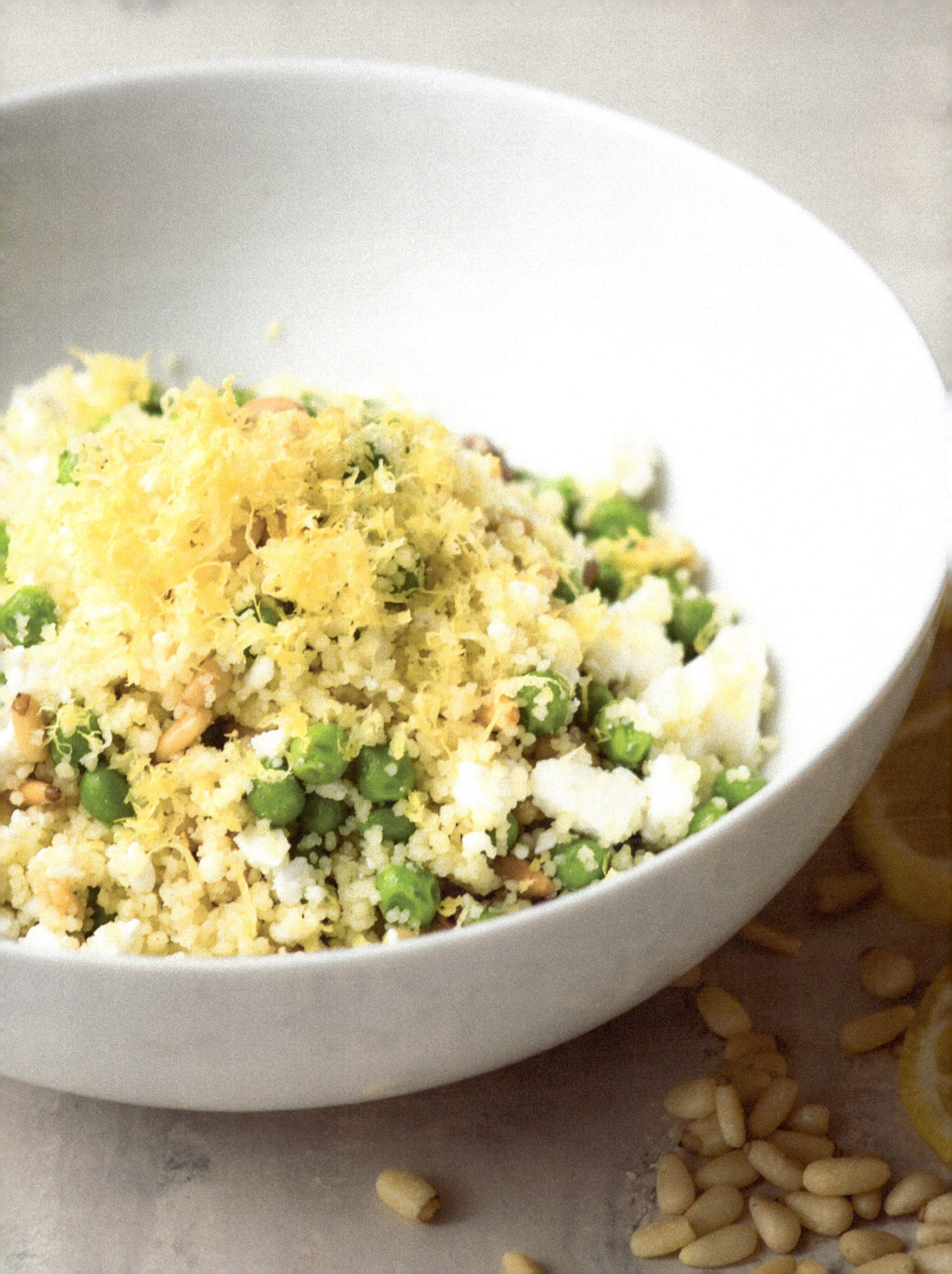

Danielle Formaro

MEDITERRANEAN COUSCOUS SALAD

This salad will make you feel like you are in dining in a small bistro over the Mediterranean sea. It is light, fluffy, and has just the right hint of salt and citrus. I love pairing this with grilled meats such as a chicken, beef, or lamb skewer. Couscous is a wonderful grain because it takes in the flavor of whatever you wish to add to it. What is great is that it is very fast cooking, which us moms always appreciate!

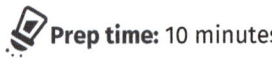 **Prep time:** 10 minutes 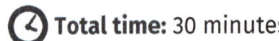 **Total time:** 30 minutes 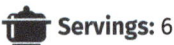 **Servings:** 6

Ingredients

- 2 tbsp. avocado oil
- ½ cup pine nuts
- 1 cup couscous
- 1¼ cup water
- juice of half a lemon
- 2 tbsp. lemon zest
- 1 cup peas
- ½ cup feta cheese
- 1 tsp. olive oil
- salt and pepper

Directions

- In a saucepan on medium heat, add 1 tbsp. of avocado oil. Add pine nuts, and cook until golden brown (a couple of minutes).
- In another saucepan, add another tbsp. of avocado oil and bring water to a boil. Add couscous, then cover, turn off the heat and let sit for 5 minutes. Fluff with a fork when done.
- In a bowl, combine couscous, pine nuts, lemon juice, lemon zest, peas, feta cheese, olive oil, and salt and pepper to taste. Toss a few times and serve.

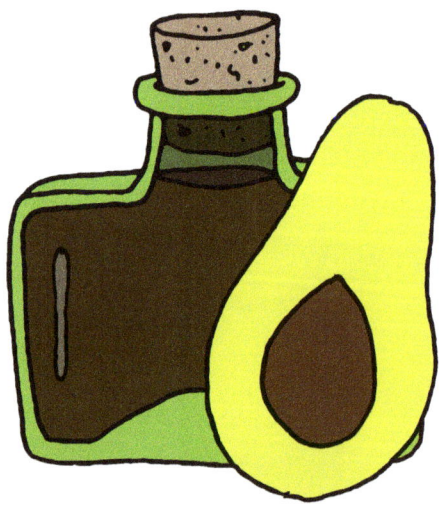

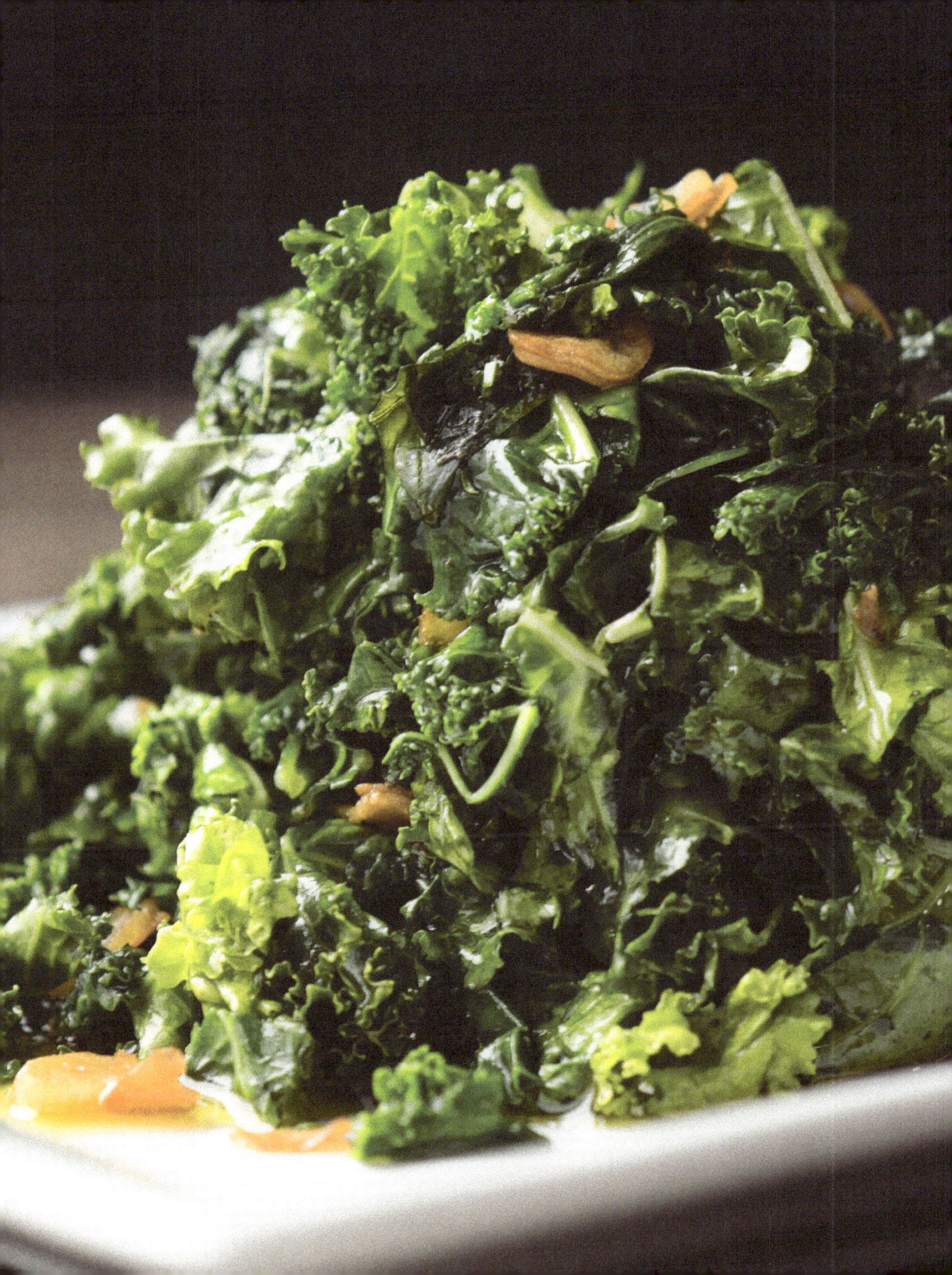

CHOPPED KALE SALAD WITH CRISPY GARLIC AND OIL

Kale is one of the world's healthiest foods. It is loaded with antioxidants, vitamin C, and vitamin K, and has been known to help fight cancer. What better than to take something so good for you and make it mouthwatering. The first time I tried this at a friend's house I was hooked. Years later, every time I make it for my friends it is always a hit!

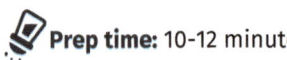 **Prep time:** 10-12 minutes   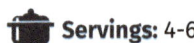 **Servings:** 4-6

Ingredients

- 10 cups kale (center ribs removed, cleaned and chopped)
- ⅓ cup light olive oil
- 2 tbsp. garlic (finely chopped)
- coarse kosher sea salt and pepper

Directions

- Place 10 cups chopped kale into a large salad bowl.
- Heat oil in a small saucepan, and then add garlic.
- Cook until garlic turns slightly darker than a golden color. You want it crispy but not burnt.
- Immediately pour hot oil and garlic over chopped kale and toss together. The hot oil will cook the kale a little. Then season with salt and pepper. I tend to be generous with the salt in this dish since kale can be a slightly bitter green.

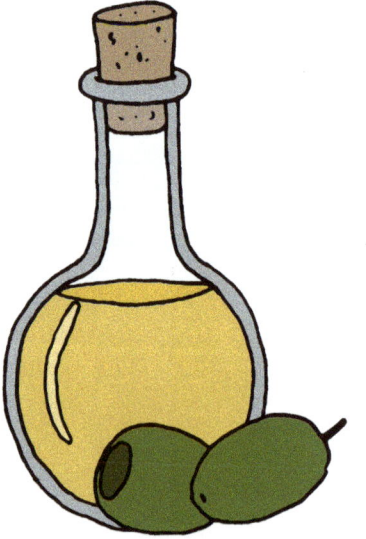

TIP:

For a little heat, a dash of cayenne pepper will kick it up a notch!

QUICK TIP:

You can also just buy a bag of pre-cleaned and chopped kale as well, this will shorten your prep time.

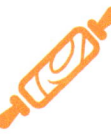

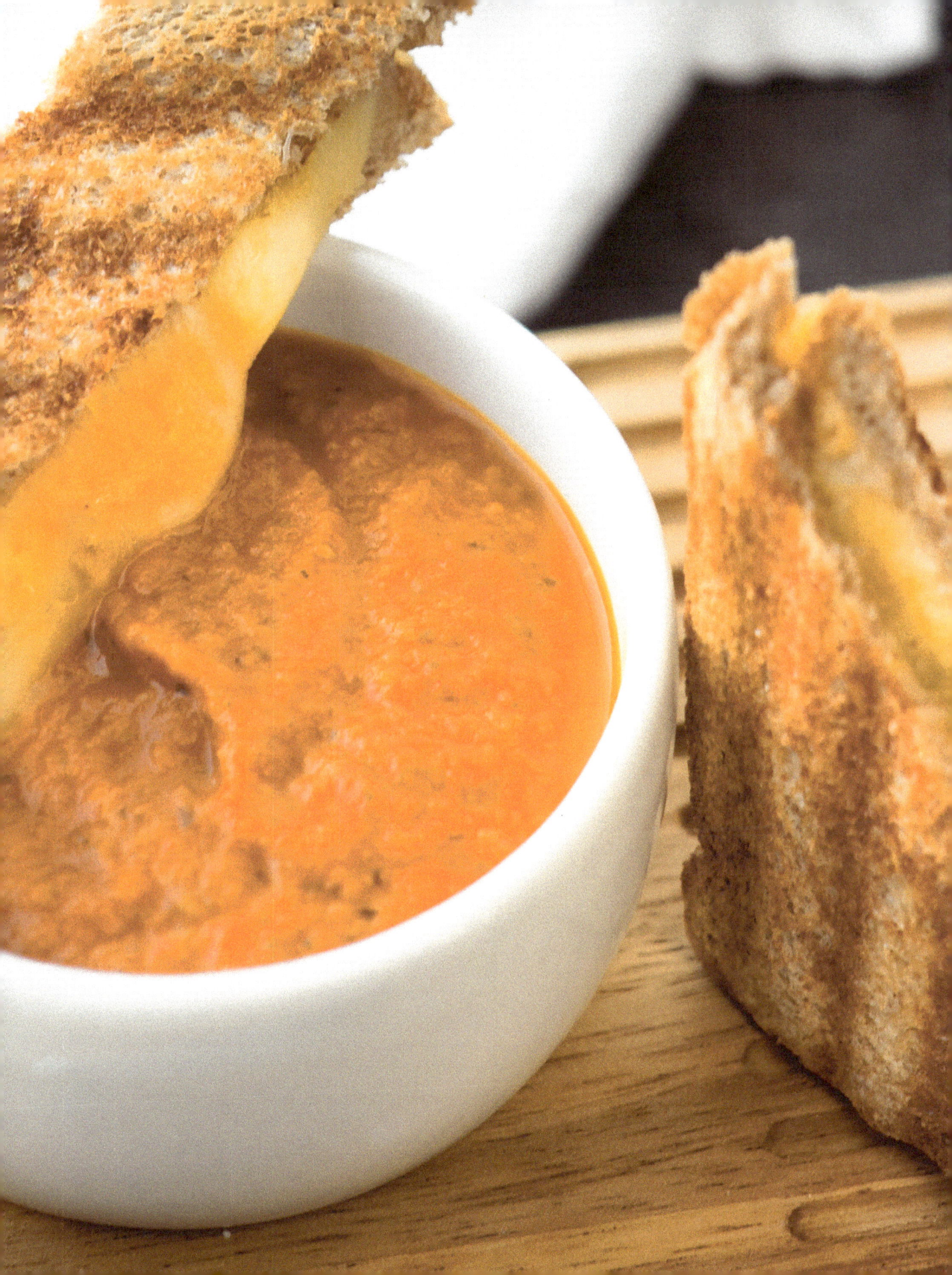

FRESH PLUM TOMATO SOUP WITH GRILLED CHEESE SANDWICHES

This was a childhood favorite for me. Eating this sandwich brings me back to elementary school, except my school's kitchen never packed this much flavor into their tomato soup. This is a much healthier option than the traditional grilled cheese on white bread loaded with butter. In this case, you will be providing whole grains, dairy, and a variety of colorful vegetables. Doesn't get better than that! The aroma alone will say it all. Yummy!

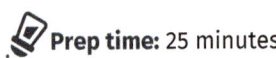 **Prep time:** 25 minutes   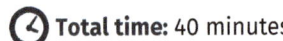 **Total time:** 40 minutes   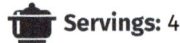 **Servings:** 4

Ingredients

- 2 tbsp. avocado
- ½ a yellow onion (diced)
- 1 celery stalk (diced)
- 1 carrot (diced)
- 1 tbsp. garlic (diced)
- handful fresh basil (minced)
- 1 tbsp. fresh oregano (chopped)
- 1½ lbs. fresh plum tomatoes (cleaned and chopped) or 1 (28 oz.) can whole plum tomatoes with juice (chopped)
- 2 cups organic or low sodium chicken broth
- salt & pepper
- pinch of sugar
- 8 slices of whole-grain bread
- 8 slices of extra sharp cheddar cheese or Swiss cheese
- avocado oil

Directions

- In a medium pot, heat oil on medium-low and add onion, celery, and carrot. Cover and cook until tender (about 5 minutes). Uncover and add garlic and cook for one more minute.
- Add basil, oregano, and tomatoes and simmer uncovered for another 10 minutes. Add broth and bring to a boil. Then lower heat to simmer and cook another 15 minutes, stirring occasionally.
- Remove from heat. In a blender, puree soup in batches until it becomes completely smooth. If you like your soup not as thick, you can add more broth to thin it out as needed. After each batch is completed, return to medium pot.
- Once you have pureed all of the soup, season with salt and pepper and add a dash of sugar. Adjust these ingredients as you feel necessary. Keep soup heated on low while you prepare your sandwiches.
- Put two slices of cheese in between two slices of bread. Brush each side of bread lightly with oil. In a skillet or grill pan on medium heat, brown the sandwiches lightly on each side or until bread is to desired crispiness and cheese is melted. Use another pan or sandwich press to help seal the bread pieces of bread together.
- Once sandwiches are done, cut into two triangles and serve with tomato soup.

THE BEST HOMEMADE CHICKEN SOUP

Ever wonder why chicken soup has, for years, been our "go-to" when we are sick? It is due to the broth! But here is the trick: you must boil the bones! Mark Sisson, author of The Primal Blueprint, actually calls bone broth a "superfood" thanks to the high concentration of minerals. He says that the bone marrow can help strengthen your immune system. In fact, ballplayers have bone broth as part of their diets due to the many nutritional benefits. Bone broth will speed up the movement of mucus in your nose simply because it's a hot fluid. That causes dilation of blood vessels, which causes increased blood flow and allows the mucus to flush everything out. Soups are also hydrating, which is particularly important when fighting off an infection. My biggest piece of advice is to freeze some of the broth each time you make it, for emergencies—times when you get a quick onset of illness, and you are too tired and weak to make this. It will be a lifesaver; you will thank me later!

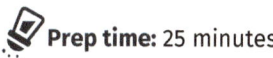 **Prep time:** 25 minutes   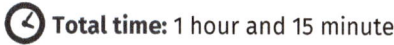 **Total time:** 1 hour and 15 minutes   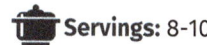 **Servings:** 8-10

Ingredients

- 1 x 4 lb. whole chicken (skin removed)
- 2 cups organic chicken broth
- 4 large carrots (chopped)
- 4 large celery stalks with leaves (chopped)
- 1 medium-sized white onion (diced)
- ½ tsp. garlic powder
- ½ tsp. celery salt
- ½ tsp. onion powder
- ¼ tsp. salt or to taste
- ½ tsp. ground pepper
- ¼ cup Parmesan cheese
- 1 cup ditalini pasta (dry, not cooked yet)

Directions

- Wash and remove the skin from chicken.
- Place chicken in a large pot, then fill with water until it covers the chicken by at least 3 inches.
- Boil chicken on medium heat until fully cooked (40 minutes or so).
- Carefully transfer chicken to a cutting board. DO NOT DRAIN THE WATER! This is your broth base. I like to pick my chicken out of the water with a pair of tongs from the inner cavity.
- As chicken is cooling, skim water with a strainer for any particles or foam so that it is nice and clear.
- When the chicken has cooled down about 5 minutes or so, shred the chicken by hand.
- Add organic chicken broth, shredded chicken and all other ingredients into the pot and simmer for about 20 minutes or until vegetables and pasta are softened.

LENTIL SOUP

This is one of those rainy-day types of soups. It is comforting, healthy, and very flavorful. The great thing about this soup is you can always make the lentils a day before and cut your cooking time by thirty minutes the next day. Nutritionally, lentils are high in protein and iron, and also provide antioxidants such as vitamin A and vitamin C, which bind with and destroy free radicals, reducing oxidative damage to cells. Lentils also have a high content of tannins, phytochemicals that prevent cancer growth, making them a good addition to any diet. So dive in and enjoy the benefits of this amazing legume!

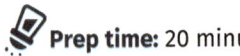 **Prep time:** 20 minutes   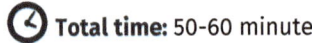 **Total time:** 50-60 minutes   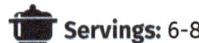 **Servings:** 6-8

Ingredients

- 2 cups water
- 1 lb. lentils (thoroughly washed and rinsed)
- ¼ cup olive oil
- 1 large white onion (diced)
- 4 garlic cloves (minced)
- 1 qt. beef broth
- 1 beef bouillon cube
- 1½ cups celery (diced)
- 1½ cups carrots (chopped)
- 1 tsp. garlic powder
- 1 tsp. salt
- 1 tsp. pepper
- ¼ cup Parmesan cheese
- 1 x 28 oz. can tomato puree

Directions

- In a large pot, add water and lentils, and bring to a boil. Cover and simmer about 30 minutes or until lentils are tender.
- In a separate skillet, sauté onions until softened (about 5-6 minutes). Then add garlic and sauté one more minute. Set mixture aside for later.
- Once lentils are tender, add all remaining ingredients to that pot and simmer for 30 minutes.
- After 30 minutes, add your onion and garlic mixture to the lentil mixture and cook another 5 minutes or until your vegetables are tender.
- Season with additional salt, pepper, and cheese to taste. You may also add more water if you wish to thin it out a little.
- Serve immediately.

EXTRA YUMMY TIP:

Serve with a nice piece of toasted baguette. It makes for yummy dippings!

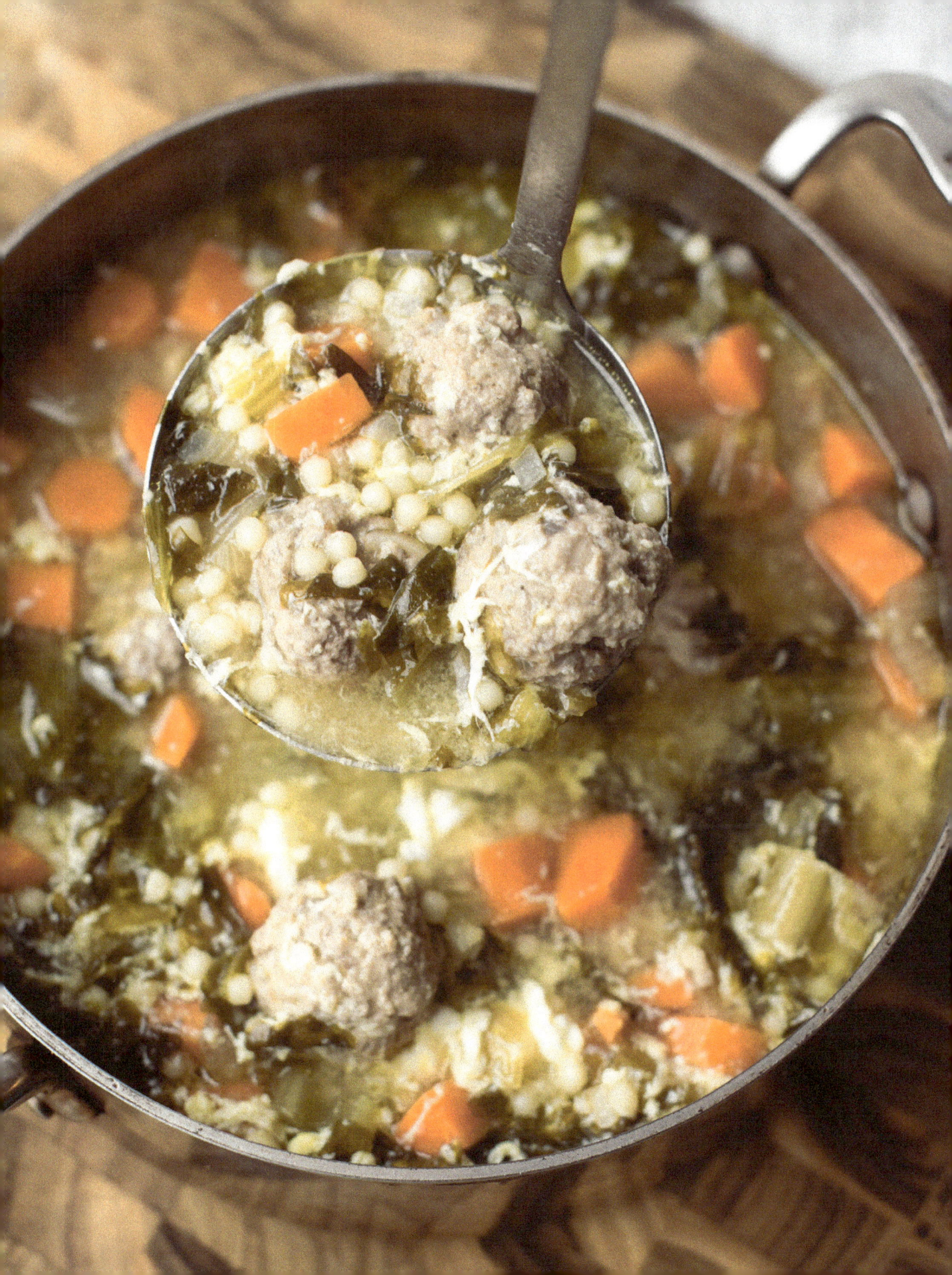

ITALIAN WEDDING SOUP

Many people may think this soup got its name due to being served as a traditional wedding soup at Italian weddings, but it is sort of the other way around. From what I have been told, this soup became a wedding tradition because of its name. The name is a mistranslation of "minestra maritata" (married soup). The Italians use this term to describe how well vegetables and grains go together in a soup. It's a good "marriage" of ingredients. In some parts of Italy, the traditional soup contains meat, and in others, it does not. Bet you didn't know that, did you?

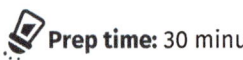 **Prep time:** 30 minutes   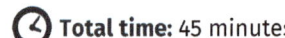 **Total time:** 45 minutes   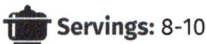 **Servings:** 8-10

Ingredients

The Meatballs
- 1 lb. 95% lean ground beef
- 1 lb. pork
- 1 medium-sized onion (minced)
- 2 garlic cloves (minced)
- 1½ tsp. salt
- 1 egg
- ½ cup plain bread crumbs (or you can process one piece of whole grain bread)
- ¾ cup Pecorino Romano cheese
- 1 cup fresh Italian flat-leaf parsley

The Soup
- 4 qts. low-sodium or organic chicken broth
- 2 carrots (peeled and chopped)
- 3 celery sticks (chopped)
- 1 cup pearl couscous (uncooked) or other small pasta such as acini de pepe
- 1 lb. escarole (chopped)
- 3 tbsp. of Pecorino Romano cheese
- 3 eggs
- salt and pepper to taste

Directions

- In a large bowl, combine all meatball ingredients. Mix together with your hands until well blended and then form 1-inch-diameter meatballs (about a tsp. and a half) and place on a tray and set aside.
- In a large Dutch oven or large soup pot, bring chicken broth to a boil.
- Reduce heat to medium and add meatballs, carrots, celery, and pearl couscous. Let cook for 6 minutes, giving a stir occasionally.
- Then add escarole, and let cook another 5 minutes.
- In a small bowl, beat eggs and Parmesan cheese together.
- Slowly pour egg mixture into the hot soup, stirring constantly with a fork to create small egg strings. The eggs will look slightly scrambled; that is ok!
- Season with salt & pepper to taste.
- Cook another 5-10 minutes on low-medium heat or until meatballs are cooked all the way through.

CANNELLONI BEAN, GARLIC, BASIL & LEMON SOUP

What gives this soup its hidden punch is the lemon you add at the very end. This is the ingredient that will prompt people to ask you what is in the soup when they eat it. You will be handing this recipe out like this today's paper.

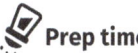 **Prep time:** 10 minutes 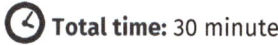 **Total time:** 30 minutes 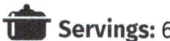 **Servings:** 6

Ingredients

- ¼ cup avocado oil or light olive oil
- 1 large sweet yellow onion (diced)
- 6 cloves garlic (minced)
- 1 (28 oz.) can crushed tomato
- 1 (28 oz.) can cannelloni beans (rinsed and drained)
- 4 cups homemade or organic chicken broth
- 2 cups fresh basil (loosely packed)
- ¼ cup lemon juice
- ⅓ cup Pecorino Romano cheese
- salt and pepper to taste

Directions

- Heat oil in Dutch oven or heavy soup pot on medium heat.
- Add onions and sauté until tender (about 10 minutes).
- Add garlic and sauté one minute.
- Add tomatoes and a dash of salt and pepper, and cook for another 10 minutes.
- Add beans and chicken broth and simmer on low for 12 minutes. At the 10-minute mark, add your basil, lemon juice, and Romano cheese, so it flavors but does not overcook in the soup.
- Remove from heat and serve with a sprinkle of Parmesan cheese.

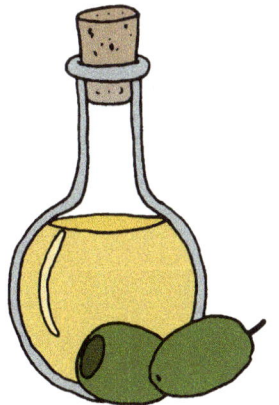

> **EXTRA YUMMY TIP:**
>
> Serve with a nice piece of toasted baguette. It makes for yummy dippings!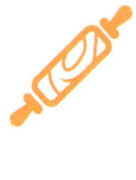

MINESTRONE SOUP: PASTA AND BEANS

The name of this soup originally came from the old Italian word "minestrare," which means to "dish up" or "serve." This was my Italian grandmother's favorite soup. She loved her pasta and beans, and every time I have a spoonful of this recipe, I get a warm, fuzzy feeling inside. The great thing about this soup is you can get creative with your vegetables. You will see many recipes with all different types, but this is the one I enjoy the most.

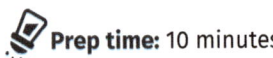 **Prep time:** 10 minutes   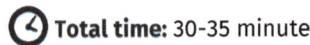 **Total time:** 30-35 minutes   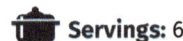 **Servings:** 6

Ingredients

- 3 tbsp. avocado oil
- 1 large white onion (finely chopped)
- 2 carrots (chopped)
- 1 medium-sized zucchini (chopped)
- 1 stalk celery (chopped)
- 3 garlic cloves (minced)
- ½ tsp. salt
- ½ tsp. pepper
- 1 tbsp. fresh chopped oregano
- ¼ tsp. ground dried thyme
- 1 (15 oz.) can diced tomatoes in sauce
- 8 cups organic vegetable broth
- 1 (15 oz.) can white navy beans (drained & rinsed)
- 1 (15 oz.) can kidney beans (drained & rinsed)
- 4 cups spinach (lightly packed)
- handful of fresh chopped basil (about 8-9 leaves)
- 1 cup whole-wheat medium shell pasta (dry)
- ¼ cup Pecorino Romano cheese

Directions

- In a large soup pot on medium, heat oil.
- Add onions, carrots, zucchini, and celery and cook until a little softened (about 2 minutes).
- Add garlic and cook for one minute.
- Add salt, pepper, oregano, and thyme and stir to combine ingredients.
- Add tomatoes in juice, vegetable broth, beans, spinach, basil, and pasta to pot and raise heat to high until the soup comes to a boil.
- Once it reaches a boil, lower heat to low and simmer until pasta is cooked (about 10-15 minutes). Remove soup from heat.
- Last, add Pecorino Romano cheese. You may also season again with a little salt and pepper to taste if you feel it is needed.
- Serve immediately with a sprinkle of Pecorino Romano cheese.

Add THIS to Your Plate!

Leaving a Legacy at the Dinner Table

Dinnertime was probably the most routine and regimented event in my family. My mother had dinner on lockdown. Without being a minute late, dinner was on the table every night at 5:30 sharp. My mother, brother, and I sat patiently at the dinner table waiting for dad to come up the basement steps from his long day at work, and man did that guy hustle. He is still hustling to this very day! When I was a kid, there were no cell phones, iPads, or video games (except Atari and Nintendo, and those were in our bedrooms). At our dinner table, we had only each other to entertain us. The television wasn't on, and if the phone rang, it was not answered. My mom was a real drill sergeant about that. If someone called during dinnertime, they are what she called "ignoramuses." That word always cracked me up! She had a name for every type of person that rubbed her the wrong way; it was hysterical.

The point of the story above is that the ritual of dinner and the importance of eating together as a family is sometimes overlooked in today's busy, late-in-the-day-working society. Families are dining out and not only eating unhealthier, but they are missing the family table experience that would create memories to last a lifetime. Nothing compares to eating in your own home with your family. This is what makes a house a home.

I tend to say that phrase a lot, but it is all the little things that paint the big picture. I find that the families who stay together are the ones who eat together. Most divorced couples have one thing in common: they were not getting the *little things* out of the marriage. You hear it every day; the wife or husband says, "He was never home," or "She never spent quality family-time with us." Eating together at night was always one of the things lacking in these families, I noticed. Now I am not going to say that if you don't eat dinner together your family will fall apart, but what I am saying is that eating dinner together will create a glue that will provide each family member with that sense of love and affection we all desire as humans. It is a chance to give everyone the recognition they need, as well as a sharing of each other's daily activities so that everyone is involved in everyone's life. It should be a place where everyone can feel valued.

It is too often you see families acting like roommates and not family members. Take this time together seriously, and set the tone like my mother did. This had a big part in my immediate family's success. Although my family was not perfect, we had a very strong family bond, and as a family, we were ONE. I attribute it to unbroken family traditions, especially the most important one of all: dinnertime. This is how you will leave a legacy.

Dinner

MOM'S CLASSIC HOMEMADE TOMATO SAUCE: A SUNDAY TRADITION

Maybe this is just the Italian in me, but in my opinion, every woman of the house should know how to make a special family sauce. Although most families never share their recipes (claiming theirs to be the best, of course), I am going to share mine with you. I know, I know, you have probably heard this before, but seriously, my family makes the best sauce around. Oh, and by the way, it's called "sauce" in my house, not "gravy." We save gravy for Thanksgiving (just saying).

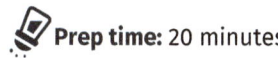 **Prep time:** 20 minutes 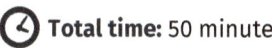 **Total time:** 50 minutes 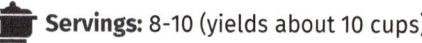 **Servings:** 8-10 (yields about 10 cups)

Ingredients

- ¼ cup olive oil
- 1 medium-sized yellow onion (diced)
- 5 medium-sized garlic cloves (sliced)
- 1 can tomato paste
- 2 (28 oz) cans of crushed tomatoes
- 1 (28 oz) can water
- salt and pepper to taste
- ¾ cup Pecorino Romano cheese
- handful of fresh basil, (about 10-12 leaves) (chopped)
- 7 fresh medium-sized mint fresh leaves (chopped)
- ¼ tsp. thyme
- 1 tsp. oregano
- 1 tsp. Italian seasoning
- 1 tsp. garlic powder (optional if you want more flavor)

TIP:

Freeze any leftover sauce as this recipe yields a lot! You can defrost for that emergency quick meal in the future. I normally save the sauce for a future lasagne or eggplant parmesan dish.

- 1 tsp. onion powder (optional if you want more flavor)

Directions

- Heat oil in a medium-sized non-stick saucepan on a medium flame.
- Once the oil is heated, add onion and cook until tender, stirring occasionally (about 5 minutes or so).
- Add garlic to the pan and cook for one minute with onion.
- Lower heat to medium-low, and add the tomato paste. Cook about 1-2 minutes, stirring and being careful not to burn it.
- Add two cans of crushed tomato sauce.
- Fill up one of the empty tomato cans with water, and add to the mixture.
- Add remaining ingredients (Pecorino Romano cheese, salt, pepper, basil, mint , thyme, oregano, Italian seasoning, garlic powder, and onion powder) —and stir with a little love.
- Bring sauce to a light boil, stirring frequently. Then reduce heat to low and simmer for 50 minutes.
- Be sure to stir your sauce occasionally; you don't want to burn the sauce on the bottom of the pan.
- When finished, add more salt and pepper if needed.
- Add to any pasta of your choice!

Meat Option: To make this a meat sauce, simply add 2 lbs. of 90% beef to the pan after you add your onion and garlic and sauté until nice and browned (about 15-20 minutes). Then continue the rest of the recipe as listed above

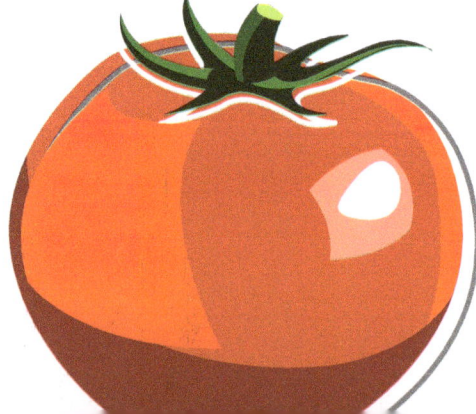

A TRADTIONAL BOLOGNESE SAUCE WITH TAGLIATELLE

Bolognese is a meat-based sauce originating from Bologna, Italy, hence the name! What makes this sauce so delicious is the combination of beef and pork, making you go in for just one more bite. Although traditionally, tagliatelle pasta is used, you can use another flat pasta such as fettuccine or pappardelle. They will go just as well. This is one of my favorite sauces; enjoy!

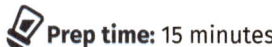 **Prep time:** 15 minutes   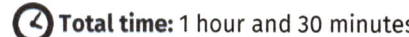 **Total time:** 1 hour and 30 minutes   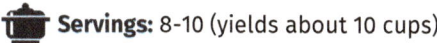 **Servings:** 8-10 (yields about 10 cups)

Ingredients

- ¼ cup olive oil
- 2 carrots (diced)
- 1 celery stalk (diced)
- 1 small onion (diced)
- 3 oz. pancetta (diced)
- 1 lb. lean ground beef (90%)
- 1 lb. ground pork
- ½ cup dry red wine
- 1 (28 oz.) can crushed tomato
- 2 tbsp. tomato paste
- 2 cups beef broth
- 1 cup whole milk
- sea salt and freshly ground pepper
- ½ tsp. nutmeg
- 1 lb. fresh or dried tagliatelle pasta

Directions

- In a medium non-stick saucepan over medium-low heat, heat your olive oil.
- Raise flame to medium-high and add carrots, celery, onion, and pancetta and cook for about 25 minutes, stirring occasionally, until all ingredients are nice and browned. If it browns too much, you can add a little water to deglaze the pot.
- Add beef and pork and stir well, combining with the vegetable and pancetta mixture. Break up meats with a wooden spoon and cook until lightly browned, about 20 minutes.
- Add wine and deglaze the pan, scraping bits off the bottom of the pan. Cook wine about 2 minutes until evaporated.
- Then add the can of crushed tomato, tomato paste, broth, milk, salt and pepper to taste, and nutmeg, and stir with love.
- Bring sauce to a simmer, then reduce to simmer for about 45 minutes to an hour, stirring occasionally. If the sauce becomes too thick, you can add more beef broth or a little water.

The Pasta

While the sauce is cooking, bring a large pot of water to a boil (three-quarters full), and add a teaspoon of salt to the water. Once water is boiling, add your pasta and cook until al dente (check after 3 minutes for the right firmness or follow package instructions). Once sauce is done, you can combine your sauce and pasta. Just remember you want to coat your pasta with your sauce, not drown it. Add a little at a time until you feel it is coated just right.

CASA ROMANA SAUCE WITH ELBOW PASTA & PARMESAN

This sauce was served to me in the kitchen of my first true love (and still to this day) or his father Leonardo's kitchen, I should say. He is first-generation Italian, so when I would visit him at his dad's house, I would also get to enjoy Leo's cooking. He would always make me this sauce with elbow pasta, and although you can serve this tomato sauce with another type of pasta, there is just something about serving it with elbow pasta that makes it extra special. Maybe it is because you can use a spoon to shovel it in!

Although garlic is used in most Italian recipes, this one it does not call for it. In fact, onion and carrot is the main flavor to marry with your tomatoes. Although I never added ground beef to this sauce, I would imagine it would also taste incredible. Leonardo told me the secret to this sauce was to simmer it on low—never let it bubble. He said take your time with Italian cooking; the longer and slower it cooks, the more enjoyable the food. He was right.

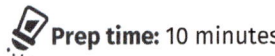 **Prep time:** 10 minutes   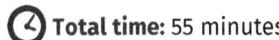 **Total time:** 55 minutes   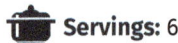 **Servings:** 6

Ingredients

- ¼ cup olive oil
- 4 carrots (grated)
- 1 white onion (diced)
- ¼ tsp. black pepper
- pinch of crushed red pepper
- 1 beef bouillon cube
- 1 (14.5 oz.) can tomato puree
- Parmesan cheese for serving
- 13.25 oz. elbow pasta (1 box)

Directions

- In a medium-sized saucepan, heat oil on a low-medium flame.
- Add carrots, onions, black pepper, crushed red pepper, and beef bouillon cube and cook for 5 minutes.
- Reduce to simmer, cover, and cook for 20 minutes.
- Then add tomato puree, and stir together. Uncovered, simmer for another 20 minutes, stirring occasionally.
- While sauce is cooking, prepare your pasta.
- Bring 4-6 quarts of water to a boil. Add a little dash of salt. Add pasta to water and cook for about 6 minutes or until al dente. (or follow instructions on the box)
- Serve with a sprinkle of Parmesan.

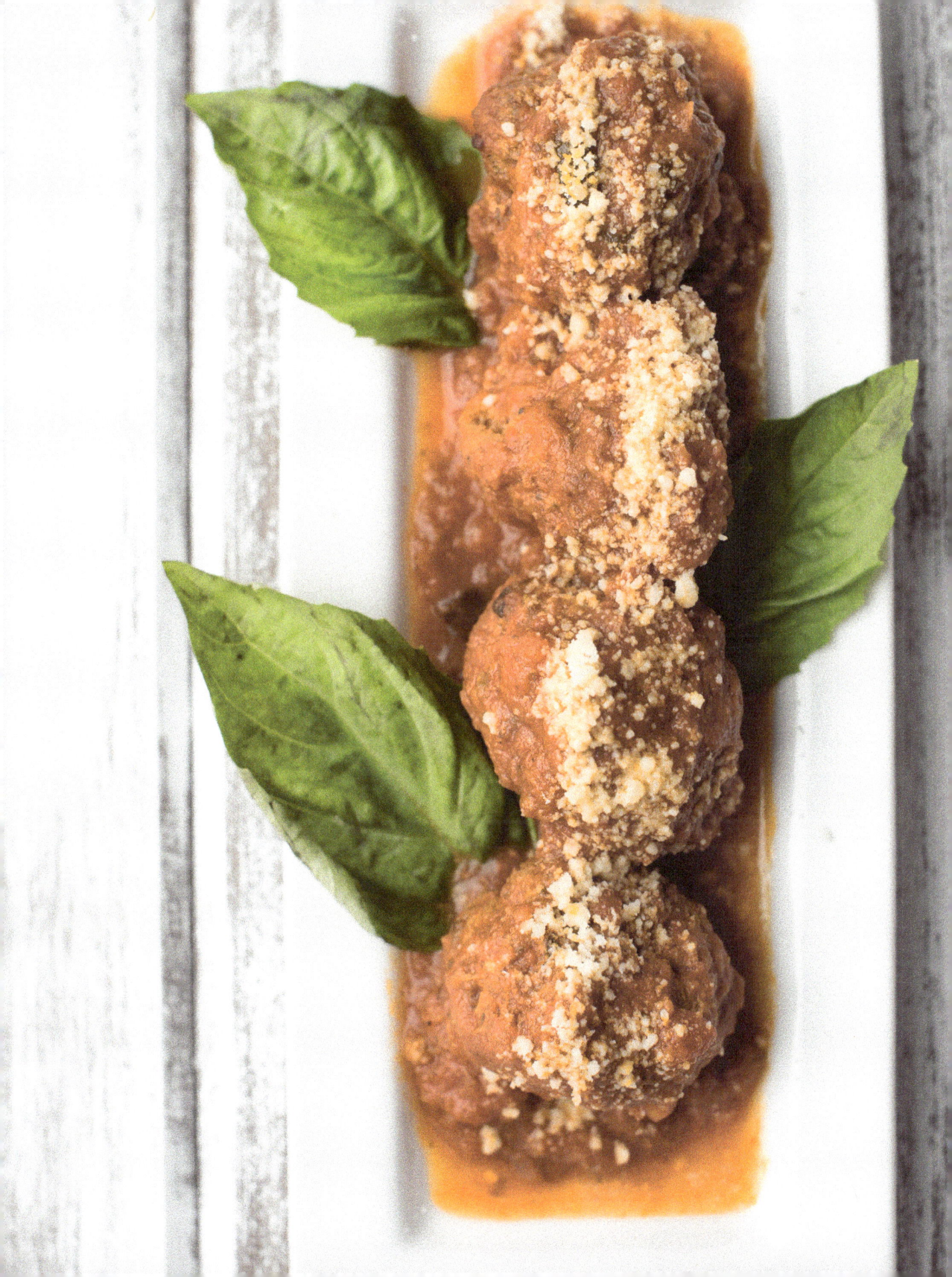

MAMA D'S MEATBALLS

Everyone claims that their mom makes the best meatballs. But guess what, I am going to tell you that not only does my mom make the best meatballs, but mine are even a little better. Shhhhh! Don't tell her, but even my grandmother, the pickiest woman in the world, whispered this into my ear one night while at the dinner table. It was pretty funny, I must say.

But getting down to what makes a great ball, in my opinion, is the meat you use, and also a few key ingredients. This recipe is my mother's recipe with a few additions inspired by other recipes I have tried in the past. For me, it is a requirement to have three types of meat in your balls. I like veal, pork, and beef. A lot of stores sell a meatloaf mix which is already conveniently ground and mixed for you. The other HUGE secret to my meatballs is not only freshly chopped basil, but are you ready? Wait for it... MINT!

Yes, MINT! It is the ingredient that makes my meatballs so special and taste so fresh. This is what will make your meatballs different from everyone else. I was asked by friends when I decided to add this if I was really going to give this recipe away, and I said, "I would be committing a crime if I didn't." Now I am not going to lie, this will be a full-day preparation. This is a sauce you make on a rainy Sunday afternoon. Or you can make this the day before and serve the next evening if you have company coming over. It is not the preparation that takes a long time, but the low simmer on the sauce. Some people sauté their meatballs or bake them first, which you can and it will cut your cooking time down since the balls will be cooked, but they will not soak into the sauce and have the tenderness that this recipe will. If you make this meal a Sunday tradition, I promise you will leave a legacy.

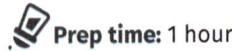 **Prep time:** 1 hour   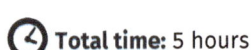 **Total time:** 5 hours   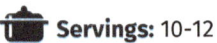 **Servings:** 10-12

> **TIP:**
>
> If you do not have 5 hours to make this recipe, you can sauté your meatballs in a pan with some oil, browning all sides so that they half way cook. Then you can add to your sauce and let simmer in the sauce for about an hour. I just happen to be really bad at sautéing meatballs! Honest truth, but you can try both ways!

Ingredients

Meat
- 2 oz. Fontina cheese
- 2 oz. Pecorino Romano cheese
- 2 oz. sharp Provolone cheese
- 2 oz. Asiago cheese
- 1 lb. ground lean ground beef (such as 90% lean)
- 1 lb. ground veal
- 1 lb. ground pork
- 1 egg (beaten)
- 1 cup Italian bread crumbs (see eggplant recipe for fresh made bread crumb recipe)
- handful of fresh basil (chopped)
- ¼ cup fresh mint (chopped)

Vegetable Mixture
- 1 medium carrot (coarsely chopped)
- 1 celery stalk (coarsely chopped)
- 1 medium onion (coarsely chopped)
- 6 cloves garlic
- 1 handful fresh Italian flat leaf parsley
- 1 handful fresh basil
- 3 tbsp. olive oil
- 1 tsp. salt
- 1 tsp. pepper
- a couple of pinches of crushed red pepper

Sauce
- ¼ cup olive oil
- 1 (6 oz.) can tomato paste
- 6 (28 oz.) can crushed tomato
- 1 (28 oz.) can water
- salt and pepper to taste
- ½ cup Pecorino Romano cheese
- handful of fresh basil (chopped)
- ½ tsp. thyme
- ½ tsp. oregano
- ½ tsp. Italian seasoning

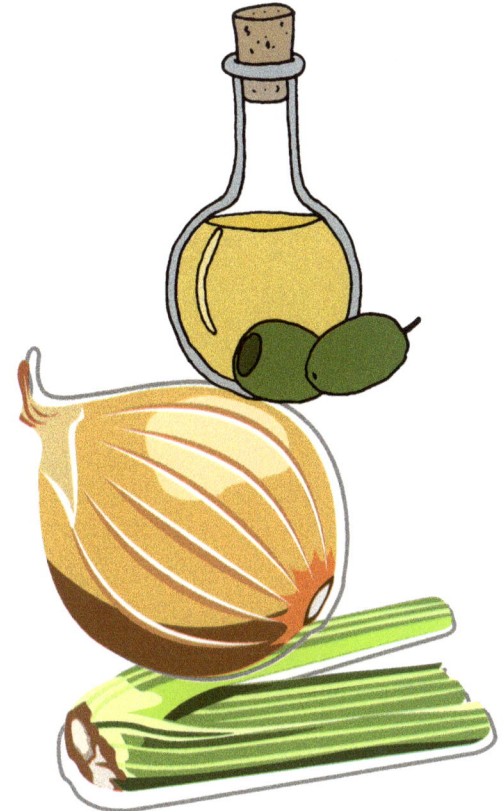

TIP 2:

Do not attempt to use a crockpot for this recipe, although we are slow cooking, the meatballs will have a funny texture from the heat distribution. Trust me, I tried it!! No bueno

Directions

- In a food processor, combine all the cheeses until very fine.
- In a large bowl, combine all the meats together and then mix in the cheeses with your hands.
- Add the egg, breadcrumbs, mint, and basil to meat and continue to use your hands to combine all the ingredients. Do not over-handle the meat. Cover meat mixture, and put in the refrigerator until it is ready to form into balls.
- Prepare your vegetable mixture. In a food processor, add your carrot, celery, onion, garlic, parsley, basil, olive oil, salt, black pepper, and red pepper. Process until it becomes well blended. It should be on the smooth side, but not overly pureed. About 15 seconds or so should do it.
- In a large pasta pot (at least an 8-9 quart), heat 1/4 cup olive oil and add vegetable mixture to the pan. Season with salt, pepper, and red pepper and cook for about 8 minutes, stirring occasionally.
- Remove meat mixture from refrigerator and add half of the cooked vegetable mixture to meat mixture and combine. Leave the other half of the vegetable mixture in the pan for your sauce.
- Add 1/4 cup olive oil to your pasta pot and then add your tomato paste and sauté for 3 minutes with remaining vegetable mixture.
- Add all cans of crushed tomato, take one of the 28 oz. empty tomato cans and fill it with water and add to the sauce mixture.
- Then add your seasonings (salt, pepper, Romano cheese, basil, thyme, oregano, Italian seasoning) and stir with lots of love. Let sauce simmer on low for 20 minutes until it gets nice and hot. Stir occasionally.
- While your sauce is cooking, start forming 3-inch meatballs until complete.
- Once sauce is nice and hot, add raw meatballs right to the hot sauce. Be sure the sauce is fully covering all the meatballs, and let them cook on a low simmer for 30 minutes. IMPORTANT: Do not stir the sauce for 30 minutes or the meatballs could fall apart. After 30 minutes, gently give the sauce and meatballs a stir, and then let simmer on low for 4 hours, stirring occasionally so sauce does not burn on the bottom of the pan.

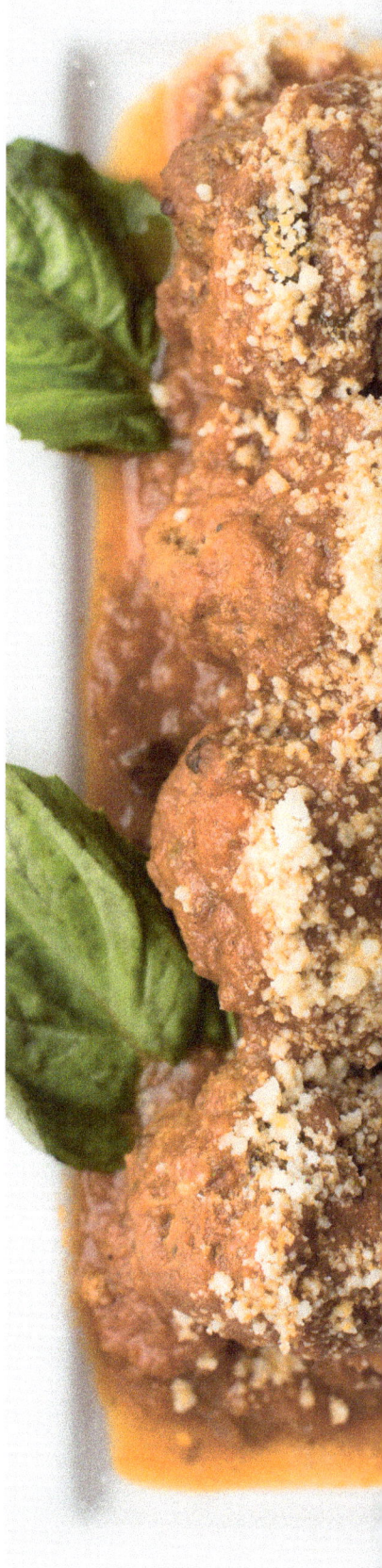

A HEALTHIER EGGPLANT PARMESAN

What is one of the biggest complaints about this dish? People complain it is not healthy. This version is the opposite; if done correctly is very nutritious! I made a few small changes which I believe make a big difference.

Yes, you can bake the eggplant, but I can promise you, it will not taste the same as sautéing it over the stove. However, we will use the correct type of oil to sauté in order not to damage the nutritional value of our eggplant, ok?

A few things I did to lighten this up: we will be making our very own fresh bread crumbs with whole-grain bread rather than store-bought bread crumbs loaded with preservatives and made with white bread, which has less nutritional value. Next, I replaced white flour for dredging your eggplant with whole-wheat flour, again for the same reason. Lastly, when we sauté our eggplant, we are going to use avocado oil, not olive oil. As we learned earlier in this book, avocado oil has a very high smoke point and will be safe to use on that high flame.

With this said, when you do eat this dish, be sure to stay within your portion control because of the cheese content. When you slice it, a portion of this should be the size of your fist. That is one portion! So don't over indulge; moderation is the key, especially with cheese, which we know is very high in saturated fat.

Now that we got that out of the way, enjoy! This is a crowd pleaser.

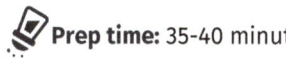 **Prep time:** 35-40 minutes   **Total time:** 1 hour and 10 minutes   **Servings:** 6-8

Ingredients

The Sauce

See Mom's Classic Homemade Tomato Sauce page 142

The Bread Crumbs

- 3 cups whole-wheat bread crumbs (about 8 slices fresh, whole-wheat bread, or if you can't eat wheat, any whole-grain bread is ok too!)
- 1 tbsp. garlic powder
- 1 tbsp. onion powder
- 1 tbsp. Italian seasoning
- 1 tsp. salt
- 1 tsp. pepper

Eggplant Layers

- 1 cup organic wheat flour
- 6 eggs (beaten)
- 2 large eggplants (cut into about ¼-½-inch thick rounds)
- 1½ cups avocado oil or grapeseed oil (must be a high smoke point oil)
- 3-4 cups shredded mozzarella cheese
- Fresh basil (a big handful, about 16 leaves)
- ¾ cup Parmesan cheese

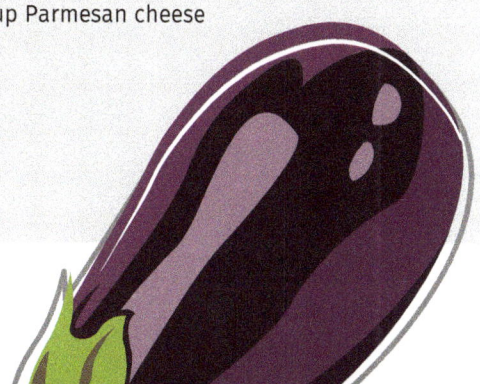

Directions

- First, prepare your breadcrumbs. In a blender or food processor, simply break the bread into pieces with your hands and process until it becomes fine crumbs. You might need to do it in batches depending on the blender or processor size.
- Once bread has been made into crumbs, place in a medium-sized bowl and add other dry ingredients (garlic powder, onion powder, Italian seasoning, salt, and pepper) and stir together with a fork until fully blended. Put aside.
- Have a few trays lined with paper towels ready to rest each finished sautéed eggplant on.
- All next to each other in 3 separate bowls, have your beaten eggs, wheat flour, and fresh breadcrumb mixture ready to start the eggplant preparation. It will look like an assembly line.
- In a large skillet on a medium-high flame, heat about ½ inch of oil. Oil should be about 380-400°F.
- Take one piece of eggplant and lightly coat each side with wheat flour.
- Dip the entire eggplant into the egg mixture, remove, and let the remaining egg drip off.
- Coat each side generously with your homemade breadcrumb mixture.
- Place eggplant down into heated skillet, and repeat this process until you run out of room in the pan. Cook eggplant until golden brown, about 2 minutes on each side. You can use a pair of tongs to flip it over.
- When finished, remove from pan and place on tray layered with paper towels to dry up oil drippings. Repeat this process until all of the eggplant is all cooked. (This takes the longest.)
- Next, you will start the layering process. Have a 9 x 13 non-stick baking pan ready.
- Spoon about 1 cup of tomato sauce on the bottom of pan. Top with a layer of the fried eggplant. The slices can overlap a little. Top with 1 cup of shredded mozzarella. Top with a layer of torn basil leaves. Repeat this process 2 more times (should be 3 layers high, end with a layer of mozzarella on top).
- On the last layer, sprinkle Parmesan cheese over the top of the mozzarella.
- Place in middle rack of oven, and cook on 350°F for 30-35 minutes until cheese is slightly browned, melted, and bubbly.
- Enjoy this heavenly dish.

SPINACH, ARTICHOKE, AND MUSHROOM RISOTTO

Risotto is a favorite northern Italian rice dish cooked in a broth to a creamy consistency. The texture of risotto, if done correctly, should be creamy and al dente, not sticky and gluey. Risotto is excellent with vegetables and seafood.

Prep time: 10 minutes **Total time:** 35 minutes **Servings:** 4-6

Ingredients

- 5 tbsp. high smoke point cooking oil like avocado oil
- 2 cups mushrooms (diced)
- 1 (14 oz.) can artichoke hearts (drained and diced)
- 3 cups spinach (chopped)
- salt and pepper
- 2 shallots (minced)
- 3 garlic cloves, minced (or 1 tbsp)
- 1 cup Arborio rice
- 4 cups organic chicken or vegetable stock
- ¼ cup Asiago cheese
- Parmesan cheese for sprinkling

Directions

- Heat 3 tbsp. oil in a skillet on medium heat.
- Add artichokes, spinach, and mushroom to the pan and continue to cook on medium-high heat until softened and mushrooms have released their fluids (about 10 minutes). Stir occasionally, so vegetables do not stick to the pan. Season with salt and pepper.
- In a separate, medium-sized saucepan, heat the remaining 2 tbsp. oil on a medium flame and add shallots. Sauté until soft (about 3-5 min).
- Add garlic and cook one more minute.
- Add rice and cook for about 1 minute to absorb flavors of garlic and shallots.
- Raise flame to medium-high, and add one cup of vegetable broth and stir frequently until all liquid is absorbed into the rice. Be careful to not have rice stick to the pan.
- Add another cup of the vegetable broth, and repeat the same steps as above. Repeat this until all stock is gone. If needed, add the remaining broth until rice is cooked through.
- Once all is absorbed rice should be tender with a little bite to it (al dente).
- Add cheese last, and stir into risotto.
- Add vegetable mixture to risotto and stir to combine.
- Serve immediately and sprinkle with Parmesan cheese.

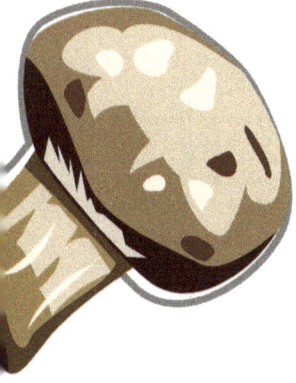

CLASSIC HOMESTYLE CHILI

Chili is an amazing comfort food. It is nutritious, has exciting bursts of flavor, and gives you a swift kick right before the game. The best chili is the kind you can make from scratch, so that is just what we are going to do. Forget buying pre-packaged chili mix loaded with sodium, who needs all that salt? Not us! We are going to season from scratch and heat this bad boy up with a variety of peppers that will set your party on fire. It goes well over brown rice too!

Prep time: 25 minutes   **Total time:** about 2 hours   **Servings:** 8

Ingredients

- ¼ cup avocado or grapeseed oil (or other high smoke point oil)
- 1 jalapeño (diced)
- 1 Anaheim pepper (diced)
- 1 red bell pepper (diced)
- 1 large white onion (diced)
- 4 garlic cloves (minced)
- 2 lbs. of 93% lean ground beef
- 1 tbsp. chili powder
- 1 tsp. coriander
- 1 tsp. cumin
- 1 tsp. garlic powder
- 1 tsp. onion powder
- 1 tsp. paprika
- 1 tsp. salt
- 1 tsp. pepper
- ⅓ cup tomato paste
- 1 (15 oz.) can kidney beans (drained and rinsed)
- 1 (15 oz.) can black beans (drained and rinsed)
- 1 (15 oz.) can pinto beans (drained and rinsed)
- 1 (28 oz.) can ground peeled tomatoes
- 2 cups beef broth
- shredded cheddar cheese (for serving)

Directions

- In a large pot or Dutch oven on medium-high flame, heat oil. Add your jalapeño pepper, Anaheim pepper, red bell pepper, and onion. Sauté until softened, about 5 minutes. Add garlic and cook one more minute.
- Increase flame to medium-high, and add ground beef to pot. Cook until nice and browned (about 10 minutes).
- Combine all dry spices to the meat mixture (chili powder, coriander, cumin, garlic powder, onion powder, paprika, salt, and pepper) and then mix in tomato paste. Cook another 5 minutes.
- Add kidney beans, black beans, pinto beans, ground peeled tomatoes, and beef broth to pot. Stir very well to blend all ingredients.
- Lower heat and simmer for 1 ½ hours.
- Serve with cheddar cheese.

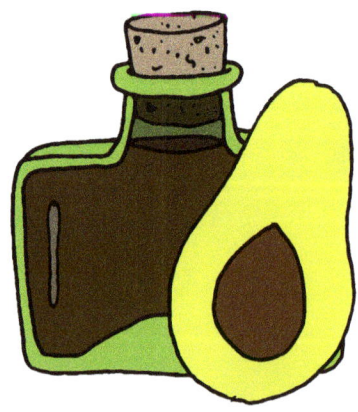

MOM'S LASAGNA

There are a lot of types of lasagna: with meat, without meat, with red sauce, béchamel sauce, and the list goes on. For this book, I am going to stick with my family's traditional lasagna; you can lighten it up a little by replacing the white egg pasta with whole-wheat pasta. This will add some nice whole grains to your dish and will also provide you with some great fiber. Cheese gets a bad rap because of the saturated fat content, but when served in moderation, it is a nice source of calcium and nothing to feel guilty about. One serving should be the size of your fist.

The key to having this dish come out great is to let it rest after you remove it from the oven. As I mentioned before, Italian food requires time and love. So give this love a 20-minute rest before serving.

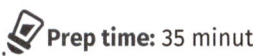 **Prep time:** 35 minutes   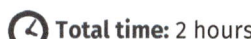 **Total time:** 2 hours   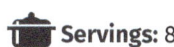 **Servings:** 8

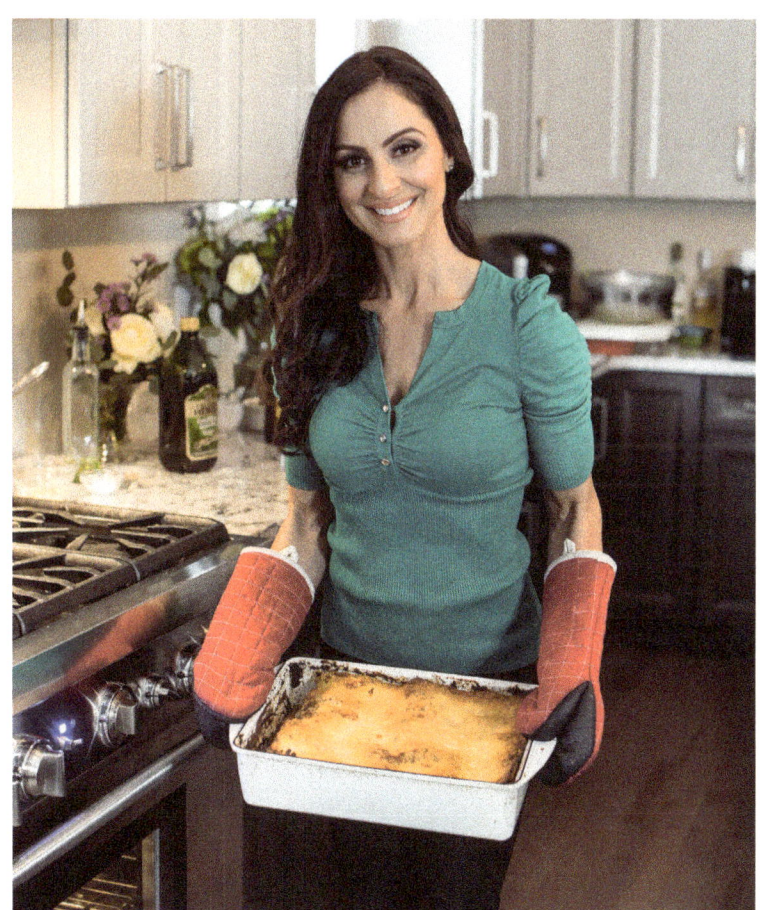

TIP:

I like to make my sauce a few days ahead. Sauce always tastes better the next day and saves you an hour of time in the kitchen!

Ingredients

- 16 oz. lasagna (you can substitute whole-wheat lasagna for a healthier option)
- 2 (32 oz.) containers of part-skim ricotta cheese (water drained if any in packaging)
- 16 oz. package of mozzarella cheese
- 5 eggs (beaten)
- handful fresh chopped parsley (about a ½ cup)
- black pepper (about a ½ tsp.)
- 1½ cups Parmesan cheese

Sauce

- See Mom's Classic Homemade Tomato Sauce, page 142 (optional: add meat to sauce)

Directions

- Pre-heat oven 350°F on bake.
- Boil lasagna just until it bends (8 minutes or so, or follow package instructions) Remove from pan, separate with cool water, and lay out flat on a cooling tray.
- In a bowl, hand mix ricotta cheese, eggs parsley, and pepper.
- You will need at least a standard 13 x 9 lasagna dishpan.
- To assemble, spread 1½ cups of sauce onto the bottom of the pan. Arrange a layer of lasagna over the sauce. It is ok over to overlap the noodles on the edges. You can also arrange noodles in the opposite direction at the end of the pan if there is extra space.
- With a large serving spoon, scoop 3 mounds of the ricotta cheese mixture across each strip of lasagna (about 1¾ cups or so). Spread with a spatula. It should be just enough to cover the lasagna. Take about 1½ cups of sauce and spread over the ricotta cheese mixture and spread with spatula. Again, this should be a thin layer; just enough sauce to coat the cheese.
- Spread about a cup of shredded mozzarella cheese over the sauce. Continue this process until you are done. Sprinkle 1 cup Parmesan cheese over the last layer of mozzarella cheese.
- Place aluminum foil over the pan to cover, and bake lasagna on 350°F for about 35 minutes or until bubbly and tender.
- Remove and be sure to let it rest for a minimum of 20 minutes before serving in order to congeal the contents. This is a super important step so it does not fall apart.

> **TIP:**
>
> Tip: I always buy an extra box of lasagne just in case something goes wrong while cooking it, such as letting it over cook by accident. This will save you an emergency store run if you have a back up. It has happened to all of us!!

SHEPHERD'S PIE

It's America's classic comfort casserole, and it is still one of my favorites. This is such a simple dish, but it always has me going back for seconds. I had this dish one time with a creamy mushroom combo and when I reviewed the recipe, it had cream of mushroom soup in it. My eyes widened as I read the sodium content on the can. Wow! To re-create that creamy goodness without all the sodium and preservatives, I added my own fresh mushrooms and some mascarpone cheese, which is a great cream substitute. Save this recipe for a snowy day.

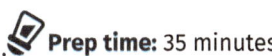 **Prep time:** 35 minutes   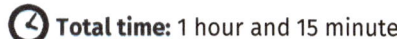 **Total time:** 1 hour and 15 minutes   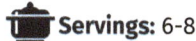 **Servings:** 6-8

Ingredients

- 2 lbs. mashed potato (see sides for mashed potato recipe, page 197)
- 3 tbsp. avocado oil or other high smoke point oil
- 1 cup onion (diced)
- 1 cup carrots (peeled & diced)
- 1 cup mushrooms (cleaned, stems removed and chopped)
- 1½ lbs. lean beef (such as 90%)
- ½ tsp. salt
- ½ tsp. pepper
- 1½ tsp. Worcestershire sauce
- 1 tomato (diced)
- 1 cup beef broth
- 1 tsp. fresh or dried rosemary
- ½ cup mascarpone cheese
- ½ cup peas
- ½ cup corn

Directions

- Place a rack in the upper part of the oven, about 6-8 inches from broiler. Pre-heat oven on broil (high).
- Prepare potatoes: recipe listed in sides section. Page 197
- In large sauté pan on a medium flame, heat 3 tbsp. of oil. Add onions, carrots, and mushrooms and cook for about 5 minutes or until they soften a bit.
- Increase the flame to medium-high, and add meat to the pan. Cook until nice and browned (about 10 minutes).
- Add salt, pepper, and Worcestershire sauce to meat.
- Add tomato, beef broth, and rosemary to meat mixture, and cook another 5 minutes. Add the mascarpone cheese and cook another 5 minutes, stirring occasionally.
- Add peas and corn to mixture, and combine all ingredients.
- Remove meat mixture from pan and transfer to a 9 x 13 casserole dish.
- Spoon potato mixture on top of the meat mixture as the second layer. You can fluff the potato with a fork to give it some design.
- Place dish in the oven on the top shelf and broil for about 5 minutes or until the potatoes have browned on top. Remove and enjoy.

TIP:

Pairs well with mushroom gravy recipe. Page 194

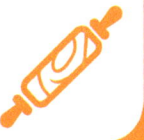

CLASSIC PORK TENDERLOIN TOPPED WITH SAUTÉED SWEET ONIONS

When it comes to cooking the perfect tenderloin, there are a few steps and rules to abide by. The first step is to sear it before it goes into the oven. What this does is creates a crust around the meat, which then locks in the juices as it cooks in the oven, creating a more succulent piece of meat. Remember never to cut into your meat until you let it set. If you cut into it too early, you will release all the juices, causing a dry piece of meat.

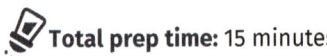 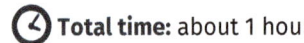 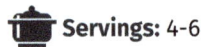

Total prep time: 15 minutes **Total time:** about 1 hour **Servings:** 4-6

Ingredients

- 1 (1 lb.) pork tenderloin
- 2-3 garlic cloves (cut into slivers)
- ½ tsp. salt
- ¼ tsp. pepper
- ½ tsp. onion powder
- ½ tsp. garlic powder
- 1 tbsp. fresh or dried rosemary
- 7 tbsp. avocado oil
- 1 large sweet onion (sliced)

Directions

- Position rack in middle of oven, and preheat to 400°F on bake.
- Use a paring knife to cut small ½-inch holes about an inch apart along the top of the entire length of the tenderloin. Stuff each hole with a sliver of the garlic and repeat for each hole.
- In a small bowl, combine salt, pepper, onion powder, garlic powder, rosemary, and 4 tablespoons of oil. Mix with a spoon, and then use a brush to coat the tenderloin thoroughly with the herb seasoning. Be sure to coat all sides.
- In a large skillet, on a high flame, brown the tenderloin on all sides using a pair of tongs (about 2 to 3 minutes).
- Transfer into a baking dish and bake in the oven until the internal temperature of the thickest part reaches 155°F, about 20 to 35 minutes, depending on your oven. When finished, let rest for about 8 to 10 minutes.
- While the tenderloin is cooking, start sautéing your onions.
- On a medium-high flame, heat the oil. Add onions and sauté until very browned and softened (about 12 to 15 minutes). Then season with a little salt and pepper.
- Carve tenderloin into 1½-inch-thick slices, top with onions, and enjoy!

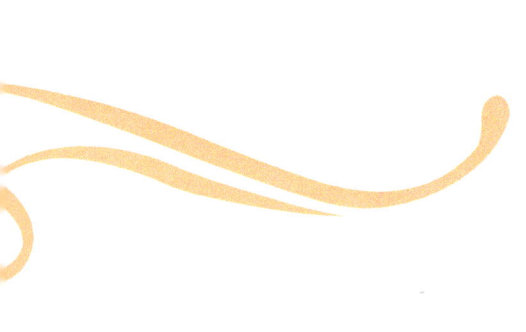

Add THIS to Your Plate!

BUTTERNUT SQUASH MAC 'N' CHEESE

Who doesn't like mac 'n' cheese? I remember boxed mac 'n' cheese being one of the first things I learned how to cook. I was about twelve years old and thought I was a pro. Boy, was I wrong. I tasted that stuff recently and wow, have my tastebuds changed. No offense!

I love nothing more to than to add nutrition to a dish. To do this, I added butternut squash, replaced whole milk with almond milk, and replaced the pasta with whole-wheat pasta and breadcrumbs for added fiber. Making these small changes to this classic lightens this dish up, making you feel excited to serve it to your family. This mac 'n' cheese will be mature enough for an adult and yet still desired by your kids.

Total time: 1 hour and 30 minutes   **Servings:** 6-8

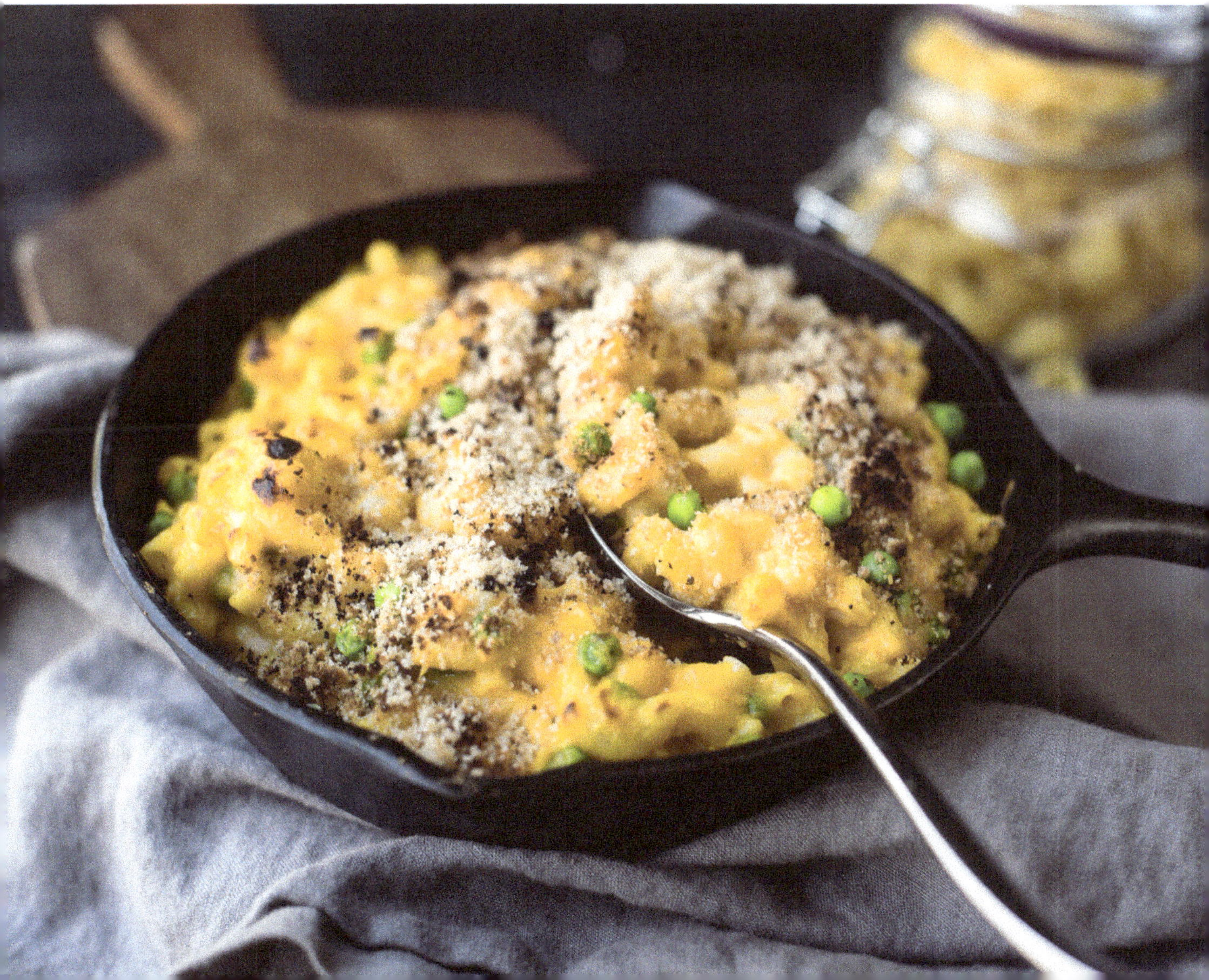

Ingredients

- ½ cup whole-wheat or whole grain bread crumbs (about 2 slices of bread)
- 1 large butternut squash
- 5 cups cooked whole wheat shell pasta
- 2 cups non-sweetened almond milk
- 2 tbsp. wheat flour
- 1 garlic clove (sliced)
- 3 cups very sharp cheddar cheese
- 1 tbsp. Dijon mustard
- ½ tsp. salt
- ¼ tsp. pepper
- ⅛ tsp. crushed red pepper (or more if you like it spicy)
- ½ cup peas
- olive oil for drizzling

Directions

- Prepare breadcrumbs.
- Take bread and break up into small pieces. Then place in a blender or food processor and process until it turns into fine crumbs and then put aside for later.
- Prepare squash.
- Fill a baking pan with about 1-2 inches of water. Cut the squash in half, remove the seeds, and place face down onto the pan, skin facing up.
- Bake 375°F for about 40-60 minutes. You will know it is done when the skin looks wrinkled and browned and is soft when pressed.
- Scrape out the squash meat into a bowl, and put aside.
- Set oven to broil and position a rack on the upper half of oven, about 6-8 inches from broiler.
- Prepare your shell pasta. Follow instructions on box for an al dente preparation.
- In a medium-sized saucepan on medium heat, whisk together almond milk, flour, and garlic. Continue to whisk until nice and hot, but not boiling.
- Add squash to the liquid mixture. Use a hand mixer or blender to combine and puree. Careful not to splash because it will be hot.
- Once mixture is pureed, add cheese, mustard, salt, black pepper, and red pepper, and stir until cheese melts.
- Add pasta and peas to the sauce and combine.
- Transfer to a casserole dish (be sure to spray with a non-stick spray) and then sprinkle breadcrumbs over the top. Get a little olive oil and drizzle lightly over the top for browning.
- Broil on upper rack for about a minute or until golden brown and crispy.

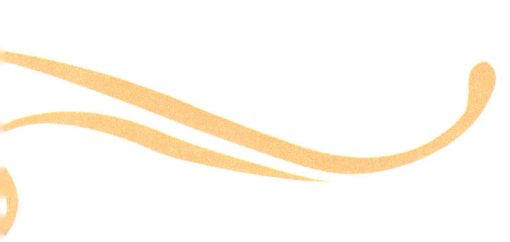

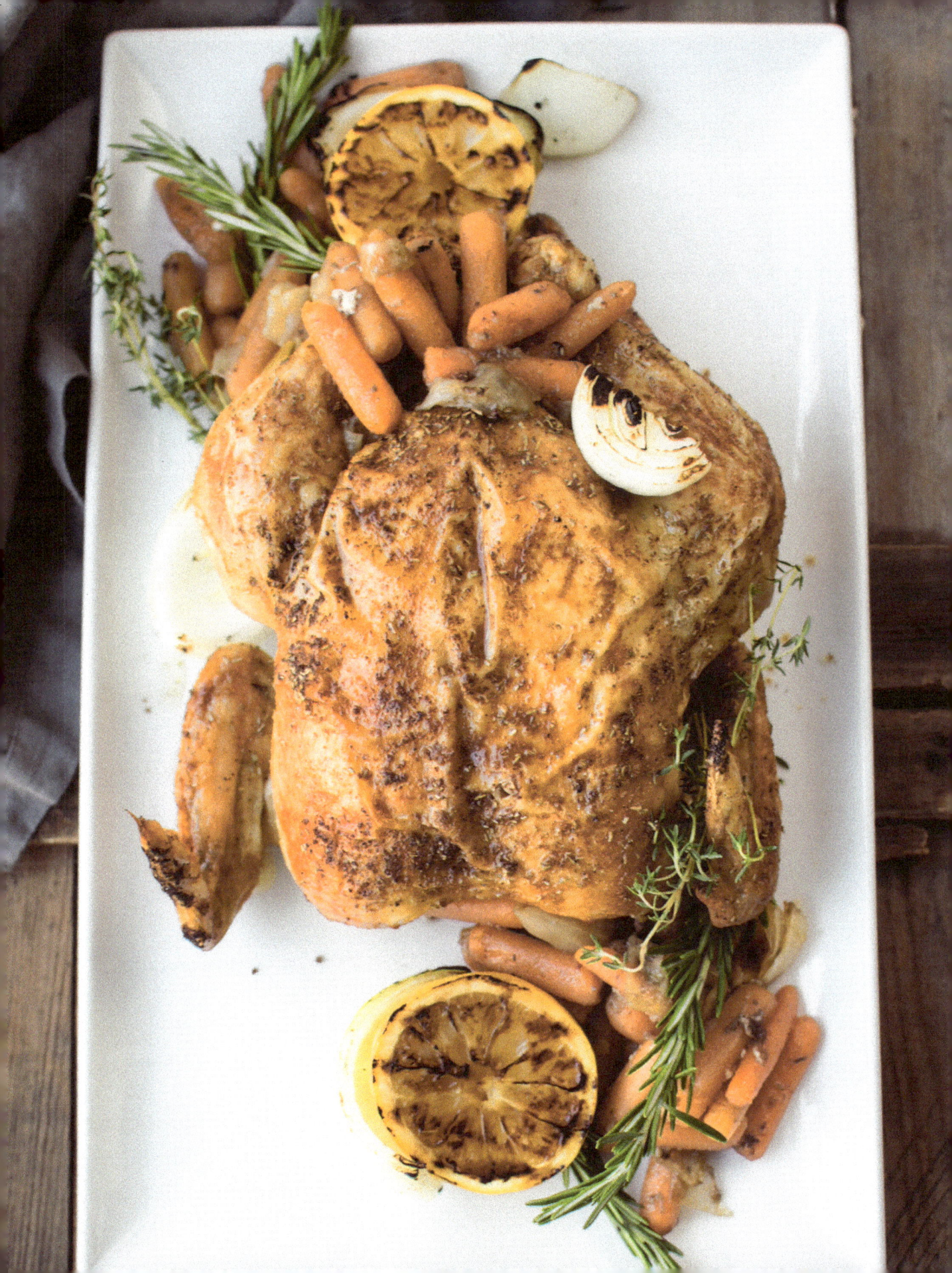

LEMON, GARLIC, AND HERB ROAST CHICKEN

Everyone should know how to make a roast chicken. If you don't, you will now! It is a staple meal, so I had to make sure you knew how to make a standard tasty bird. It is so easy but looks so impressive when you remove it from the oven. When I remove a bird from the oven I always get the same reaction from whoever is in the room, a big, "Wow, that looks good!" I almost wait for the reaction now.

The trick to creating a flavorful chicken is to be sure to season the inside and the outside of your bird. Adding a fresh herb bundle and some vegetables to the cavity will really provide a beautiful bouquet to your meat.

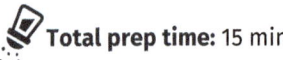 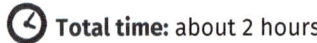 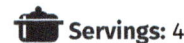

Total prep time: 15 minutes   **Total time:** about 2 hours   **Servings:** 4

Ingredients

- 1 (5 lb.) whole chicken
- 5 medium-sized yellow onions (chopped)
- 6 cups carrots (chopped)
- olive oil
- salt and pepper
- ½ lemon
- 4 garlic cloves
- fresh herb bundle (thyme & rosemary)
- about a ½ cup avocado oil or other high smoke point oil.
- 1 tsp. dried oregano
- 1 tsp. dried thyme
- 1 tsp. garlic powder
- 1 tsp. onion powder
- 2 tbsp. dried or fresh rosemary

> **MOISTER TIP:**
>
> Every half hour you can take baster and extract juice from the bottom of the pan and squeeze into the center cavity of the chicken. This will help keep it moistened. You can also squeeze some over the tops of the chicken as well.

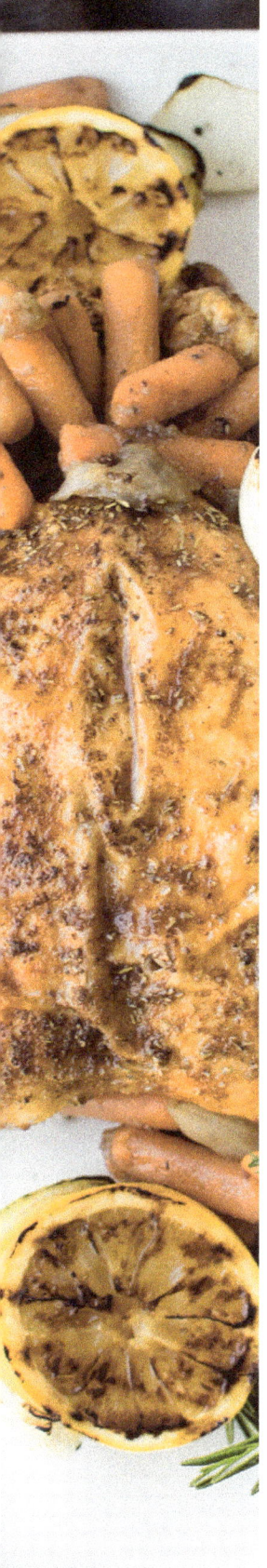

Directions

- Pre-heat the oven to 450°F.
- Place a rack in the lower-middle of the oven.
- Clean your chicken. First, start by removing the giblets. Reach inside the cavity of the chicken, and remove the bag of giblets. Then rinse the inside cavity of chicken with water. I literally fill it up with water and then dump it out to rinse out the blood.
- Pat the chicken dry with paper towels. Make sure to absorb any liquid behind the wings or legs. Blot inside the body cavity too, getting the chicken as dry as you can, inside and out.
- Cut your onions and carrots, and toss with a little bit of oil and salt and pepper.
- In a small bowl combine oregano, thyme, garlic powder, onion powder, and rosemary. Pour ⅓ cup of oil into mixture, and stir to combine herb mixture. Brush the herb mixture all over the outside and inside of the chicken.
- Place lemon, garlic, and a fresh bundle of herbs inside the cavity. Then fill the rest of the cavity with some chopped carrots and onions. Tie legs together with some baking string.
- Put about 4 cups water in the bottom of the roasting pan. Add the remaining chopped carrots and onions to the bottom of the pan. (You want to have a few inches of water in the pan, you can use chicken broth too.)
- Place the chicken breast-side up in the pan. Bake at 450°F for 15 minutes. Lower the temperature to 350°F. Cook 20 minutes per pound of chicken. For this recipe, for example, we will check the chicken after 1 hour and 40 minutes.
- Once finished, check the chicken. The chicken is done when it registers 165°F in the thickest part of the thigh, when the wings and legs wiggle loosely, and when the juices run clear.
- If it does not appear done, continue roasting the chicken and checking it every 10 minutes until it is done. Once finished cooking, transfer the chicken to a cutting board and let it rest for about 10-15 minutes. You can take the juices from the pan to create a nice gravy or just use the natural juice straight from the pan.
- Carve the chicken into the breasts, thighs, and drumsticks, and serve with cooked onions and carrots from the roast pan and top with natural juice.

BROILED SALMON FILLET

This is as simple as it gets. Salmon is such a flavorful fish that not much is really needed other than salt and pepper. My biggest secret to a tasty salmon is to broil it. Broiling it will give it a nice crust on top and also removes some of the fishy taste from the fish. It will give you a more well-done piece of fish, but that is how I prefer it. If you like it rarer, you can bake the fish on 350°F for 20 minutes or so and then just broil it the last 2 minutes for a little crusting.

If you wish to have a little seasoning, one of my favorites is to mix a little low-sodium soy sauce with ground ginger, and you can just brush it over the top. That will also be a delicious way to have your salmon. I find re-heating salmon the next day makes it fishy, so instead you can throw it onto a salad cold, which is a nice way to be creative with your leftovers.

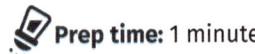 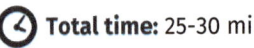 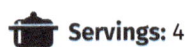

Prep time: 1 minute   **Total time:** 25-30 minutes   **Servings:** 4

Ingredients

- 2 lb. salmon fillet
- coarse sea salt
- freshly ground pepper

Directions

- Set the oven to broil.
- Season salmon with salt and pepper, about ½ teaspoon of each.
- Place salmon on a broiler pan. Place in oven on the top shelf about 6 inches from broiler.
- Broil for about 25-30 minutes. The top will have a nice crust on it and will have a flaky texture.

TASTY TIP:

Try combining ¼ cup of soy sauce or liquid coconut aminos with a teaspoon of fresh pureed ginger and rubbing over the top of salmon before you broil it. It is a very delicious variation.

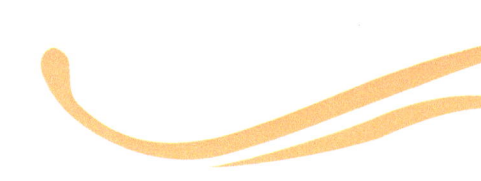

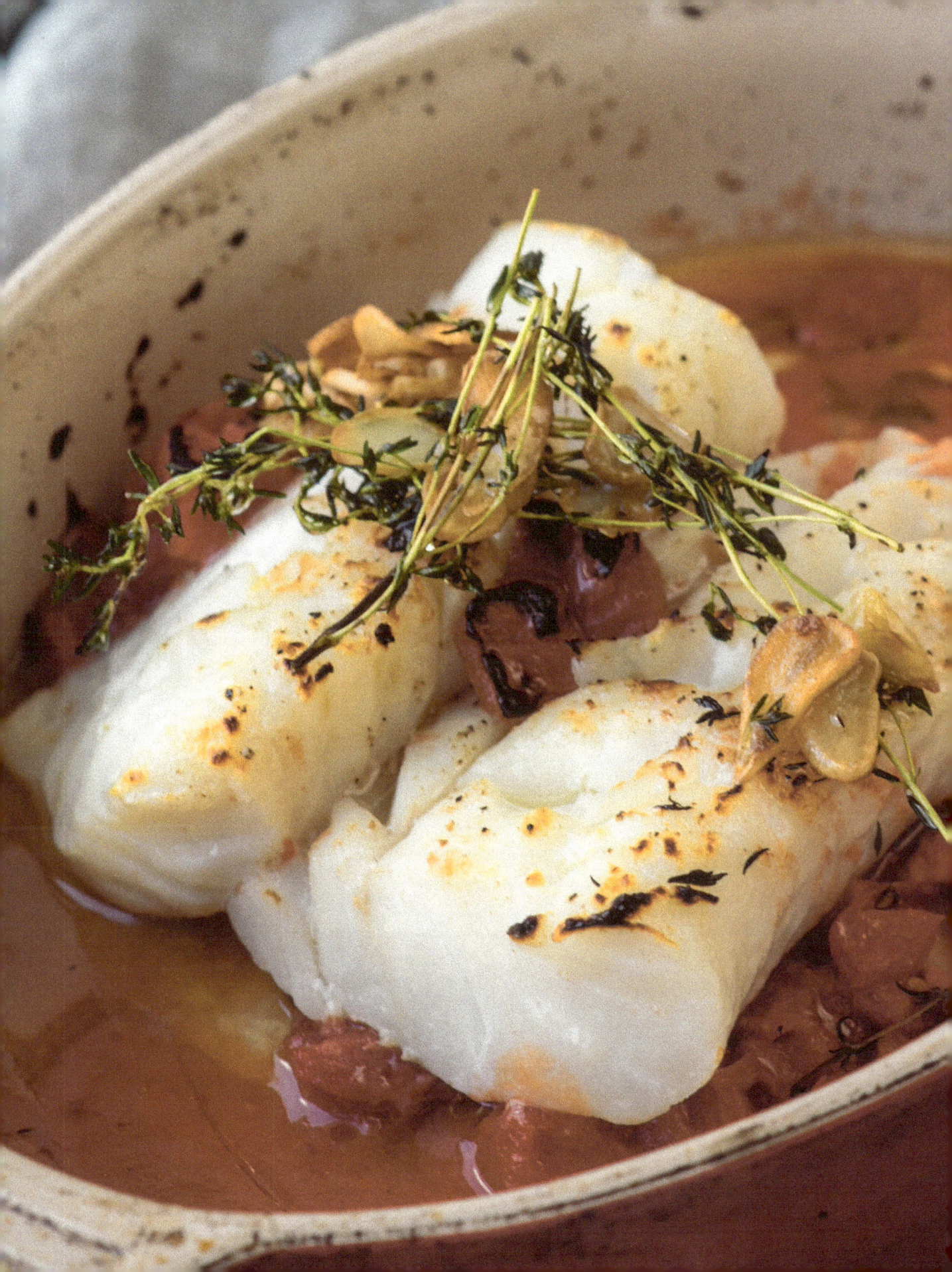

Danielle Formaro

A SIMPLE-YET-DELICIOUS BAKED COD

This is my quick go-to healthy recipe. When my fellow mom friends ask me for a quick, healthy recipe, this is the one I always email them, and they all love it. I always keep a nice 1-pound cod fillet in my freezer for when I need a quick, no-fuss, easy clean-up dinner. With a few steps, this is a basic yet tasty way to prepare your cod. Although you can buy smaller cod fillets, I prefer one large piece as it is less likely to get dry, and it is easier to prepare one large piece than a few smaller pieces.

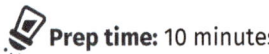 **Prep time:** 10 minutes   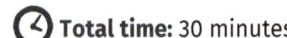 **Total time:** 30 minutes   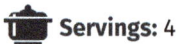 **Servings:** 4

Ingredients

- 1 lb. cod fillet
- olive oil
- ¼ tsp. salt
- ¼ tsp. pepper
- ¼ tsp. garlic powder
- ¼ tsp. onion powder
- ¼ tsp. oregano
- 1 (14.5 oz.) can chopped tomatoes or 3 freshly chopped Roma tomatoes
- 2 lemons (cut into quarters)

Directions

- Preheat oven to 350°F on bake.
- Arrange cod fillet in a single layer on a medium baking pan. Combine all dry ingredients in a bowl—salt, pepper, garlic powder, onion powder, and oregano.
- Drizzle olive oil, and then sprinkle dry herb mixture over the fish. Spoon chopped tomato right over the top of the fillet.
- Place cod into the oven and cook for about 20 minutes. (When you see the fish start to flake apart a little, you can tell it is done).
- Squeeze some lemon on top and enjoy.

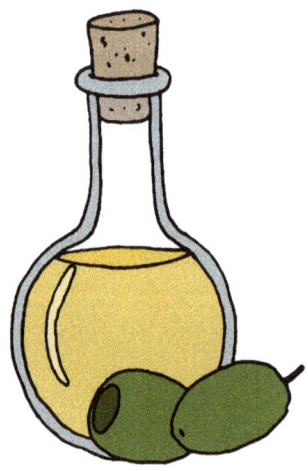

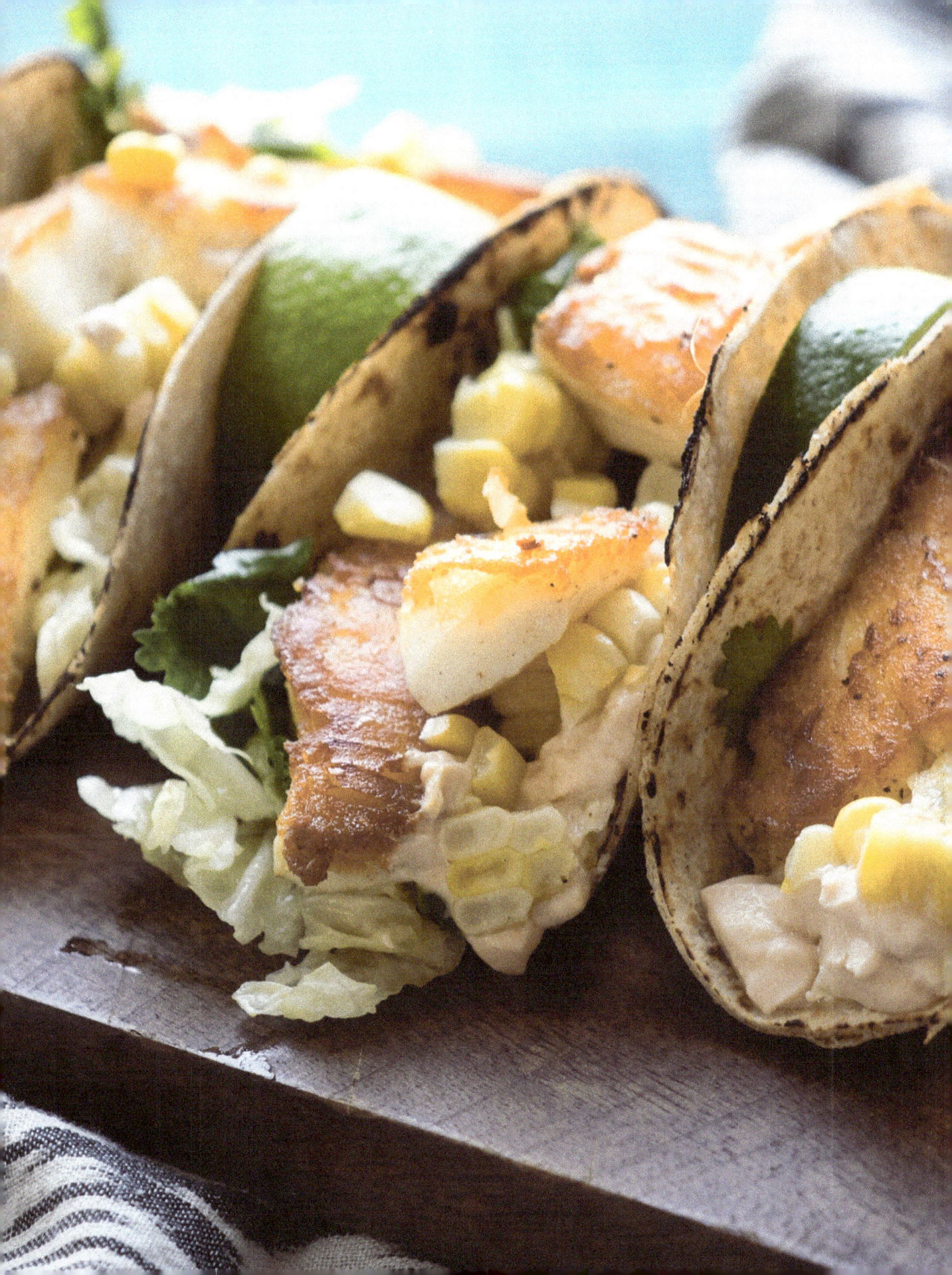

FISH TACOS WITH CHIPOLTE-AVOCADO AIOLI

You don't have to go to Baja, California to get great fish tacos; you can make them in your own kitchen, I promise! I know a lot of people fry the fish, but because we are keeping our recipes on the light side, we are going to avoid the fryolator and use a grill pan instead. You will find the sweet corn and hot chipotle aioli really complementing each other in this dish. Bursting flavors in every direction will have your mouth watering with each bite.

Prep time: 12-15 minutes   **Total time:** 20-25 minutes   **Servings:** 3-4 (about 1-2 tortillas each)

Ingredients

The Chipotle-Avocado Aioli
- 1 pepper in adobe sauce (minced)
- 6 oz. Greek yogurt (0% fat)
- 3 oz. sour cream
- ½ avocado (pureed or mashed well)

The Fish
- 3 tbsp. of light cooking oil such as avocado oil
- 2 lbs. white fish such as mahi mahi, tilapia, or cod
- salt and pepper
- juice of 1 lime
- 6-inch round, whole-wheat tortillas

The Toppings (set aside for serving)
- 2 cups napa cabbage (shredded or chopped)
- 2 cups cooked sweet corn (shucked)
- 2 cups cilantro (cleaned and chopped)

Directions

- In a small bowl, mix together pepper in adobe, yogurt, sour cream, and avocado. Set aside.
- On a medium-high flame, heat oil.
- Add fish to the pan and season with salt and pepper.
- Cook fish on medium-high for about 4 minutes on each side or until solid white.
- When fish is finished, squeeze lime juice over fish and remove from heat.
- Prepare tacos. Spread a 1 tsp. or more to your liking of aioli on a wheat tortilla, then add your fish and top with cabbage, corn, and cilantro.
- Enjoy!

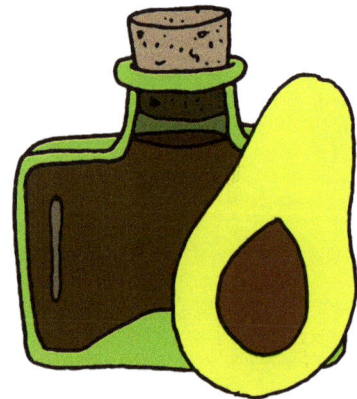

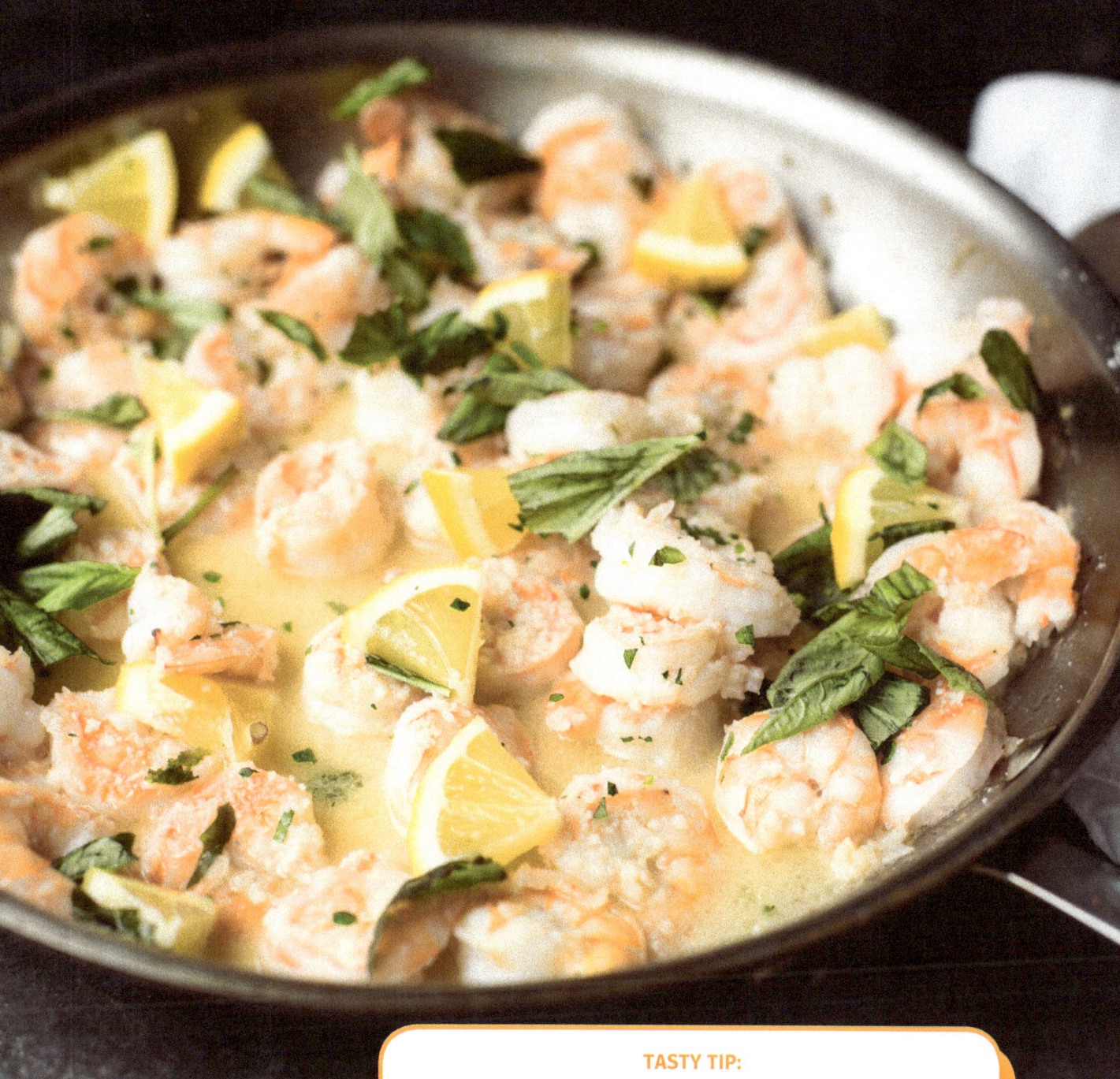

TASTY TIP:

Pairs well over a serving of angel hair pasta. See packaging for correct serving size. You can get white or brown rice pasta for a healthier option. Just be mindful not to go overboard with the pasta portions as it does absorb oil quickly and you do not want a dry dish. I would recommend four portions of cooked pasta can be tossed with this entire dish in the pan without drying it out.

SHRIMP SCAMPI

This is a classic Italian-American dish, meaning the Italians who came to America created a newer version of this classic. Scampi are in fact tiny, lobster-like crustaceans with pale pink shells (also called langoustines). One traditional way of preparing them is to sauté them with olive oil, garlic, onion, and white wine. Italian cooks in the United States swapped shrimp for scampi, but kept both names, which is how we got the name "shrimp scampi!" There are many variations such as adding bread crumbs or tomato, for example. I personally love to cook it the traditional way, but I add fresh chopped basil and lemon to mine. It just gives it that little extra something.

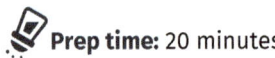 **Prep time:** 20 minutes   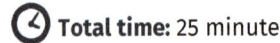 **Total time:** 25 minutes   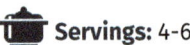 **Servings:** 4-6

Ingredients

- ¼ cup avocado oil or oil with high smoke point
- 5 cloves garlic (minced)
- 2 cup dry white wine
- 4 tbsp. butter
- pinch of red pepper
- 2 lbs. large raw shrimp (peeled, tails removed and cleaned)
- salt and pepper to taste
- 1 whole lemon (juiced)
- 2 cups fresh basil, plus a little extra for garnishing (lightly packed)
- ⅓ cup Pecorino Romano cheese

Directions

- In a large sauté pan, heat oil. Add garlic and sauté one minute.
- Raise flame to medium-high, add wine, and let simmer for 2 minutes.
- Lower flame to medium, add butter and a pinch of red pepper, and mix until melted.
- Add shrimp and season with a little salt and pepper. Then sauté each side until it turns pink, about 1 minute each side.
- Drizzle lemon juice over all the shrimp, and add the 2 cups of chopped basil.
- Sprinkle half of your Pecorino Romano cheese over the top.
- With a set of tongs or utensils, give the entire mixture a toss to combine all ingredients.
- Just before serving, top each with some Romano cheese and chopped fresh basil.

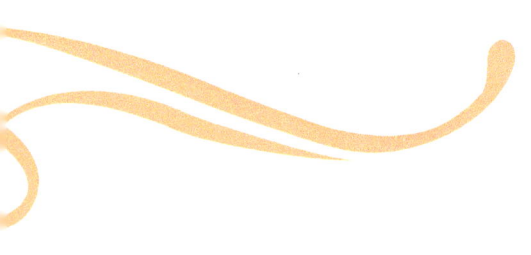

SHRIMP FRIED RICE BOWL

Chinese-American food gets a bad rap due mostly to the high MSG (monosodium glutamate) and sodium content, as well as the high calories caused by frying many of their dishes—yes, even the vegetables. Ever wonder why a Chinese restaurant's green beans have a crunch? Now you know!

What I love about this dish is that I can enjoy the flavors of one of my go-to Chinese food items without the guilt. This is also a well-balanced meal to serve your family. It is the perfect blend. It is high in protein, complex carbohydrates, fiber, and loaded with vitamins and nutrients. Not bad for a Chinese-food-inspired dish!

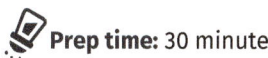 **Prep time:** 30 minutes 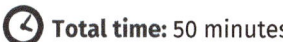 **Total time:** 50 minutes 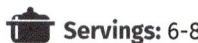 **Servings:** 6-8

Ingredients

- 6 tbsp. avocado oil or a high smoke point cooking oil
- 2 lbs. shrimp (cleaned with tails removed)
- salt and pepper
- 3 eggs (lightly beaten)
- 1 tbsp. fresh ginger (minced)
- 7 scallions (chopped)
- 2 cups peas
- 1 orange bell pepper (sliced)
- 1 cup white button mushrooms (diced)
- 3 tbsp. Asian fish sauce
- 2 tsp. rice vinegar
- ⅛ tsp. crushed red pepper
- 4 cups brown rice (cooked)
- 4 tbsp. fresh chopped cilantro

Directions

- Heat a wok or a deep, nonstick pan on medium-high heat, and add 2 tablespoons of oil. Let oil heat up for a minute.
- Add shrimp, season with salt and pepper, and cook a few minutes on each side (they will turn pink when cooked). Remove from heat and set aside. You may have to do it in batches, depending on the size of your shrimp.
- Reduce flame to medium, and add another 2 tablespoons of oil to the pan. Add eggs and cook a minute or so, gently folding eggs into each other to form large, soft curds. Continue cooking eggs until they are set (3 minutes or so), and then set aside with the shrimp.
- Increase the flame to medium-high, and heat another 2 teaspoons of oil in the pan. Add ginger and scallions. Cook until fragrant, about 30 seconds. Add peas, orange bell pepper, and mushrooms to the pan, and stir-fry until soft, about 8 to 10 minutes. Season with salt and pepper.
- In a small bowl, combine fish sauce, vinegar, and crushed red pepper.
- Return shrimp and eggs to wok and add rice and cilantro, then stir in the fish sauce. Stir fry one more minute to combine flavors. Serve hot.

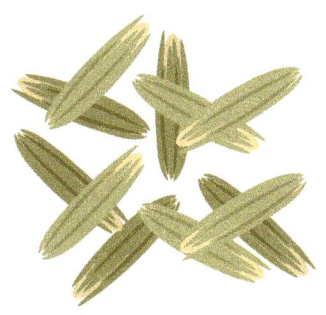

SCALLOPS FRA DIAVOLO

Fra diavolo, or "brother devil" sauce, is an Italian-American creation that some believe started in New York City or Long Island. It is a spicy sauce for pasta or seafood. Most versions are tomato-based and use chili peppers for spice, but the term is also used for sauces that include no tomato, or that use cayenne or other forms of pepper. This is a simple recipe that will certainly kick things up a notch. You can play with your amounts of pepper to figure out how much spice you can handle. You can also chop fresh red peppers into your sauce as well but I prefer to use cayenne pepper powder because I can control the heat a little easier with this recipe. You can eat this dish as an appetizer, or you can boil up some pasta and combine it with your scallops fra diavolo for dinner. It is up to you!

 Prep time: 10 minutes   **Total time:** 25-30 minutes   **Servings:** 4-6

Ingredients

- 3 tbsp. olive oil
- 2-3 garlic cloves (sliced)
- 1 (28 oz.) can crushed tomato
- 1 tsp. Italian seasoning
- ⅓ cup red wine (such as a pinot noir)
- salt and pepper
- as much crushed red pepper as you can handle
- about a 1 lb. of scallops

Directions

- In a skillet on a medium flame, sauté your garlic and oil until garlic is golden.
- Add crushed tomato, Italian seasoning, red wine, salt and pepper, and red pepper and bring to a boil.
- Simmer low for 20 min.
- Increase flame to medium and add scallops to the sauce. Let cook a few minutes on each side. (They should be medium rare in the center.)
- You can add more seasoning depending on how you like it, and test one scallop first to see if you like the temperature.

TASTY TIP:

Pairs well with a pound of linguine pasta (you can also get a whole-wheat, brown rice, or quinoa pasta to lighten it up).

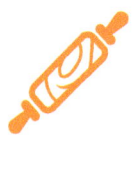

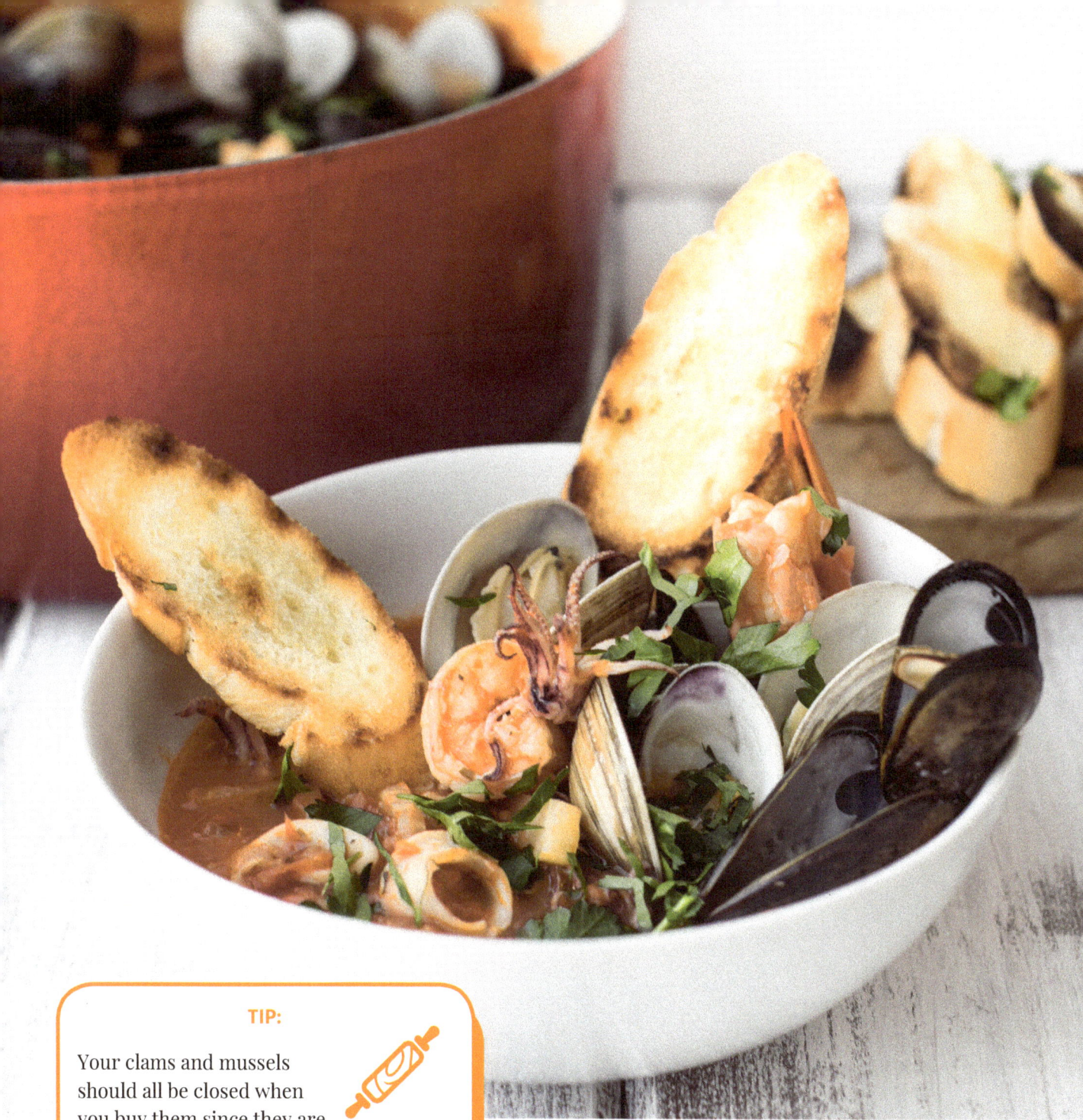

TIP:

Your clams and mussels should all be closed when you buy them since they are still alive. Sometimes clams can take a bit to open. I have steamed the clams and mussels separate to ensure that all open and then added them to the stew with the juice. Always throw away any shell fish that did not open. This means they are not good to eat!

FRUTTI DI MARE *(seafood in tomato sauce)*

Frutti di mare is a popular multi-seafood dish from along the coast of Italy. Frutti di mare literally means "fruit of the sea" and can include all types of seafood, including mussels, clams, prawns, and other shellfish. You can make it a red sauce or a white sauce; it is all preference. I personally like it in spiced tomato sauce; to add a little heat you just need a sprinkle of red pepper. Be sure to have a nice piece of bread to dip in the deliciousness.

Prep time: 20 minutes   **Total time:** 1 hour and 20 minutes   **Servings:** 6

Ingredients

- ¼ cup olive oil
- 4 garlic cloves (sliced)
- 1 small onion (diced)
- 1 fennel bulb (diced)
- 1 cup dry white wine
- 2 (28 oz.) can tomato sauce
- 1 tsp. Italian seasoning
- ½ tsp. salt
- ½ tsp. crushed black pepper
- pinch crushed red pepper (or to desired taste; for fra diavolo, or more spicy, you can increase the amount)
- 2 cups seafood stock
- 1 lb. raw clams (scrubbed and cleaned)
- 1 lb. raw mussels (scrubbed and cleaned)
- 1 lb. raw calamari with tentacles (cleaned and sliced into one-inch-thick rings)
- 1 lb. shrimp (cleaned and tail shell removed)
- 4 tbsp. fresh Italian parsley (chopped)
- 6 slices of toasted baguette bread

Directions

- In large deep sided pan, heat oil over a medium-high flame.
- Add onion and fennel bulb. Cook until soft (5 minutes).
- Add garlic, and cook one more minute.
- Pour in wine, raise flame to high, and boil off alcohol for about 2 minutes.
- Add tomato sauce, Italian seasoning, salt, crushed black pepper, and crushed red pepper and bring to a light boil. Reduce flame to low-medium and let cook for 12 minutes, stirring occasionally.
- Add seafood stock and cook on low for another 25-30 minutes, stirring occasionally.
- Bring soup to a gentle boil, and add clams and mussels. Cook covered for 5-10 minutes, or until clams and mussels start to open.
- Add shrimp & calamari, and cook covered for about 5-6 minutes or until all shells are opened, and shrimp is opaque. Discard any unopened mussels or clams. Remove from heat.
- Garnish with Italian parsley and serve with a piece of baguette bread.

QUICK & EASY BEEF BOURGUIGNON

As a former part-owner of a French restaurant, this classic is still a favorite of mine. Beef Bourguignon (or Bœuf Bourguignon, Beef Burgundy, or Bœuf à la Bourguignonne) is a well-known, traditional French recipe.

The dish originates from the Burgundy region (in French, Bourgogne) which is in the east of present-day France. It is a stew prepared with beef braised in red wine, traditionally red Burgundy, and beef broth, generally flavored with garlic, onions, and a bouquet garni, with pearl onions and mushrooms added towards the end of cooking.

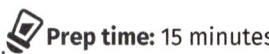 **Prep time:** 15 minutes   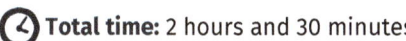 **Total time:** 2 hours and 30 minutes   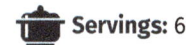 **Servings:** 6

Ingredients

- 10 pearl onions (peeled) or you can buy them frozen
- 6 tbsp. avocado oil or a high smoke point cooking oil
- 10 oz. turkey bacon (chopped)
- 1 celery stalk (chopped)
- 3 large carrots (chopped)
- 2 cups white button mushrooms (chopped)
- 2 garlic cloves (minced)
- 3 lbs. stew meat (in 2 inch cubes)
- 1 tsp. salt
- 1 tsp. pepper
- 1½ tbsp. fresh thyme
- 1 tbsp. chopped fresh or dried rosemary
- 3 tbsp. chopped fresh or dried parsley
- ½ tsp. allspice
- 2 tbsp. all purpose flour or wheat flour
- 1 tbsp. tomato paste
- 3 cups organic beef broth
- 3 cups Burgundy wine

Directions

- In small pot, bring water to a boil and add pearl onions. Boil for 2 minutes to loosen the skin. When finished, remove from heat, drain, and then remove skin from onions. Set aside.
- In a large Dutch oven on medium-high, add 2 tablespoons of oil and add turkey bacon. Cook until crispy. Remove from pan and place on a paper towel to absorb any excess oil.
- Add 2 tablespoons of oil to the pan and add vegetables (celery, carrots, mushroom, and pearl onions). Cook on a medium-high flame until softened (about 6-10 minutes). Add garlic, and cook 1 minute. Spoon out vegetable mixture and place in bowl off to the side.
- Add 2 more tablespoons of oil to the pan, and then add your meat. Season with salt and pepper. Sauté meat on all sides until browned.
- Once meat is browned, sprinkle thyme, rosemary, parsley, allspice, and flour over meat mixture and give a good few stirs.
- Add tomato paste to meat and cook for 1 more minute.
- Add vegetable mixture, turkey bacon, beef broth, and wine to the meat and give a few nice stirs to combine all ingredients.
- Bring to a boil, then cover and simmer on low for 2 hours. It is done when vegetables and meat are tender and the sauce has thickened.

CHICKEN MARSALA

Chicken Marsala is an Italian-American dish made from chicken cutlets, mushrooms, and marsala wine. The dish dates back to the 19th century when it most likely originated with English families who lived in western Sicily, where Marsala wine is produced. I have seen a lot of recipes call for pancetta, which is a fattier type of Italian cured meat, but I found turkey bacon to be a great substitute and just as good!

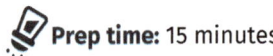 **Prep time:** 15 minutes   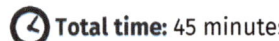 **Total time:** 45 minutes   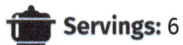 **Servings:** 6

Ingredients

- 1 cup whole-wheat flour for dredging plus 3 tbsp. for thickening agent later
- salt and pepper
- 1½ lbs. chicken tenderloin
- avocado oil or other high smoke point cooking oil
- 3 slices turkey bacon (chopped)
- ½ cup onion (diced)
- 2 cups mushrooms (cleaned, stems removed and sliced)
- 3 tbsp. wheat flour
- 1 cup sweet marsala
- ½ cup chicken stock
- 2 tbsp. unsalted butter (optional)

Directions

- Put 1 cup wheat flour in a shallow dish and season with salt and pepper. Use a fork to evenly blend together.
- In a skillet, heat about 1/4 cup of avocado oil on a medium-high flame. Take each tenderloin and dredge each side lightly with wheat flour. Place each tenderloin in the pan and cook about 5 minutes each side (should be golden brown). Once done, remove chicken tenderloins from pan, set aside in a dish, and cover to keep warm.
- Add 2 more tablespoons of oil to the pan, and add turkey bacon. Cook 2 minutes or so until crispy. Add onions and cook another 5 minutes, or until soft.
- Add mushrooms, and cook until water releases from them and they soften, about 4 to 5 minutes.
- Add 3 tablespoons of wheat flour to the pan, and mix into the mushroom mixture until well blended.
- Add sweet marsala wine, raise flame, and bring mixture to a boil. Then lower flame to medium and cook for 2 minutes. Add chicken broth, and cook until mixture thickens. If you need to adjust the thickness, you may add more wheat flour.
- Once marsala mixture thickens (4 to 5 minutes or so), add chicken back into the pan, add butter, and cook another 2 to 3 minutes. The butter creates a glassy finish.

> **TIP:**
> If you wish to serve with a pasta, whole-wheat spaghetti is nice.
>
>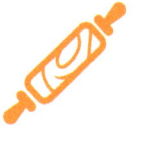

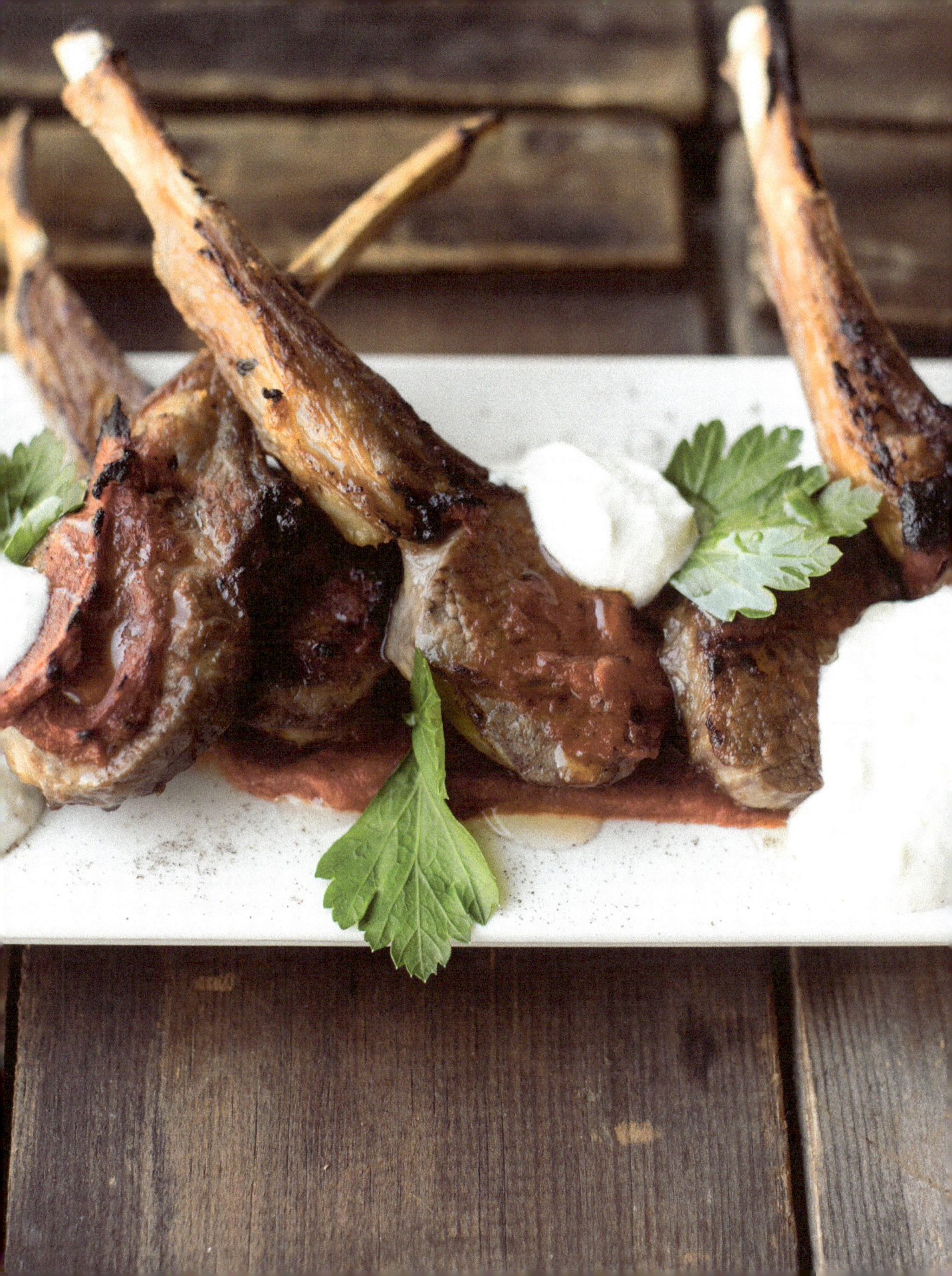

MIDDLE EASTERN LAMB LOLLIPOPS

Every culture has their specialty, and in my opinion, the Middle East has nailed it when it comes to combining spices with their meats. Some common spices used are cinnamon, cloves, cumin, and coriander. You will see what the hype is all about after you chew on this. This dish goes well with the cucumber & mint soup and wheat pilaf recipe in this book.

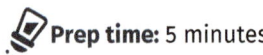 **Prep time:** 5 minutes 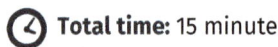 **Total time:** 15 minutes 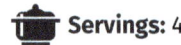 **Servings:** 4

Ingredients

- 8-9 lamb lollipops salt and pepper
- 6 tbsp. tomato paste
- 1 tsp. nutmeg
- ½ tsp. cinnamon
- ½ tsp. allspice
- ¼ tsp. ground cloves

Directions

- Pre-heat grill on medium-high or pre heat oven on broil.
- Sprinkle each side of chops with salt and pepper.
- In a small bowl, combine tomato paste, nutmeg, cinnamon, allspice, and cloves.
- Take about a ½ teaspoon of the tomato mixture and rub on one side of the chop, flip over, and do the same on the other side.
- Place on grill or in on a broiler pan in the oven on broil and cook about 4½ minutes on each side. If broiling in the oven place on top shelf, 6 inches from the top.

TIP:

This dish pairs well with the Yogurt, Cucumber, and Mint Soup recipe on page 77. I like to drizzle it right over the top.

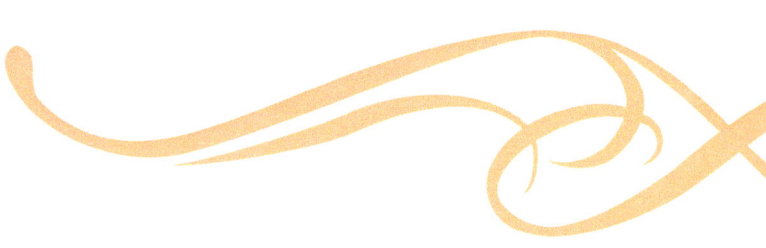

ROAST HERB BEEF TENDERLOIN

This is by far my favorite selection of meat and one that is great to serve for a crowd. It can be a little pricey, but it will melt in your mouth and is always a crowd pleaser. The tenderloin is an oblong shape spanning two primal cuts: the short loin (called the sirloin in Commonwealth countries) and the sirloin (called the rump in Commonwealth countries). The tenderloin sits beneath the ribs, next to the backbone. It has two ends: the butt and the "tail." The smaller, pointed end—the "tail"—starts a little past the ribs, growing in thickness until it ends in the "sirloin" primal cut, which is closer to the butt of the cow. This muscle does very little work, so it is the most tender part of the beef. The tenderloin can be cut for either roasts or steaks. So when you order a fillet at a restaurant, it is actually cut from the tenderloin. Pair this with a vegetable and starch and you have an elegant dinner.

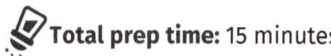 **Total prep time:** 15 minutes   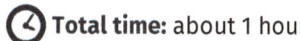 **Total time:** about 1 hour   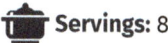 **Servings:** 8

Ingredients

- 1 (3 lb.) center-cut beef tenderloin, trimmed of silver skin and fat
- 3 medium garlic cloves, sliced
- 1 tbsp. freshly ground pepper
- 2 tsp. salt
- 1 tsp. garlic powder
- 1 tsp. paprika
- 1 tbsp. finely chopped fresh or dried rosemary leaves
- 1 tbsp. finely chopped fresh thyme leaves (or 1 tsp. dried)
- avocado oil or oil with a high smoke point
- butcher's twine, as needed
- Special equipment: a roasting pan with a rack; an instant-read thermometer

TASTY TIP:

Tenderloin is best served rare or medium rare, so use a thermometer to make sure it doesn't get cooked past 140°F in the center. If you have guests who like their meat well done, consider cutting a whole tenderloin into pieces and cooking them to different temperatures to please everybody.

SIDES:

Pair with at least one vegetable and one starch (I love mashed potatoes and Brussels sprouts).

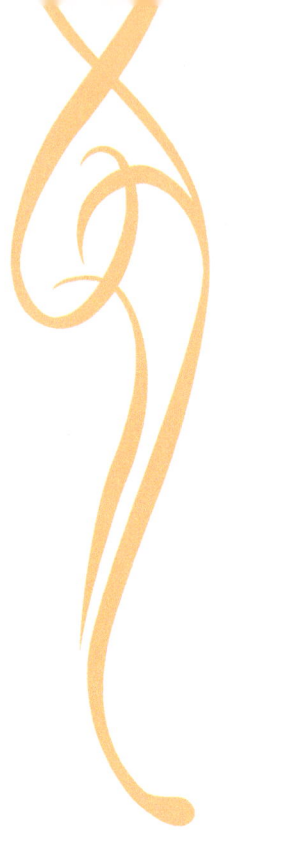

Directions

- Set oven to 475°F.
- Pat tenderloin dry.
- With a paring knife, cut about 1-inch slivers about 2 inches apart along the entire top of the tenderloin. Stuff a slice of garlic in each hole you made across the top of your tenderloin. This will add extra garlic flavor within the meat itself, rather than just the surface.
- Stir together pepper, salt, garlic powder, paprika, rosemary, thyme, and oil in a small bowl.
- Brush herb mixture all over the meat.
- A whole beef tenderloin has a thinner, tapered end. Tuck this end under itself and then tie the whole thing up (if needed) so that it is the same thickness all the way around. This will help it cook evenly.
- Put tenderloin onto the roasting pan and then place in oven and roast 10 minutes.
- Then reduce oven temperature to 425°F and cook until thermometer inserted diagonally into center of meat registers 130°F.
- Check your meat after 20 minutes to see what your temperature is, as you want to see how close you are to your desired temperature. Depending on your oven, I find mine takes about 40-45 minutes or so, but I always do a temperature test after 20 minutes just in case.
- Let beef set for about 15 minutes before serving. Just cover lightly with some aluminum foil to keep warm in the meantime. This gives the meat a chance to redistribute and reabsorb all the juices. If you cut it too soon, you will let all the juices escape the meat and it can become dry with less flavor.

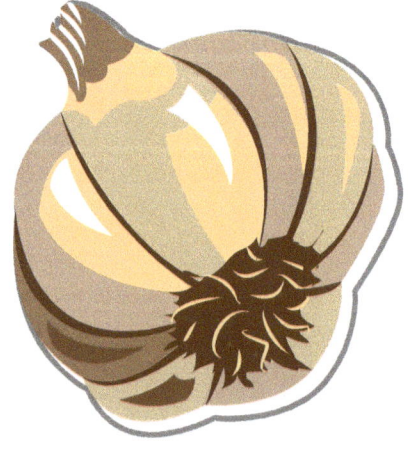

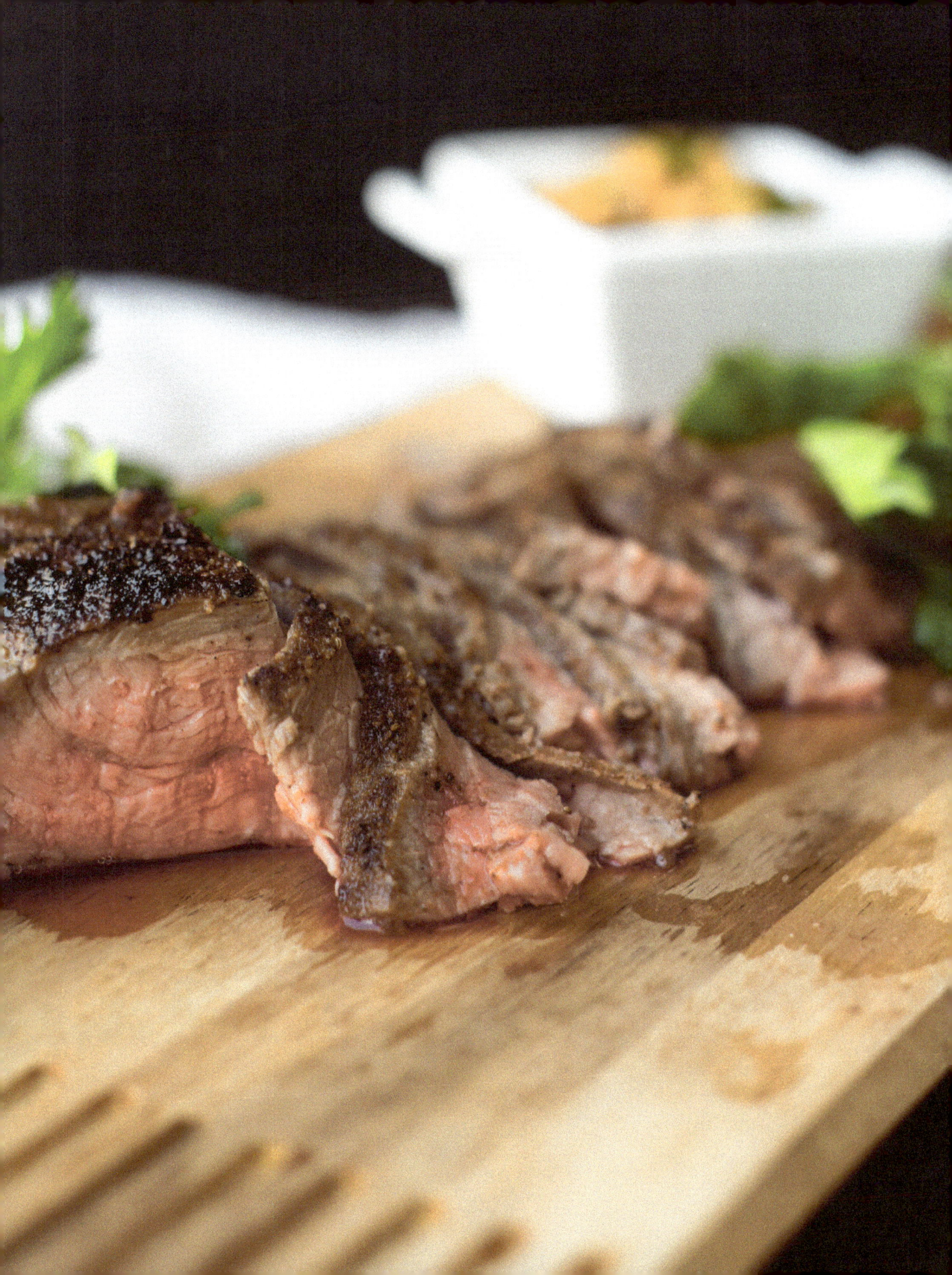

HERB-SEASONED FLANK STEAK

A relatively long and flat cut, flank steak is used in a variety of dishes including London broil and as an alternative to the traditional skirt steak in fajitas. It is very flavorful and can be can be grilled, pan-fried, broiled, or braised for increased tenderness. When searching for a nice piece of flank steak, look for one with a bright red color. Because it comes from a strong, well-exercised part of the cow, it is best sliced against the grain before serving to maximize tenderness. I personally like to broil mine; I feel it comes out just right. Pair with a vegetable and starch side for your family.

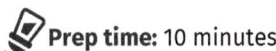 **Prep time:** 10 minutes   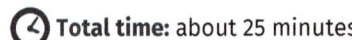 **Total time:** about 25 minutes   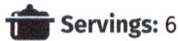 **Servings:** 6

Ingredients

- 2 lb. flank steak
- 4 tbsp. avocado oil or high smoke point cooking oil
- ½ tsp. coarse sea salt
- ½ tsp. fresh ground black pepper
- ½ tsp. thyme
- ½ tsp. nutmeg
- ½ tsp. Worcestershire sauce
- 1 tsp. garlic powder
- 1 tsp. onion powder
- 1 tsp. fresh or dried oregano
- 1 tsp. fresh or dried rosemary

Directions

- Set oven to broil.
- Place a rack in middle of oven.
- In a small bowl, combine and mix together the oil and all your herbs (salt, pepper, thyme, nutmeg, Worcestershire sauce, garlic powder, onion powder, dried oregano, and rosemary) to create your steak seasoning.
- Take a brush and coat the top of the steak with your entire bowl of seasoning.
- Place steak on a broiling pan and place top rack at least 6 inches from broiler.
- Broil for about 12 minutes for a medium-rare (bright pink center) or to desired temperature.

NOTE:

A temperature of 140°F is considered rare. Medium-rare is 145°F, medium is 160°F, and well done is 170°F. Medium-rare is recommended for beef flank steak.

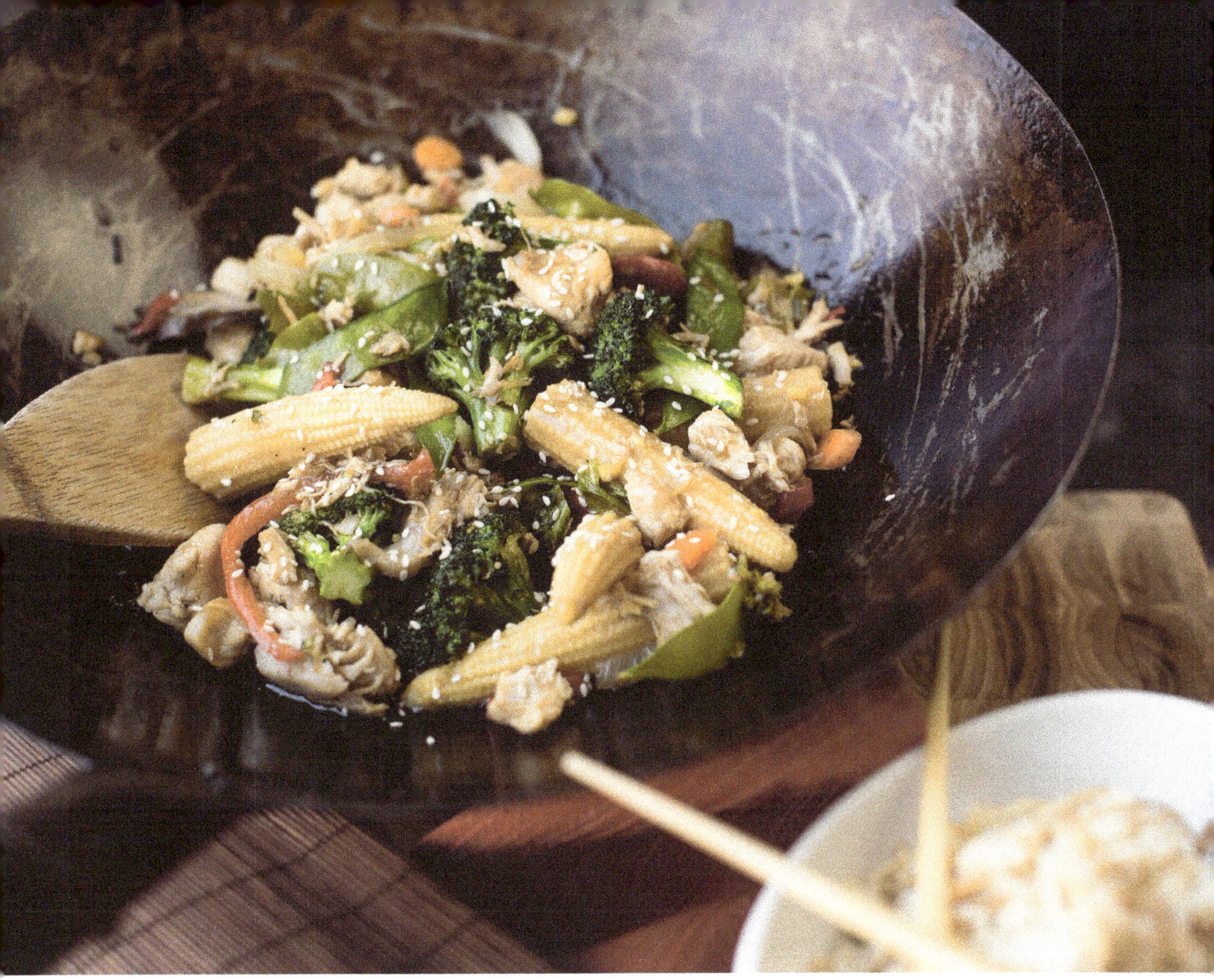

CHICKEN STIR FRY OVER BROWN RICE

One of the very first dinners I learned to cook was chicken stir-fry, but it was not from scratch. It was from the frozen food aisle and had a pre-packaged, high-sodium flavored sauce that went with it. All I had to do was cook the chicken. It may have been ok to practice on the stove, but as I got older, I wanted to learn how to create my own so that it would taste fresh and of course be healthier. Once I created this dish I was almost ashamed I had insulted my stove with the frozen version. But hey, give me a break, I was only 12! If you are not big into chicken, this recipe goes well with shrimp and beef too!

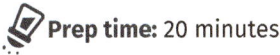 **Prep time:** 20 minutes   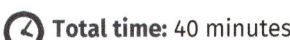 **Total time:** 40 minutes   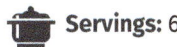 **Servings:** 6

Ingredients

The Sauce
- 1 cup organic or low-sodium beef broth
- ⅓ cup low-sodium soy sauce or coconut aminos
- 1 tbsp. dark brown sugar
- 2 tbsp. cornstarch
- ¼ tsp. Chinese ginger powder
- ⅛ tsp. crushed red pepper

The Rice
- 1 cup quick-cooking brown rice (uncooked)
- 2 cups water
- 1 tsp. avocado oil
- dash of salt and pepper
- (regular brown rice is okay as well, just follow instructions on bag)

The Chicken Mixture
- 2 tbsp. avocado or grapeseed oil
- 2 lbs. chicken breast tenderloins (cut in 1-inch pieces)
- ¼ tsp. fresh black pepper
- 3 garlic cloves, minced
- 1 tbsp. fresh ginger, minced
- 1 tbsp. sesame oil
- 3 lbs. fresh prepackaged chopped, mixed stir-fry vegetables

OR
- ½ cup carrots, sliced
- ½ cup broccoli florets
- ½ cup bell red pepper, sliced
- ½ cup white onion, diced
- ½ cup shitake mushrooms
- ½ cup baby corn
- ½ cup snow peas
- ½ cup toasted sesame seeds (optional)

Directions

- In a small bowl, combine all sauce ingredients, and whisk together.
- In a small saucepan, bring 2 cups of water to a boil. Add brown rice, oil, salt, and pepper; cover and simmer for 20 minutes.
- While rice is cooking, heat avocado oil in a wok, on medium heat.
- Add chicken and season with black pepper, then cook on high until it has a golden color (about 5 minutes).
- Add garlic and ginger; stir into chicken and cook 1 minute. Add sesame oil and toss.
- Add all vegetables to the pan, toss together, and cook for 5 minutes.
- Add sauce mixture, toss, and cook for another 5 minutes until sauce mixture thickens. Toss vegetables every 30 seconds or so to cook all vegetables evenly.
- Serve the chicken and vegetable mixture over brown rice, and sprinkle the top with toasted sesame seeds (optional).

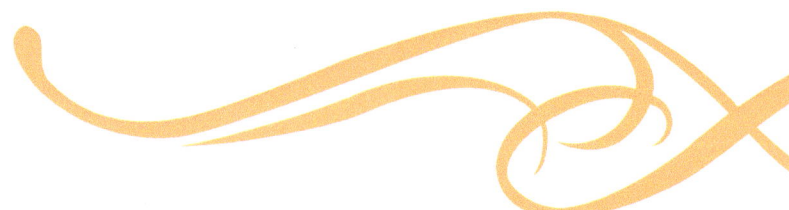

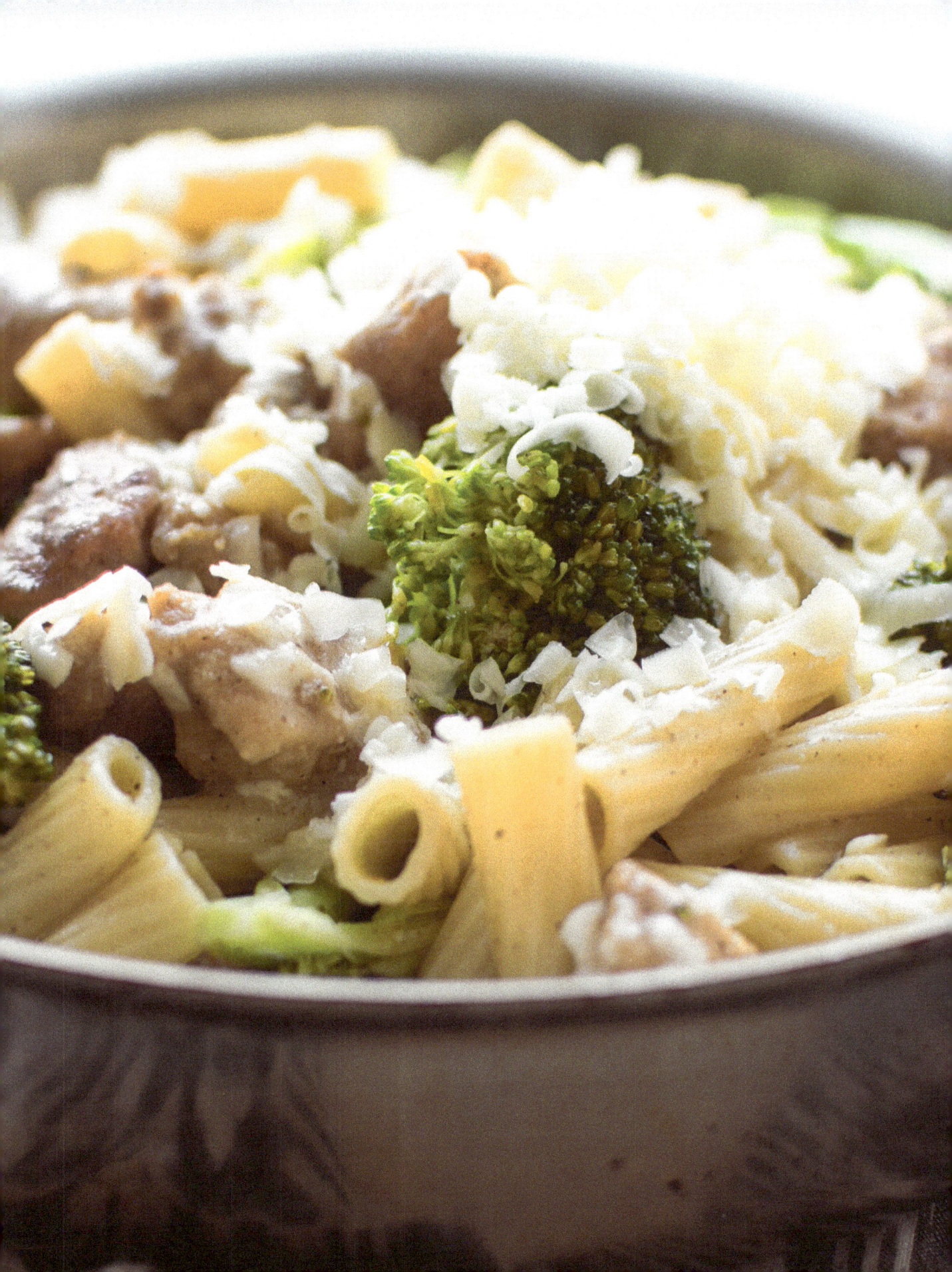

Danielle Formaro

CHICKEN, BROCCOLI, AND ZITI

This was my grandmother's recipe. She did it the best. My friends were always surprised when I told them I ate pasta quite often. They would ask me how I stayed so thin. The funny part is Italians in Italy are pretty fit for a few reasons. First, they walk a lot more than we Americans, and second, they eat their major meal for lunch, not dinner. Which means eating heavier foods such as pasta in the afternoon, and eating lighter foods in the evening with a protein-based meal such as fish and vegetables. The key with pasta and weight loss, in general, is to eat your pasta earlier in the day when your metabolism can take advantage of the carbohydrate and use it as fuel to burn it off for energy. Also stay within your portions. A portion of pasta should be the size of your first, not three fistfuls! With this said, enjoy one of my family favorites.

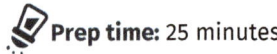 **Prep time:** 25 minutes   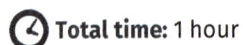 **Total time:** 1 hour   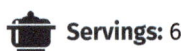 **Servings:** 6

Ingredients

- 1 lb. ziti macaroni (regular or a whole-grain pasta for a lighter version)
- ⅓ cup olive oil
- 8 cups broccoli (coarsely chopped)
- ½ cup avocado oil or another high-smoke-point cooking oil
- 2 lbs. chicken (cut into bite-sized pieces)
- 2 cups wheat flour
- 1 tbsp. paprika
- 1 tbsp. garlic powder
- 1 tbsp. onion powder
- 1 tsp. salt
- 1 tsp. pepper
- 3 garlic cloves (sliced)
- 2 shallots (minced)
- ¾ cup dry white wine (such as a chardonnay)
- 4 cups organic or low-sodium chicken broth
- 3 tbsp. cornstarch
- 3 tbsp. butter
- ¼ cup fresh squeezed lemon juice (about 1 whole lemon)
- ¼ cup Pecorino Romano cheese, plus some for sprinkling
- red pepper flakes (optional)

TIME SAVING TIP:

Once you are familiar with how long your pasta takes to cook you can save a little time by adding your broccoli to the water with the pasta just two minutes before you know the pasta will be ready, and it will blanch the broccoli for you (or cook it al dente).

Directions

- In a large pasta pot, bring water to a boil, and add pasta. Throw in a few pinches of salt and cook pasta on medium until al dente.

- Once pasta is cooked, drain the pasta, rinse with cool water to stop it from cooking more, and transfer back into large pot. Pour about ⅓ cup olive oil over the pasta and give it a quick stir to coat the pasta to prevent sticking. Set aside.

- Steam your broccoli. Place a steamer basket inside a large pot. Fill with a few inches of water. Be sure the water does not touch the bottom of the steamer basket. Bring the water to a simmer over medium-high heat. Add the broccoli florets and stems, and cover. Steam for 4 to 5 minutes, until tender. Set aside.

- In a large bowl, prepare chicken batter. Combine flour, paprika, garlic powder, onion powder, salt, and pepper. Whisk all ingredients together.

- Coat each piece of chicken in the batter on all sides, and set aside on a tray until all pieces are coated.

- In a large skillet, on medium-high, heat ⅓ cup avocado oil. Add chicken (you will need to do a few batches in order to not overcrowd the pan), and cook until golden brown on all sides, about 2 minutes on each side. Once they are done, remove and place chicken on a tray lined with paper towels, and keep covered until ready to use again. For the second batch, you may need to add another ⅓ cup olive oil to the pan.

- Once chicken is finished, add another drop of avocado oil to the pan (a few tablespoons). Add garlic and shallots. Sauté for about 30 seconds.

- Add ¾ cup of white wine, and whisk to deglaze the pan. Bring to a boil to cook off the alcohol for about 2 minutes.

- Add chicken broth, and cook on medium heat for another 2 to 3 minutes to warm broth.

- In a small bowl, whisk cornstarch with a little water, and then slowly add to the pan while whisking constantly. Increase flame to medium-high, and whisk broth mixture until mixture becomes thickened and bubbly. Add butter and stir until melted. Lastly, stir in lemon juice.

- Add the chicken and broccoli to the pan, and let all ingredients marinate each other. Cook another 2 minutes on medium. Combine chicken and broccoli mixture with pasta.

- Serve immediately and sprinkle with Pecorino Romano cheese. You can also sprinkle with some red pepper flakes if you like a little bite.

GRILLED CHICKEN PESTO OVER WHEAT LINGUINI

Pesto is a sauce originating in Genoa, the capital city of Liguria, Italy. It is a sauce of crushed basil leaves, pine nuts, garlic, Parmesan cheese, and olive oil, typically served with pasta. The name came from the Genoese verb "pestâ" (Italian: pestare), which means to pound or to crush, in reference to the original method of preparation. Strictly speaking, pesto is a generic term for anything that is made by pounding; that is why the word is used for several pestos in Italy. Nonetheless, pesto alla Genovese ("Genoese pesto") remains the most popular pesto in Italy and the rest of the world. I also love to make this sauce with shrimp.

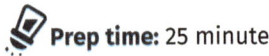 **Prep time:** 25 minutes   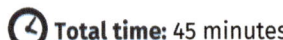 **Total time:** 45 minutes   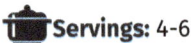 **Servings:** 4-6

Ingredients

- ⅔ cups pine nuts
- 4 cups basil (loosely packed)
- ¼ cup Pecorino Romano cheese
- ⅓ cup fresh grated Parmesan cheese
- 4 garlic cloves
- 1 tsp. salt
- 1 cup olive oil
- 1 lb. wheat linguini
- 6 boneless chicken breasts (cleaned and tenderized)
- salt and pepper
- avocado oil

TIME SAVING TIP:

If you prefer not to tenderize your chicken, you can also purchase 2 lbs. of chicken tenderloins instead since it is already a tender piece of chicken.

Directions

- Start by preparing your pesto. In a blender or food processor, combine pine nuts, basil, Pecorino and Parmesan cheeses, garlic, salt, and oil. Blend until finely chopped. Set aside.
- In a large pot, bring water to a boil. Add a few pinches of salt, and cook linguini until al dente (see packaging for estimated time to cook). Once finished, add a little olive oil and toss to avoid the pasta sticking. Set aside.
- With a meat tenderizer, tenderize each side of the chicken breasts to until about ¼-inch thick. Season each side of chicken with salt and pepper.
- Over a medium-high flame, on a grill or on a grill pan used on a stove, grill chicken for about 4 to 5 minutes on each side or until juices run clear and center is no longer pink. If using a stove, use a nonstick grill pan and add about 3 tablespoons of avocado or grapeseed oil to the pan to avoid sticking. Two batches would be needed to not overcrowd pan.
- Once chicken is finished, cut into bite-sized pieces or strips on a cutting board. In a large skillet, over a medium flame, add pesto and cook until warmed (about 1 minute).
- Add chicken to the pan, and toss to coat chicken with the pesto. Combine chicken and pesto mixture to the pot of linguini, and with a set of tongs, toss all ingredients together.
- Serve with a sprinkle of Parmesan cheese on top before serving.

CHICKEN FAJITAS

Some fun facts: fajita is a term found in Tex-Mex cuisine, commonly referring to any grilled meat usually served as a taco on a flour or corn tortilla. The term originally referred to the cut of beef used in the dish, which is known as skirt steak. Popular meats today also include chicken, pork, shrimp, lamb, and all cuts of beef, as well as vegetables instead of meat. For this recipe, I just happen to prefer chicken.

This is another one of those recipes most people do not know how to make from scratch so they buy pre-packaged mixes loaded with sodium and preservatives, making us feel bloated and lousy at the end. This is actually a nutritious meal, so why ruin it with a pre-packaged mix when fresh ingredients and love are all it needs?

 Total prep time: 20 minutes   **Total time:** 40 minutes   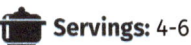 **Servings:** 4-6

Ingredients

For the Chicken

- 2 lbs. boneless skinless chicken breast or chicken tenderloins (cut into strips)
- 2 tbsp. avocado oil or light cooking oil with a high smoke point
- juice of one lime
- ½ tsp. salt
- ¼ tsp. fresh black pepper
- ⅛ tsp. crushed red pepper
- 1 tsp. oregano
- 1 tsp. paprika
- 1 tsp. chili powder
- ½ tsp. garlic powder
- 2 garlic cloves (minced)
- sour cream for serving
- cilantro for serving

For the Vegetables

- 3 tbsp. avocado or light cooking oil with high smoke point
- 1 green bell pepper (julienned)
- 1 red bell pepper (julienned)
- 1 yellow bell pepper (julienned)
- 1 large red onion (thinly sliced)
- 2 garlic cloves (minced)
- 8 whole-wheat tortillas (for serving)

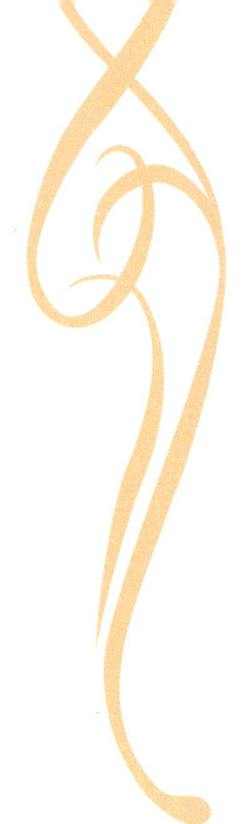

Directions

- In a bowl, combine chicken with all ingredients listed, *except* the garlic, sour cream, and cilantro. Be sure to combine well so it will marinate the flavors. Cover and put in fridge.
- In a large skillet or grill pan, heat oil and add bell peppers and onion, and season with salt and pepper.
- Continue to cook on a high flame until vegetables become soft and look roasted. This will take about 12 minutes or so, tossing about every 3 minutes with a set of tongs. If the bottom of the pan starts to burn a little, you can add a little water to deglaze the pan.
- Once vegetables are done, lower heat, remove the vegetable mixture, and put in a bowl. Cover with aluminum foil to keep warm and set aside.
- Add a little water to the pan to deglaze it again, if needed. This helps get up all the brown bits stuck to the bottom of the pan. Those brown bits are called "fond," and that is where all the flavors are.
- Add chicken to the pan and cook on a medium-high flame until golden brown on all sides and the middle of the chicken has no pink color, about 4 to 5 minutes each side.
- Add garlic and give it a quick stir into the meat. Then immediately add vegetable mixture back into the pan, give it a toss, and let cook 1 more minute.
- Serve on 8-inch, whole-wheat flour tortillas. Top each with a teaspoon of sour cream and cilantro.

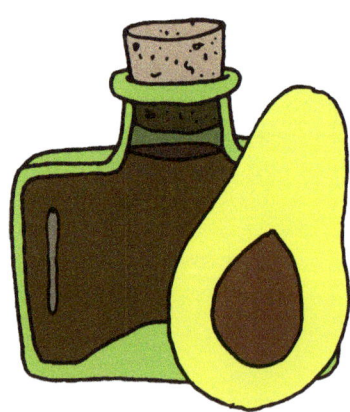

TIP:

I like to warm up my tortillas in the oven before serving. You can pre-heat your oven to 200°F before you start cooking. Once your meal is almost done, you can lay several tortillas on a large baking pan and let heat for 5 minutes or so in the oven, just enough to warm them but not heat them too much or they will get hard. You can also give them a quick, 10-second nuke in the microwave.

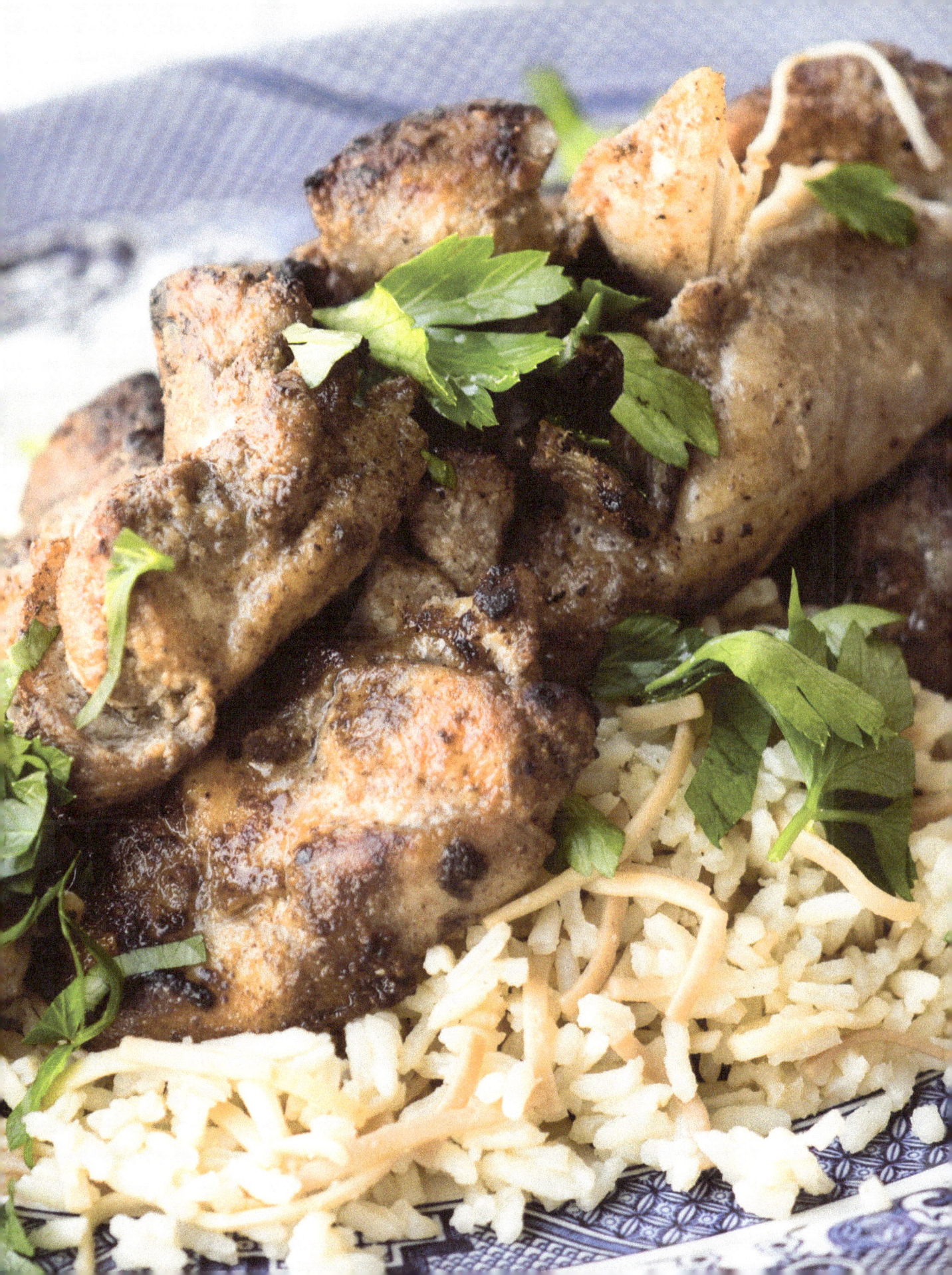

ARMENIAN-INSPIRED GRILLED CHICKEN THIGHS

This is a grilled favorite at any BBQ. In America, most of us are brought up eating the chicken leg or breast, but the thighs, in my opinion, are the juiciest and the tastiest, especially when grilled. The secret blend in this recipe that gives this chicken its unique flavors is the cumin, cinnamon, cloves, and nutmeg. The thigh is a very flavorful part of the chicken, so when you combine these two together, your guests will ask, "Hey where did you get this chicken?" And you can proudly say, "Me! I made it!" It pairs very well with Mediterranean grilled vegetables and family-style rice pilaf in this book.

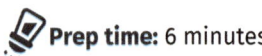 **Prep time:** 6 minutes   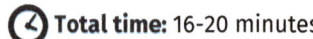 **Total time:** 16-20 minutes   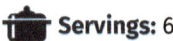 **Servings:** 6

Ingredients

- 3 lbs. skinless, boneless chicken thighs
- 1 tsp. cinnamon
- ¼ tsp. ground cloves
- 1 tbsp. cumin
- ½ tsp. nutmeg
- ½ tsp. allspice
- 1 tsp. garlic powder
- 1 tsp. onion powder
- ½ tsp. salt
- ½ tsp. pepper
- juice of half a lemon
- ¼ cup avocado oil

Directions

- In a large bowl, combine chicken with all ingredients. Cover and refrigerate for 2 hours to let chicken marinate in the spices.
- Pre-heat grill to medium-high. Brush grill with oil. Add marinated chicken and grill about 5 minutes on each side, or until cooked through.
- If you do not have a grill you can also broil them on high as well. It will give you the same effect. Be sure to use a broil safe pan.

TIP:

This dish pairs well with the Yogurt, Cucumber, and Mint Soup recipe on page 77. I like to drizzle it right over the top.

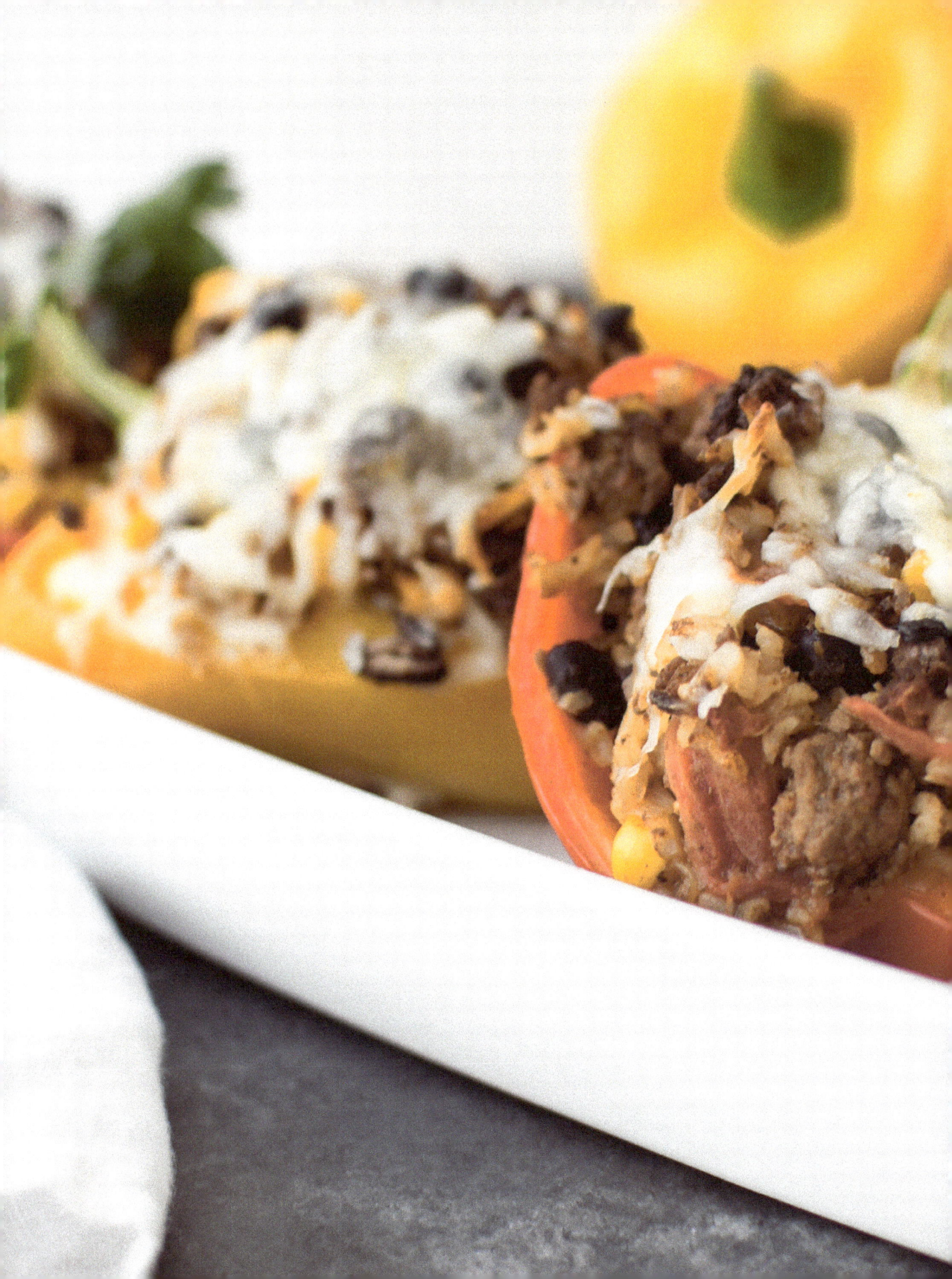

GROUND BEEF STUFFED BELL PEPPERS

Stuffed peppers not only have a ton of nutrition, but they can be made so many different ways. Once you have the right recipe, you can sub out different meats and fillers to change it up each time. You can also use quinoa as a healthy and lighter filler option as well. I just happen to like brown rice because it keeps me feeling full longer and it's a hearty whole grain.

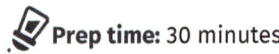 **Prep time:** 30 minutes   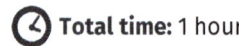 **Total time:** 1 hour   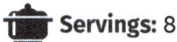 **Servings:** 8

Ingredients

- 1 cup brown rice (uncooked)
- water
- 8 bell peppers, assorted colored (cleaned, cut in half, seeds removed)
- 3 tbsp. high smoke point cooking oil like avocado oil
- 1 medium-sized Spanish onion (diced)
- 2 shallots (diced)
- 4 garlic cloves (minced)
- 2 lbs. 90% lean ground beef
- 1 tsp. salt
- ½ tsp. black pepper
- ⅛ tsp. cayenne pepper
- 2 tbsp. chili powder
- 1 tbsp. cumin
- ½ tsp. paprika
- ½ tsp. coriander
- 1 (14.5 oz.) can diced tomatoes in juice
- 1 (15.5 oz.) can black beans (drained and rinsed of starch)
- 2 cups corn (frozen or fresh and shucked)
- 1 cup shredded Monterey Jack cheese

Directions

- Start by preparing your rice. Follow instructions on the packaging. When finished, set aside.
- Wash peppers, slice in half, and clean out the center of seeds. Place in large baking pan, and set aside (you will probably need a couple of baking pans).
- In a large skillet or large deep pan, heat oil on a medium-high flame and add onions and shallots. Sauté until translucent (about 5-8 minutes).
- Add garlic, and cook one more minute.
- Add beef to the pan and combine with shallots, onions, and garlic.
- Add all spices (salt, black pepper, cayenne pepper, chili powder, cumin, paprika, and coriander) and combine with meat. Cook until meat is nice and browned (about 10-12 minutes). You can check the heat of the spice after the meat is cooked. If you feel you wish to have more heat you can add more cayenne pepper.
- Add can of tomatoes, and cook another 2 minutes.
- Combine beans, corn, and rice and turn off heat.
- Take a spoon and generously fill each half pepper to the top. Let it spill over the pepper. Repeat this for each pepper. Any remaining filling you can just pour right over the top of all the peppers.
- Bake on 375°F for 30-35 minutes until peppers are soft.
- Sprinkle cheese over the top of all peppers and bake another 3 minutes or until the cheese is melted.

BEEF SIRLION MEATLOAF WITH MASHED POTATOES AND MUSHROOM GRAVY

I feel meatloaf does not get as much credit as it should. It is definitely underrated as it can be quite an impressive offering if you have a great recipe. I personally like ground sirloin with this dish; it molds better with the ingredients since ground sirloin is a leaner meat than ground beef. Adding Anaheim pepper gave this loaf a nice little bite. I love when you get a little surprise with your bite—and it does just that. This is a great meal during the cold winter months with a nice glass of red wine.

 Prep time: 25 minutes   **Total time:** 1 hour and 25 minutes   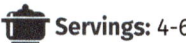 **Servings:** 4-6

See sides for mashed potato recipe.

Ingredients

Meatloaf
- 2 lbs. ground beef sirloin
- 3 eggs (beaten)
- ½ cup Anaheim pepper (minced)
- 1 cup yellow onion (diced)
- ½ cup fresh parsley (chopped)
- 4 garlic cloves (minced)
- 2½ tsp. Dijon mustard
- 1½ tsp. Worcester sauce
- 1½ tsp. salt
- 1 tsp. pepper

Mushroom Gravy
- 1 tbsp. olive oil
- 2 shallots (minced)
- 1 cup mushrooms (thinly sliced)
- 2 cups organic or low sodium beef broth
- ¼ tsp. garlic powder
- ½ tsp. fresh or dried parsley
- salt and pepper to taste
- ¼ cup mashed potato
- ¼ cup cornstarch

Mashed Potatoes
- See recipe on page 197

Directions

Meatloaf

- Preheat oven to 350°F.
- In a large bowl, combine all ingredients.
- Place meat mixture into a 9.25 x 5.25 x 2.75-inch baking dish, coated with nonstick spray.
- Bake on middle rack for one hour, or until meat thermometer reaches 165°F.
- Prepare Mashed Potatoes, then serve with meatloaf topped with mushroom gravy.

Mushroom Gravy

- In a small saucepan, heat oil on medium heat. Add shallots and sauté for about 2 minutes or until soft. Add mushrooms, and cook another 5 minutes, until softened.
- Pour in beef broth, and add garlic powder, parsley, and mashed potatoes. Season with salt and pepper. Bring mixture to a light boil, whisking constantly until mashed potatoes are blended and dissolved into the broth.
- In a measuring cup, combine cornstarch with about ¼ cup of warm water. Pour cornstarch into the pan, and whisk until gravy becomes thickened.

Add THIS to Your Plate!

On the Side

When it comes to sides, my rule is to prepare one or two vegetable sides and one carbohydrate, such as rice or potato, with your protein. The goal is to have most major food groups on your plate, particularly a protein, a vegetable, and a carbohydrate. Below, you can mix and match with some of the main protein dishes in the above recipes in the previous section of this book such as the salmon, cod, beef & pork tenderloins, and roast chicken.

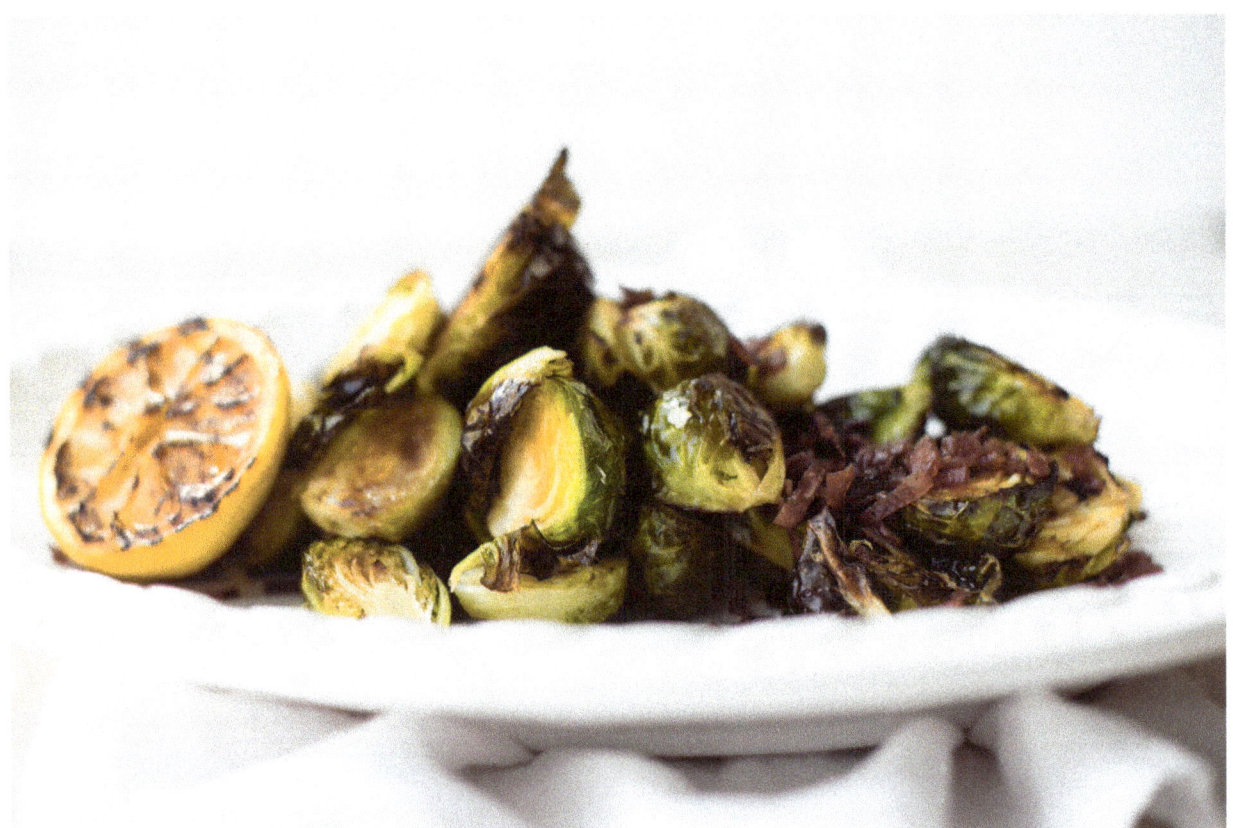

THANKSGIVING-STYLE SWEET POTATOES

The best part of Thanksgiving is all the wonderful sides to enjoy with that amazing turkey. This is a side that I prepare not only on that holiday but all through the fall and winter months. It will make the house smell so cozy and sweet. You can even replace the sweet potatoes with carrots in this recipe, and that would taste just as good!

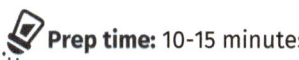 **Prep time:** 10-15 minutes   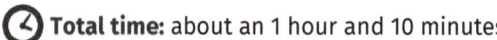 **Total time:** about an 1 hour and 10 minutes   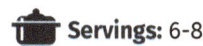 **Servings:** 6-8

Ingredients

- 5 sweet potatoes (peeled and cut into 1-inch pieces)
- ⅓ cup pure organic grade A maple syrup
- 1 tsp. allspice
- 1 tsp. cinnamon
- 1 tsp. nutmeg
- ¼ cup avocado oil
- salt and pepper

Directions

- Pre-heat oven to 400°F.
- In a deep baking dish, add all ingredients and give a few good tosses with your hands to ensure the potatoes have a good, thick, and evenly spiced coat.
- Place on middle rack of oven and bake 25 minutes. With a pair of tongs, toss the potatoes a few times to ensure the potatoes stay hydrated and re-seasoned.
- Continue to bake another 20-35 minutes or until a fork can easily pierce through the center.

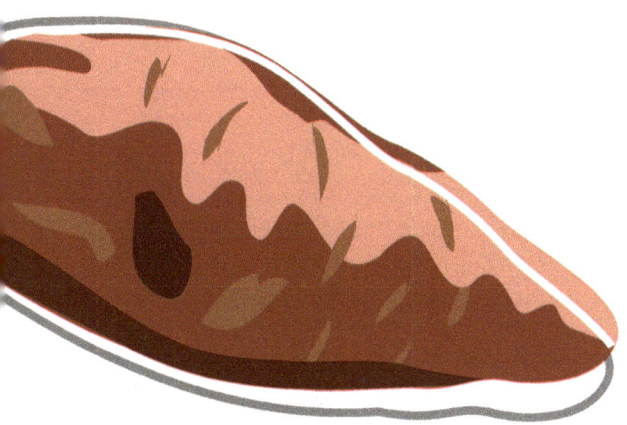

CLASSIC MASHED POTATOES

When it comes to potatoes, there is no right and wrong; it is all personal preference. Whether you want to whip them smooth or keep them lumpy is up to you. The key is to pour your liquids in a little at a time so you can control the texture and thickness of your potato. If you wanted to make these garlic mashed potatoes, all you would need to do is roast an entire bulb of garlic, and then remove the bulbs, smash them up with a fork and mix right into your potatoes. Yum!

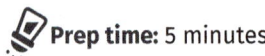 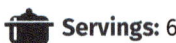

Prep time: 5 minutes   **Total time:** 30 minutes   **Servings:** 6

Ingredients

- 4 large potatoes (about 2 lbs. or so, peeled and chopped in quarters)
- ½-1 cup low-fat milk (such as 1% or 2%)
- 5 tbsp. butter
- salt and pepper
- dried parsley (for garnish)

Directions

- Place potatoes in a large pot and fill with water about 4 inches above potatoes. Add a little salt and boil on medium-high heat until soft (about 20-25 minutes).
- Meanwhile, in a small saucepan, combine milk and butter and heat on low to melt butter and combine the two ingredients.
- Once potatoes are done, strain out all the water, and then put them back into the same pot.
- First, mash them with a potato masher by hand. Then with an electric beater, whip the potatoes and slowly add the warm milk mixture until you get the desired thickness. Sprinkle a little dried parsley for garnish before serving.

TASTY TIP:

To make garlic mashed potatoes, you can add 8-9 cloves of minced garlic to the milk and butter mixture, and cook until milk is very hot but not boiling. For a stronger garlic flavor, you can roast an entire bulb of garlic, remove from casing when done, mash it and then blend that into your potatoes as well.

GARLIC-LEMON BROCCOLI

Kids never, it seems, like vegetables because they think they are boring, and you know what? Without some seasoning, they totally can be! I salute garlic with oil for enlivening vegetables without fail. Not only does my kitchen smell like heaven, but that garlic-oil mix tastes amazing poured right over my veggies. To give it a little pop, squeeze a little lemon over the top, and now you have taken your veggies to the next level.

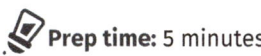 **Prep time:** 5 minutes 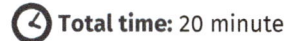 **Total time:** 20 minutes 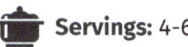 **Servings:** 4-6

Ingredients

- 2 heads broccoli (cleaned and chopped)
- ¼ cup olive oil
- 8-10 garlic cloves (sliced)
- 2-3 tbsp. freshly squeezed lemon juice
- salt and pepper

Directions

◎ Fill a large pot with about 2 inches of water and place a steam basket inside pot. Add broccoli, cover and steam on medium-high heat until soft (about 6-7 minutes or until vegetables are tender but not too soft, they should be crisp).

◎ In a small saucepan, heat oil on low-medium heat, add garlic and cook until the garlic becomes golden in color. It should only take a few minutes once the oil is heated. Add lemon juice.

◎ Remove from heat and pour over broccoli. Season with salt and pepper to taste.

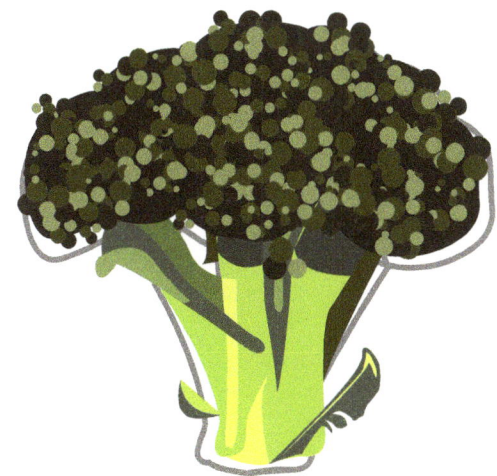

SWEET AND SPICED GLAZED CARROTS

There is something so fun about playing with flavors. Opposites definitely attract in this dish. Depending on your kids' taste buds, you may want to lighten up on the red pepper as it is not supposed to be hot, but rather a little zing with your sweet carrots.

Total time: 15 minutes **Servings:** 4-6

Ingredients

- 1½ lbs. baby carrots
- 3 tbsp. olive oil
- 1 tbsp. agave nectar or raw organic honey
- crushed red cayenne pepper
- Chopped fresh parsley for garnish

Directions

- Rinse carrots under cold water, and put in a medium saucepan. Cover with water. Bring to a boil. Reduce heat to medium-low, cover, and continue cooking for about 10 minutes, or until tender. Drain and set aside.
- In a bowl, combine oil, agave nectar or honey, and carrots.
- Stir carrots so that they are coated with ingredients.
- Give a dash or two of cayenne pepper (or more if you like it spicier).
- Sprinkle with parsley, toss, and serve.

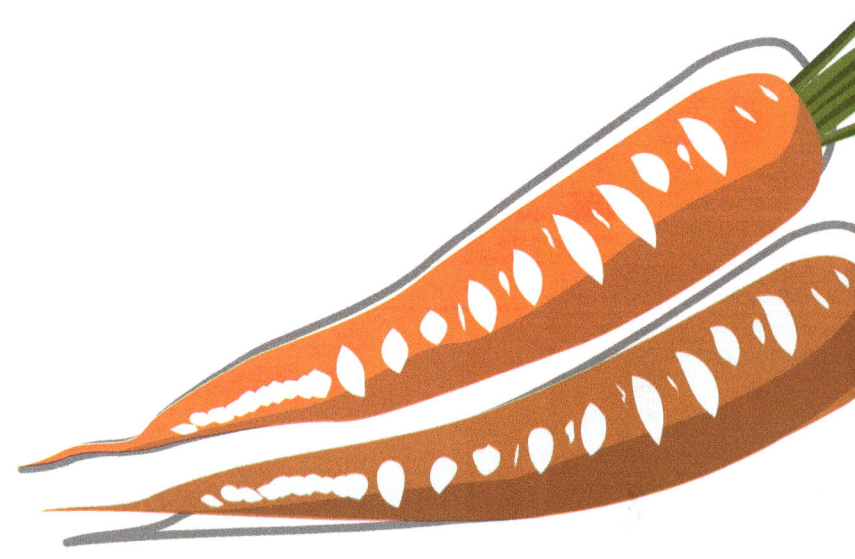

Add THIS to Your Plate!

MEDITERRANEAN STYLE GRILLED VEGETABLES

Nothing beats the easy clean-up of grilling. The grill will also give your vegetable a nice hint of smoke and will make for a delicious, colorful side. Just be careful not to overcook them; they do cook pretty fast.

Prep time: 20 minutes **Total time:** 30 minutes **Servings:** 6–8

Ingredients

- 1 eggplant (sliced in ½-inch-thick wheels)
- 1 zucchini (sliced in ½-inch-thick wheels)
- 1 yellow squash (sliced ½-inch-thick wheels)
- 2 beefsteak tomatoes (pitted, sliced ½-inch-thick wheels)
- 2 carrots (sliced ¼ inch thick on an angle)
- ¾ cup avocado oil
- 2 tbsp. balsamic vinegar
- ½ tsp. thyme
- ½ tsp. oregano
- ½ tsp. fresh or dried basil
- ½ tsp. onion powder
- ½ tsp. garlic powder
- salt
- pepper

Directions

- Pre-heat grill on medium-high heat.
- Prepare vegetables, and lay them down on a large tray.
- In a small bowl, add all ingredients (except salt and pepper) and stir together.
- With a brush, coat the tops of each vegetable with oil seasoning (3 coats).
- Place vegetables seasoned side down on the grill and close cover for about 4 minutes.
- With a brush, coat the remaining side 3 times and flip to cook the other side, for about another 4 minutes until well-marked and soft. Remove from heat and season with salt and pepper.

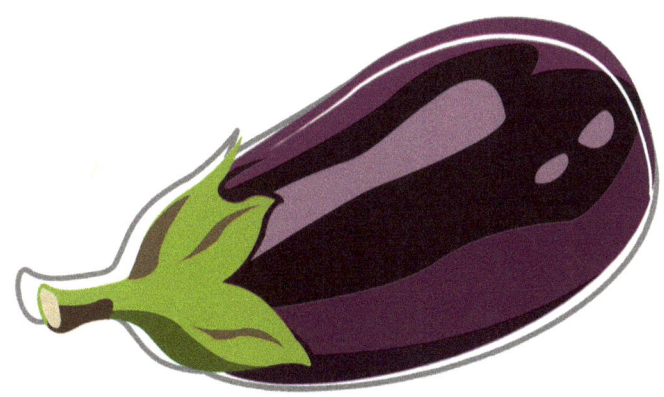

ROASTED BABY POTATOES WITH ONIONS AND HERBS

A dinner table staple. This traditional recipe is always needed, as it goes with everything. When I make my beef Bourguignon and roast chicken, this side is a must.

 Total prep time: 10 minutes   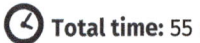 **Total time:** 55 minutes   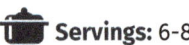 **Servings:** 6-8

Ingredients

- 1 lb. assorted colored baby potatoes (halved)
- 2 Vidalia onions (chopped)
- 3 tbsp. Greek seasoning
- ½ tsp. coarse sea salt
- ½ tsp. pepper
- ⅓ cup olive oil

Directions

- Pre-heat oven to 375°F.
- Rinse and wash potatoes thoroughly. Pat dry and put into a large bowl.
- Add Greek seasoning, salt, pepper, onions, and olive oil to bowl and toss to combine ingredients.
- Transfer to a baking pan, and bake for 45 minutes (until you can put a fork through the potato).
- If you like them more well done and crispy, you can then broil them for about 3-5 minutes. Be careful not to burn.

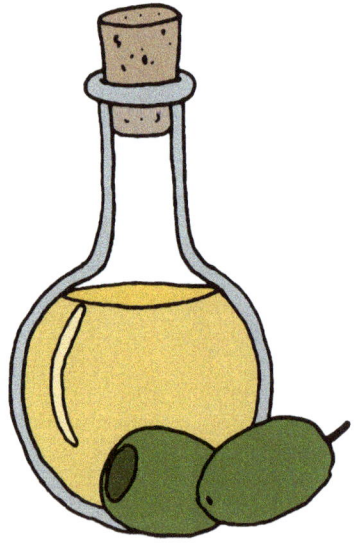

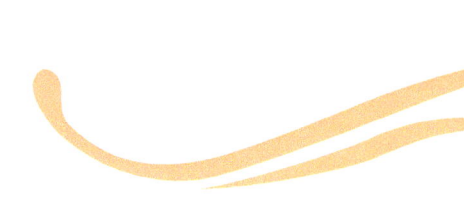

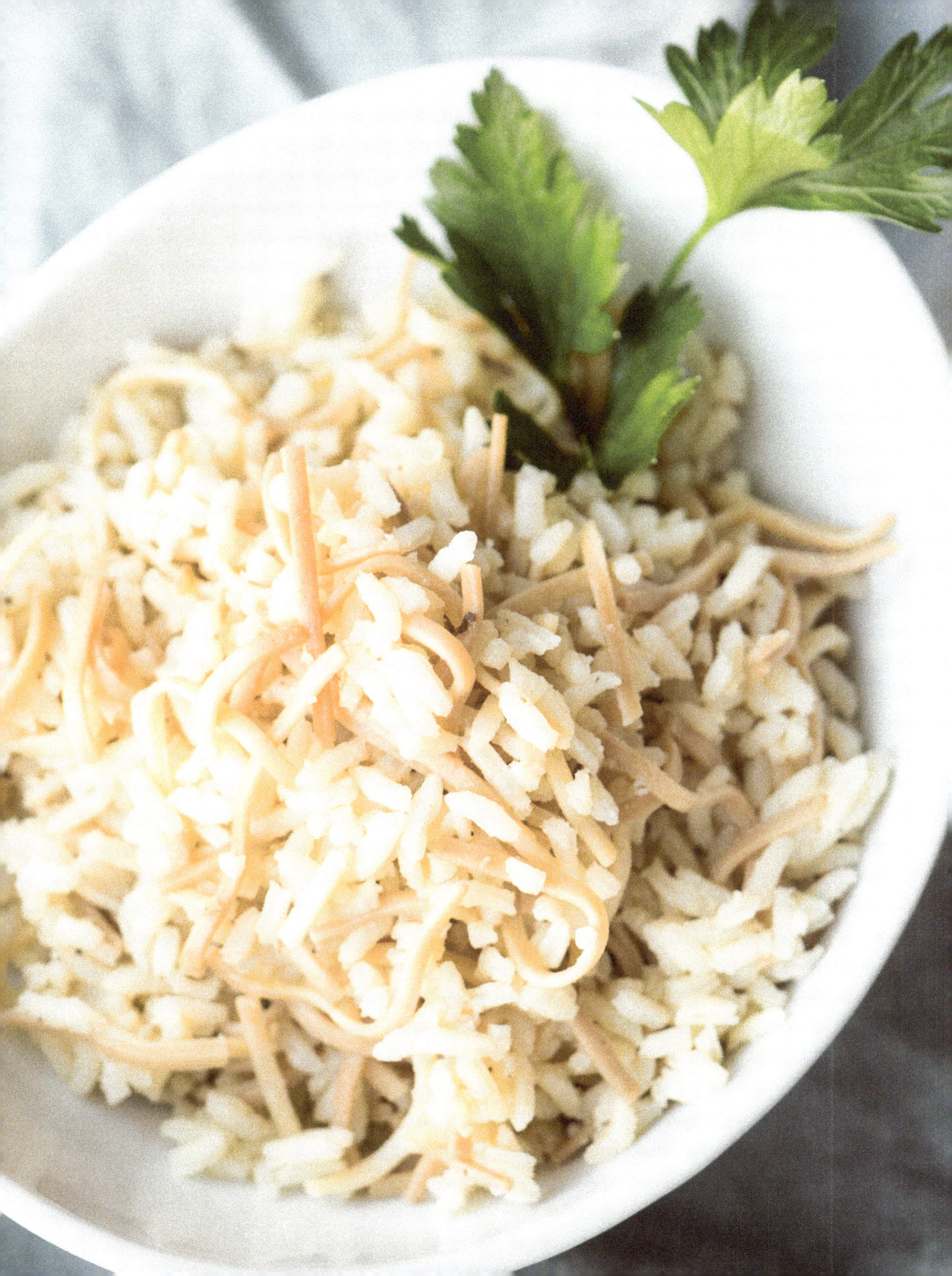

ARMENIAN RICE PILAF

This is my family's secret rice pilaf recipe and I am sharing it with you. Guess it's not much of a secret anymore! I am a little partial when I say that Armenians make the best rice pilaf. So what does "pilaf" mean anyway? Pilaf is a dish in which rice is cooked in a seasoned broth. The combination of the long rice grain and the sautéed noodles is what makes it so likable and delicious. This will be a recipe the entire neighborhood will want and the best part is, it's so easy to make.

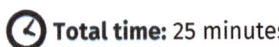 **Total time:** 25 minutes 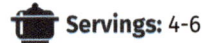 **Servings:** 4-6

Ingredients

- 2 tbsp. butter
- ½ cup fine egg noodles
- ground black pepper
- 1 cup white rice (medium grain)
- 1 chicken bouillon cube
- 2 cups low sodium chicken broth

Directions

- In nonstick medium-sized rice pan, melt butter.
- Add egg noodles, and cook in butter until golden brown (about 3 minutes; be sure to stir with wooden spoon to avoid burning). Sprinkle some pepper onto the noodles.
- Add white rice and chicken bouillon cube, and stir contents together.
- Add chicken broth, and bring to a boil. Then cover and simmer for 20 minutes.

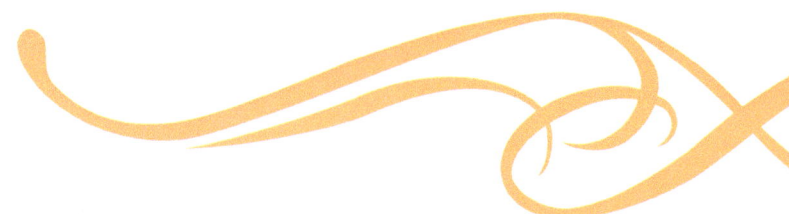

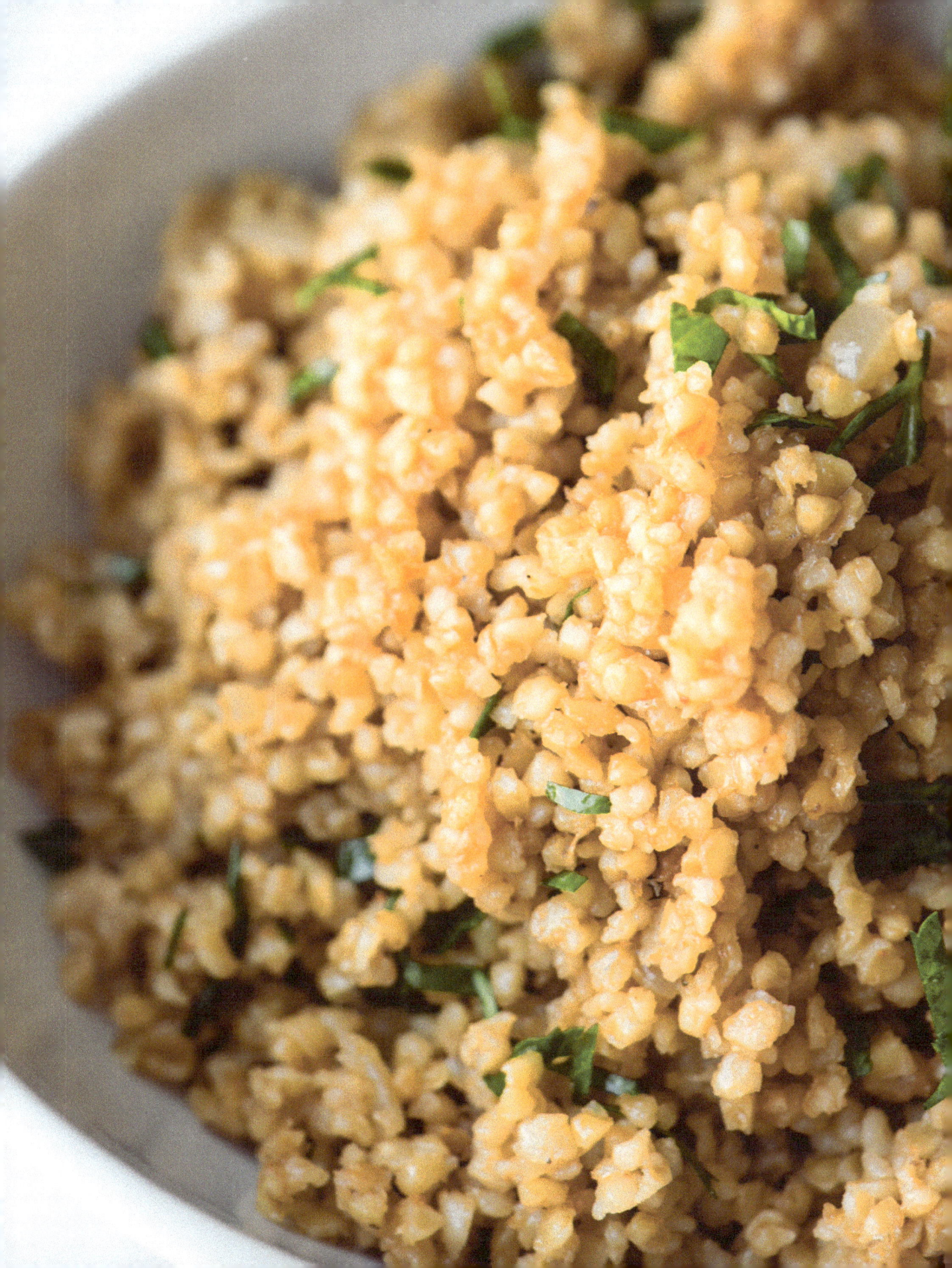

SPICY BULGUR WHEAT PILAF

Are you ready to kick it up a bit? Remember, you can control the heat for your family by staying light with your red pepper. This dish packs a punch, not only in terms of spice but in nutrition. Bulgur wheat is a whole wheat grain that has been cracked and partially pre-cooked. As a whole grain, it is a naturally high-fiber, low-fat, low-calorie, vegetarian, and vegan food ingredient. Though bulgur wheat is most commonly found in tabbouleh salad, you can use it just like rice or couscous, or any other whole grain, such as barley or quinoa. One thing to notice when you are purchasing it is the size of the grain as it comes in fine, medium, and coarse.

 Total time: 25 minutes   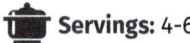 **Servings:** 4-6

Ingredients

- 2 tbsp. butter
- 1 medium-sized onion (diced)
- 1 cup coarse bulgur wheat
- 1 tbsp. tomato paste
- black pepper
- dash of crushed red pepper
- 1 small beef bouillon cube
- 2 cups low sodium beef broth

Directions

- In a medium-sized saucepan on medium heat, melt butter.
- Add onion and sauté until soft, about 5-6 minutes.
- Add bulgur wheat and blend with onion.
- Add tomato paste, black pepper, red pepper, and beef bouillon and stir together.
- Pour in broth, bring to a boil, then cover and simmer on low for 20 minutes.

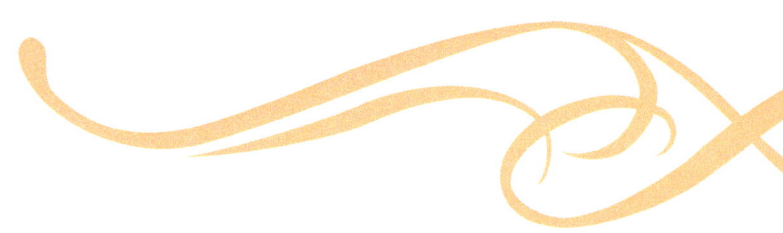

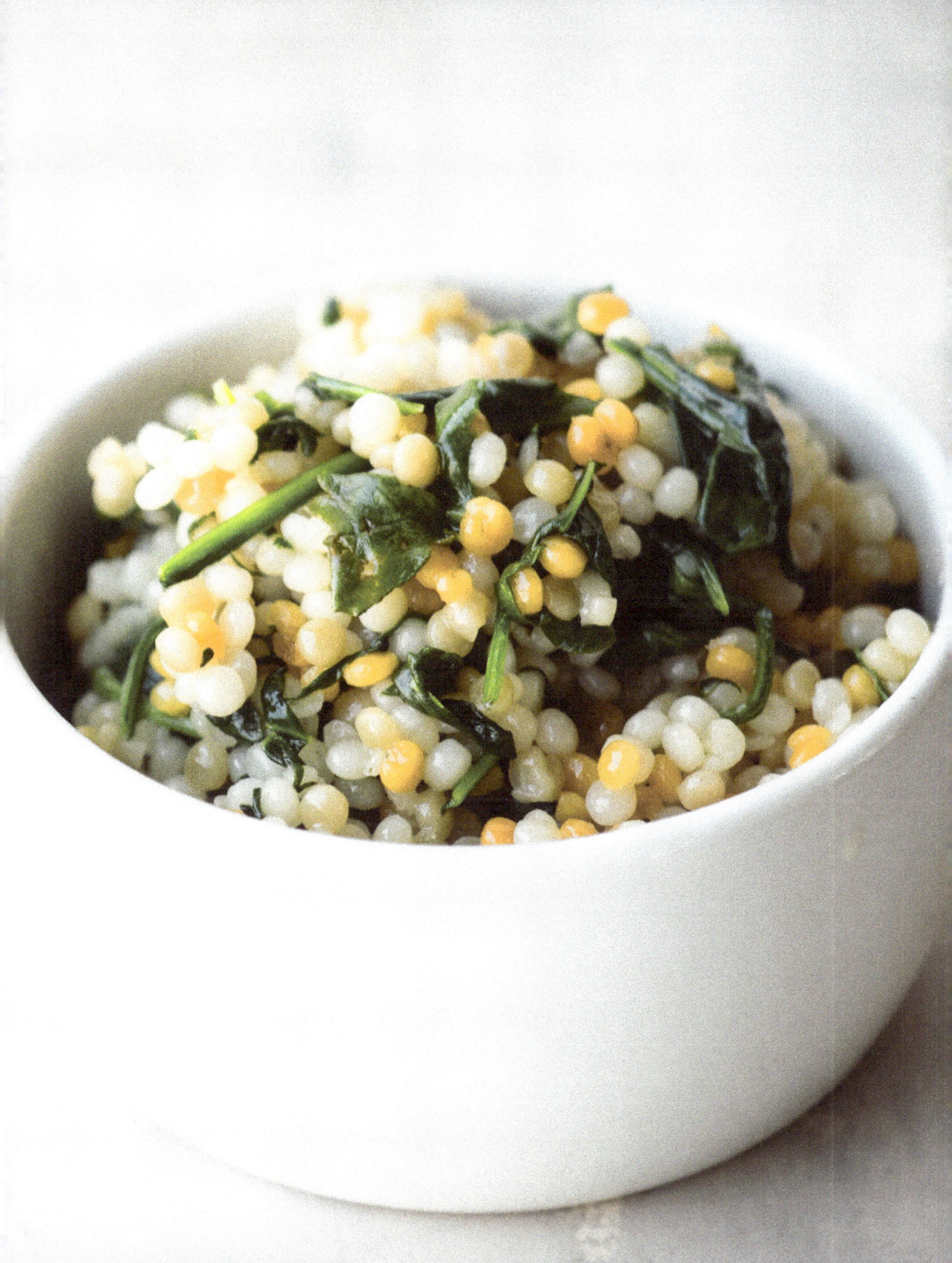

Danielle Formaro

PEARL COUSCOUS WITH SPINACH, GARLIC, AND OIL

Couscous is a type of North African semolina in granules made from crushed durum wheat. These days, it is made by machine: coarsely ground wheat (semolina) is moistened and tossed with fine wheat flour until it forms little round balls. (Think of the coarse bits as the core of a kind of wheat-flour snowball.) It can be used many different ways: in stews, salads, and as fillers in meats and baked goods.

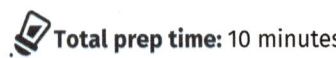 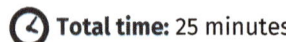 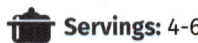

Total prep time: 10 minutes   **Total time:** 25 minutes   **Servings:** 4-6

Ingredients

- 2 cups water
- 1 cup pearl couscous
- ⅛ tsp. salt
- pinch of black pepper
- ¼ cup avocado oil
- 3 garlic cloves (sliced)
- 3 cups spinach (loosely packed)

Directions

- In a medium saucepan, add water, couscous, salt, and pepper. Bring to a boil.
- Cover, and lower heat to simmer for 15 minutes. When finished, fluff gently with a fork.
- While couscous is cooking, start garlic and oil mixture. In a small saucepan, heat the oil on a low-medium flame. Add garlic, and sauté until garlic is golden in color.
- Add spinach to the pan, and combine with garlic and oil. Cook for 1 to 2 minutes until spinach becomes soft.
- In a bowl, combine the garlic, oil, and spinach mixture to the couscous. Gently toss with a fork and serve.

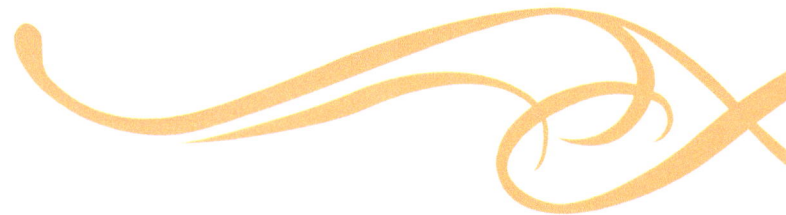

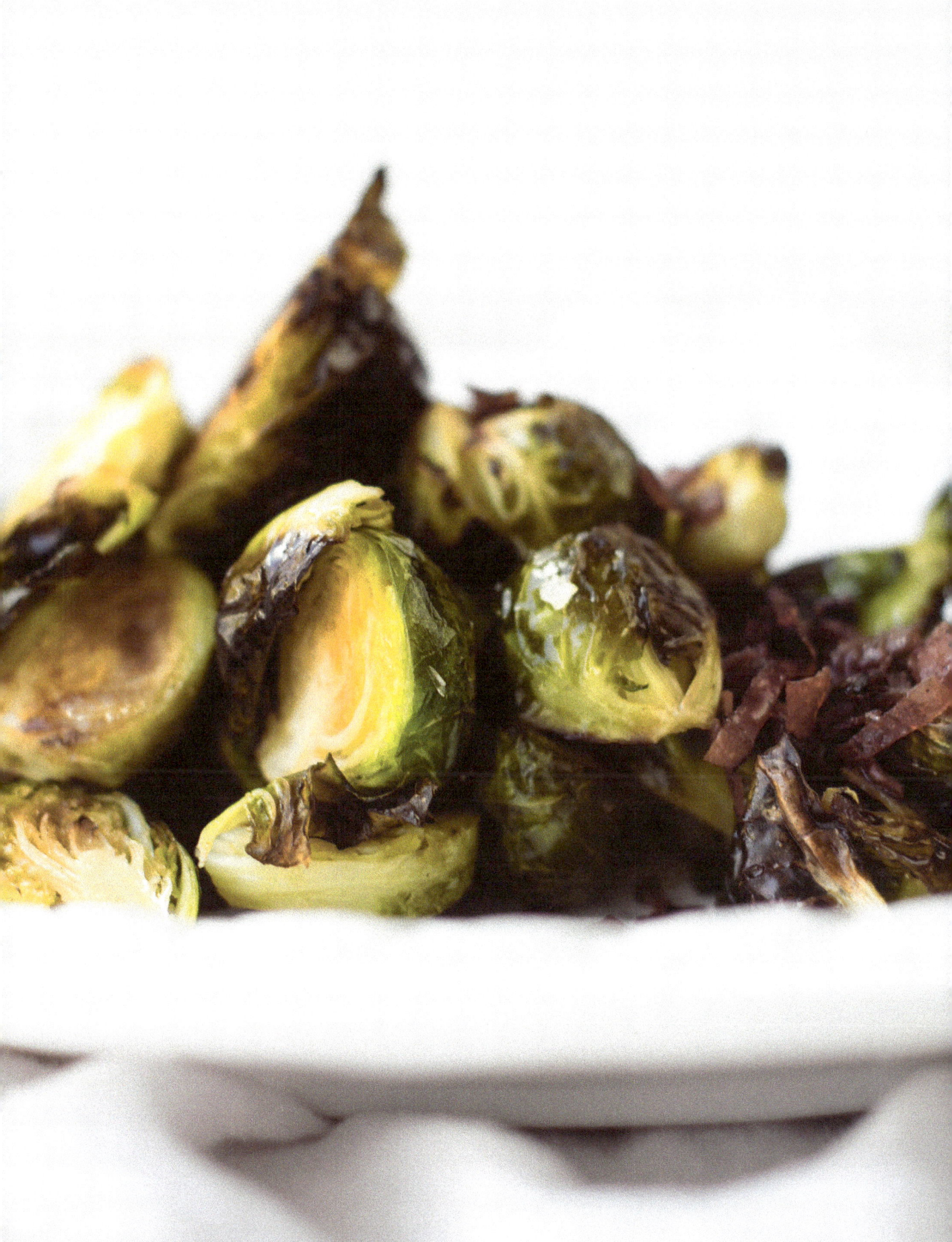

BRUSSELS SPROUTS WITH TURKEY BACON

Brussels sprouts have really won hearts over in the past few years. I can remember old TV shows where the kids would complain about having to eat Brussels sprouts. To my surprise, the first time I had them I was delighted by their flavor despite what I had heard. They are also an excellent source of vitamin C and vitamin K and a very good source of numerous nutrients, including folate, manganese, vitamin B6, dietary fiber, choline, copper, vitamin B1, potassium, phosphorus, and omega-3 fatty acids.

Total prep time: 10 minutes   **Total time:** 55 minutes   **Servings:** 6-8

Ingredients

- 2 lbs. Brussels sprouts (ends removed and sliced in half)
- 1 large Spanish onion (chopped)
- ¼ cup olive oil
- 2 tbsp. balsamic vinegar
- salt and pepper to taste
- 8 strips turkey bacon

Directions

- Set oven to 350°F on bake.
- Combine onions and Brussels sprouts in a large mixing bowl. Drizzle oil and balsamic vinegar all over onions and Brussels sprouts. Season with salt and pepper, and give them a few tosses to combine.
- Transfer them to a large baking sheet in a single layer. Bake for 45 minutes, or until tops of sprouts are brown and crisp.
- Meanwhile, on a skillet on medium-high heat, add bacon and cook until crispy, about 2 to 3 minutes on each side. When finished, lay bacon on a paper towel to absorb any extra oil. Chop bacon into fine pieces.
- Once Brussels sprouts are cooked, remove from oven. Sprinkle the bacon bits over the top. Combine all ingredients and serve!

CORN FIESTA

This side is perfect for BBQs! A spoonful of this with grilled meats will really be a hit. Another food this fun side would complement is a nice seared piece of white fish with some freshly squeezed lime on top. Wow! I can taste it now. It is perfect for summer nights when you want to keep the plate light. Serve hot or cold!

Total prep time: 10 minutes   **Servings:** 4-6

Ingredients

- 5 ears fresh cooked or grilled corn (shucked) or 5 cups frozen corn (thawed)
- ¼ cup olive oil
- ½ cup lime juice
- ½ red bell pepper (diced)
- ½ cilantro (chopped)
- 1 tbsp. Parmesan cheese
- 1 (15 oz.) can black beans (drained)
- ¾ cup queso fresca cheese
- salt and pepper to taste

Directions

- Combine all ingredients in a bowl and toss and serve!

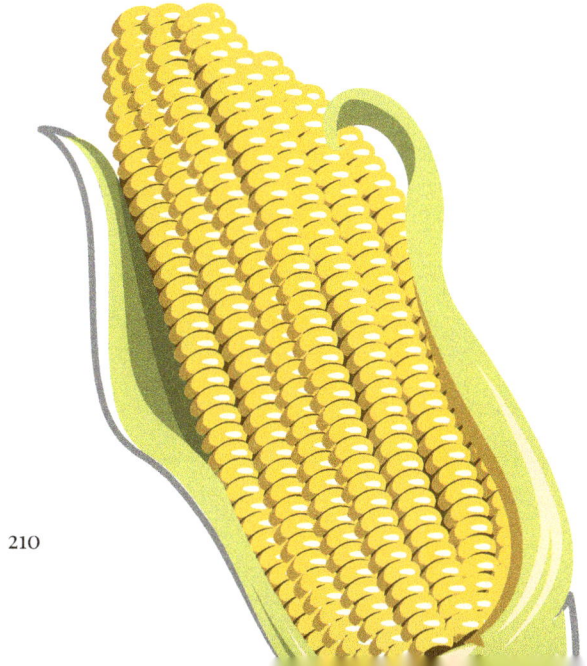

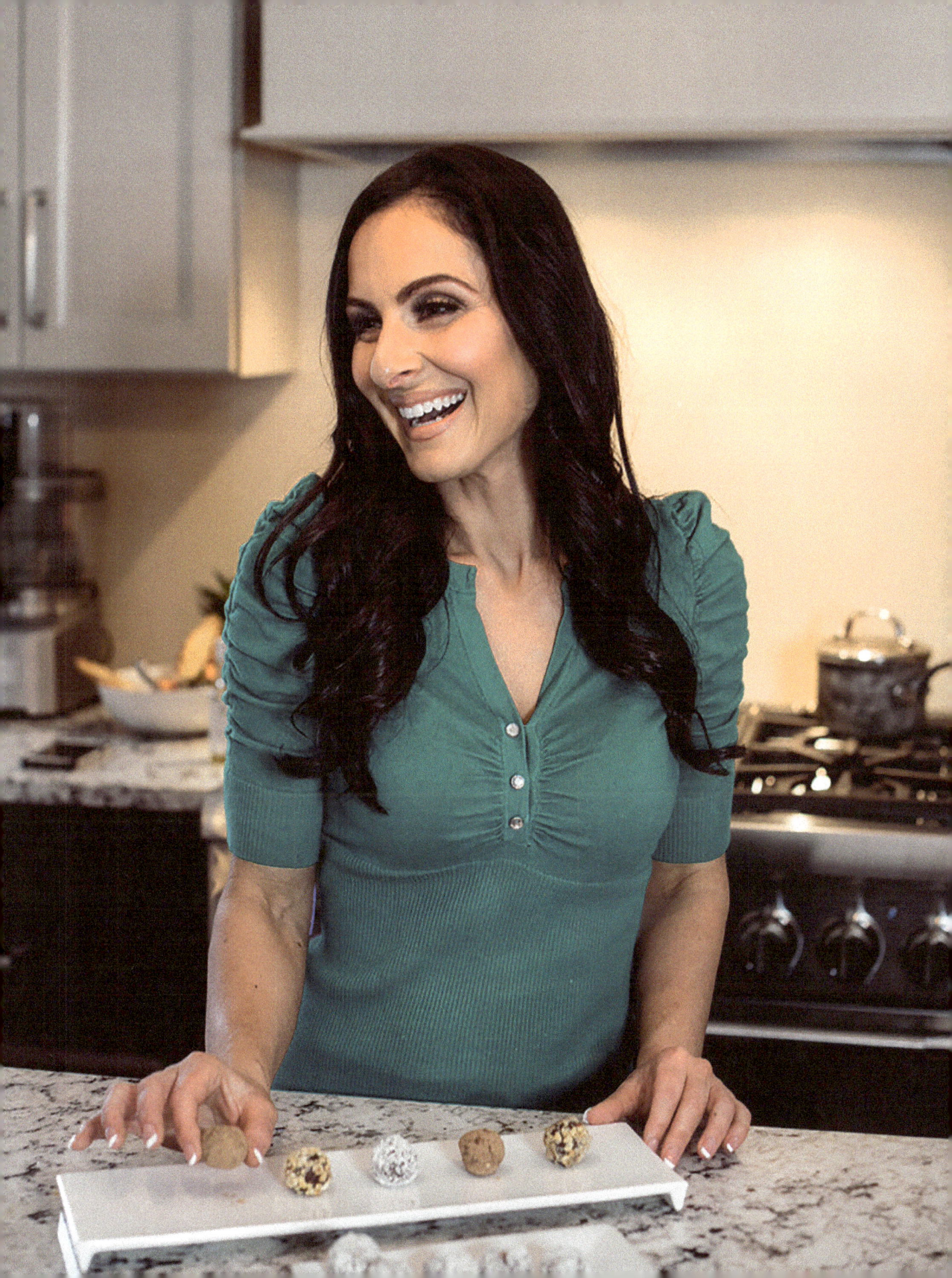

Let's Sweeten it Up a Bit!

"Once on the lips forever on the hips." Remember that one? Geez, no wonder we are all scared of dessert. It's so dramatic. I mean, FOREVER? Calm down everyone! Food should never be feared or looked at like a punishment. It should be appreciated and enjoyed with the simple rule of MODERATION. One of the biggest tips I tell my clients is DON'T DIET. Yes, you heard me, I do not believe in diets. What I do believe in is moderation. I firmly believe that if you exercise regularly, regularly eat nutritious and healthy meals, and live a healthy lifestyle overall; there is no reason you cannot enjoy sweets guilt-free once in a while. Even better, these days there are many healthy alternative recipes we can use to swap out the original, unhealthy ones.

One of my favorite quotes is from inspirational speaker Jim Rohn. He said, *"Success is nothing more than a few simple disciplines, practiced every day."* This means the opposite would apply to failure, right? The more we repeat a bad behavior, the more likely we will keep failing. I apply this rule to weight loss. If you are overeating every day and never get your tush off your couch, then sure, you may start wearing those cookies on your hips. But if you are 85-90% doing the right actions for being healthy, a sweet treat will be just that: a treat.

PROTEIN-PACKED CHOCOLATE MOUSSE

What if I told you that you could enjoy chocolate mousse without the guilt and the pounds of sugar? What if I told you that you could have a chocolate mousse that was nutrition packed and high in protein? Your wish is my command! The thickening agent in this recipe is one of the world's favorite superfoods, avocado! The great thing about avocado is it really takes on whatever flavor you add to it, so it is a great thickening agent for powdered nutrition shakes as well. To gain some of the creaminess, we added a little yogurt. And of course, what would chocolate mousse be without some real chocolate?

 Prep time: 15-20 minutes   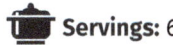 **Servings:** 6

Ingredients

- ½ cup extra-dark, bitter-sweet chocolate morsels (melted)
- 2 avocados (removed from skin)
- 1 scoop chocolate protein powder (1.5 oz.)
- ½ cup 0% fat Greek yogurt
- ½ cup almond milk
- ¼ cup agave nectar
- ¼ tsp. salt
- 1 tsp. vanilla
- 1 cup strawberries for garnish (halved)
- soy whipped cream

Directions

- In a small saucepan on low heat, melt chocolate chip morsels. Be sure to stir frequently to avoid burning.
- In a food processor or blender, combine your melted chocolate with the avocados, chocolate protein powder, yogurt, almond milk, agave nectar, salt, and vanilla. Process until smooth and creamy, about 1 minute.
- Transfer to a bowl and cover and refrigerate 4-6 hours or overnight for a firmer mousse, or you can eat right away if you just can't wait!
- Serve with a swirl of soy whipped cream and a strawberry garnish.

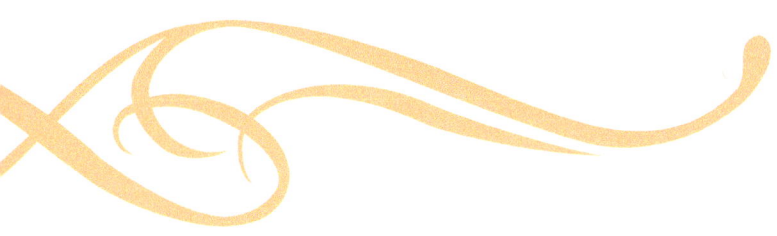

MANGO, STRAWBERRY & MINT SALAD

Can you say fresh? OMG this salad is so vibrant and refreshing it is a must at your next girls' brunch date. Make this for your guests or bring to their house, and watch them smile after each bite. The sweetness of the fruit and the freshness of the mint make this dish the perfect fruit blend.

Prep time: 15-20 minutes   **Servings:** 6

Ingredients

- 3 very ripe mangos (diced)
- 3 cups strawberries (quartered)
- ½ cup loosely packed mint (finely chopped)
- 1 tsp. freshly squeezed lemon juice
- 1 tsp. pure vanilla extract
- 1 tsp. agave nectar

Directions

- In a medium-sized bowl combine mangos, strawberries, and mint.
- Add all other remaining ingredients and toss to combine.

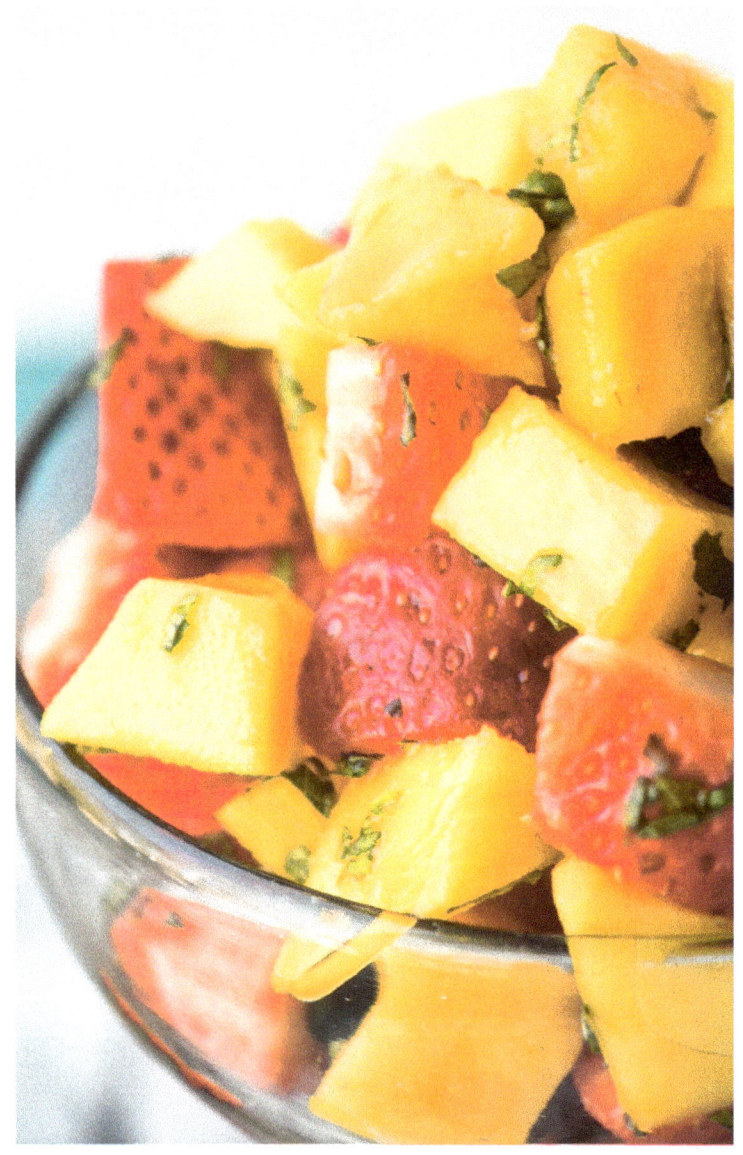

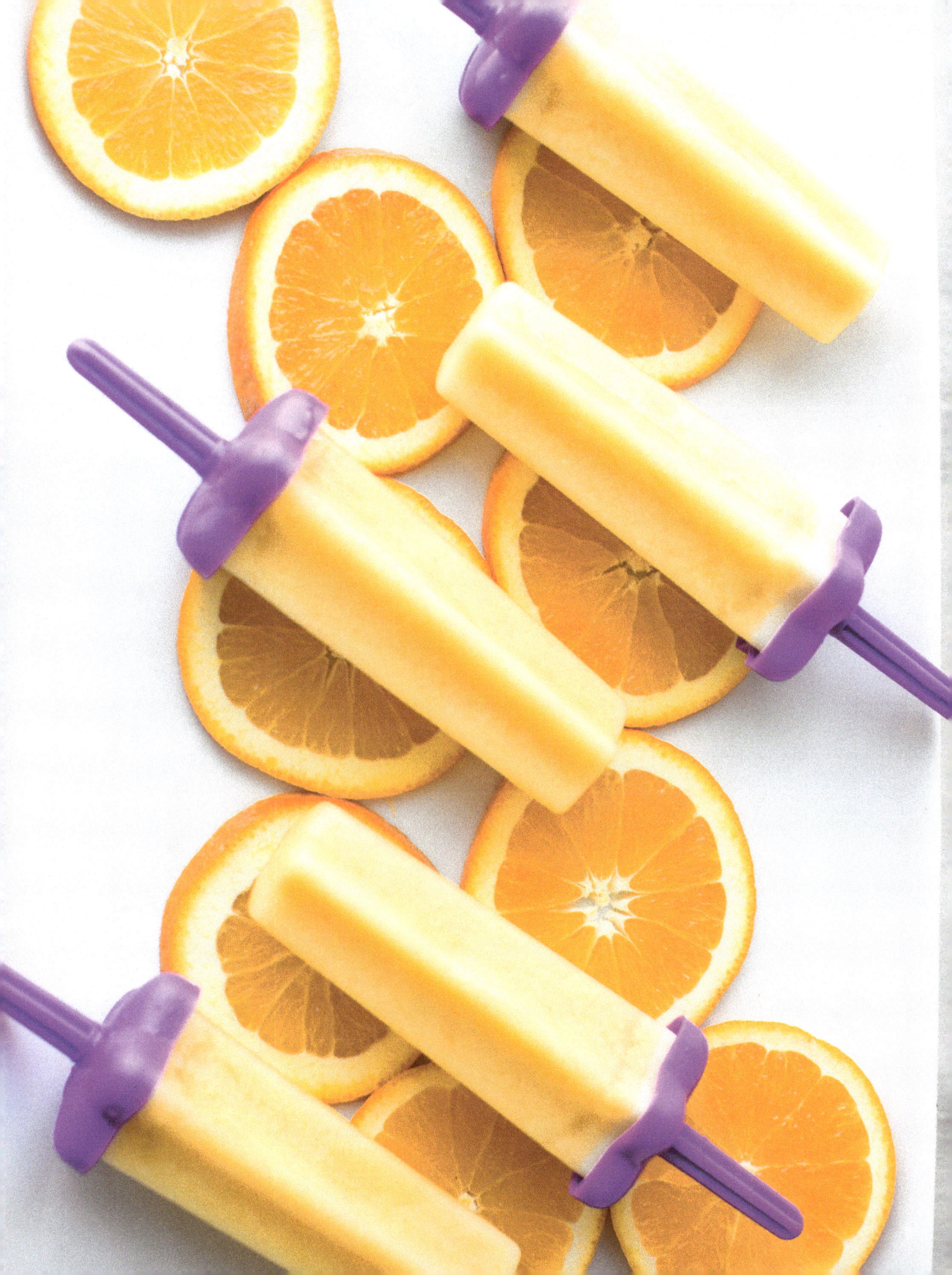

Danielle Formaro

ORANGE CREAMSICLE POPSICLES

Traditional Creamsicle recipes were made with well ... cream! The secret to lightening this up, without losing that creamy taste, is to add Greek yogurt. I tested these out on many kids, not telling them they were healthy and a great source of calcium (imagine their faces?), and to my delight they all LOVED them.

 Prep time: 15 minutes, plus overnight to freeze   **Servings:** makes 10 large popsicles or 20 small ones

Ingredients

- 6 navel oranges (juiced)
- ½ cup almond milk
- ½ cup 0% plain Greek yogurt
- 1 tsp. vanilla
- 2 tbsp. agave nectar

Directions

- Combine all ingredients in a blender, and mix well until yogurt is fully dissolved. If mixture gets a little foamy, you can skim the foam off with a spoon before pouring. Pour into popsicle molds, freeze overnight, and enjoy the next day.

> **TIP:**
>
> You can use regular orange juice but the flavor won't be as yummy as fresh squeezed juice as it is much sweeter.

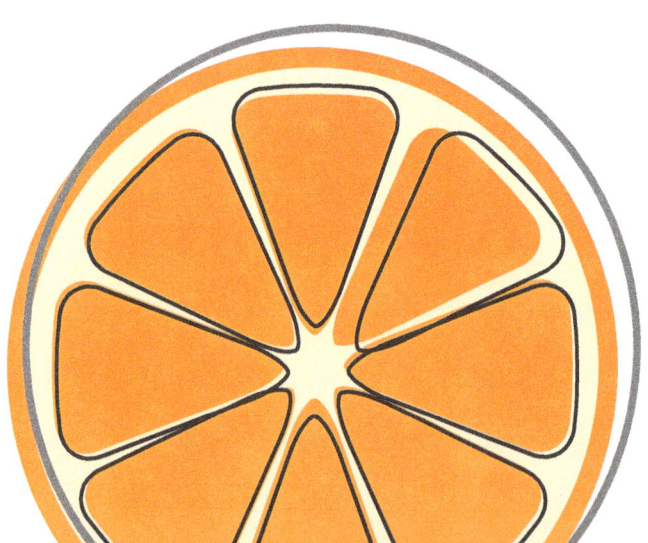

APPLE, HONEY & RAISIN

This is probably the simplest dessert you have ever seen but one of the most delectable. Apples have always been said to be nature's candy, and it's true! The natural sugar cider taste of the apple with a drizzle of honey and a sprinkle of raisins is just finger licking, sticky good!

 Prep time: 10 minutes 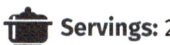 **Servings:** 2

Ingredients

- 1 apple (cored and sliced)
- raw organic honey (melted)
- ½ cup raisins

Directions

- Core and slice apple.
- Drizzle honey over slices.
- Garnish over the top with raisins.

VANILLA FROZEN YOGURT

Vanilla yogurt is always nice to have on hand simply because it goes with everything. It is a nice source of calcium and is just so refreshing on a hot summer night. Throw some fresh, homemade granola on top and you have really got something pretty yummy! The great thing about this recipe is it is actually best served right after you add it to the ice cream maker. It will be soft like a soft serve until you freeze it in the freezer.

 Total prep time: 10 minutes   **Servings:** 6-8

Ingredients

- 3 cups 0% fat plain Greek yogurt
- ¼ cup coconut milk
- ¼ cup agave nectar
- 1 tbsp. pure vanilla extract

Directions

- In a bowl, combine all ingredients. Transfer to an ice cream maker, and follow instructions from manufacturer.

BANANA AND NUTELLA MUFFINS

I couldn't write this book without one recipe containing Nutella. What is better than Nutella? Nutella and banana! These wonderful muffins will remind you of a sweet, chocolate-banana bread.

Prep time: 25 minutes   **Total time:** 40 minutes   **Servings:** 6 large muffins or 12 small muffins

Ingredients

- 2 cups organic whole-wheat flour
- 1 tsp. baking soda
- 1 tsp. baking powder
- ½ tsp. salt
- ¼ cup pure grade A maple syrup
- ¼ cup organic agave nectar
- 1 egg (beaten)
- 2 tsp. pure vanilla
- ¼ cup olive oil
- ¼ cup almond milk
- 4 very ripe bananas (mashed)
- ¾ cup Nutella (warmed)

Directions

- Pre-heat oven to 350°F.
- In a medium-sized bowl, mix together flour, baking soda, baking powder, and salt.
- In a small bowl, mix together maple syrup, agave nectar, egg, vanilla, olive oil, and almond milk.
- Slowly pour the wet mixture into the dry mixture and combine. Mix in mashed bananas.
- Spray a non-stick 12-hole muffin tin with non-stick spray, or you can line with paper muffin liners.
- Gently pour muffin mixture into each cup holder and leave a little room at the top for the Nutella drizzle.
- Be sure Nutella is melted and warm so that it is easier to swirl. Take about 1 tsp. of Nutella and pour into the center of each muffin. With a toothpick, swirl the Nutella gently through each muffin.
- Bake for 15-20 minutes, or until a toothpick comes out clean after inserting it into the center of the muffin.

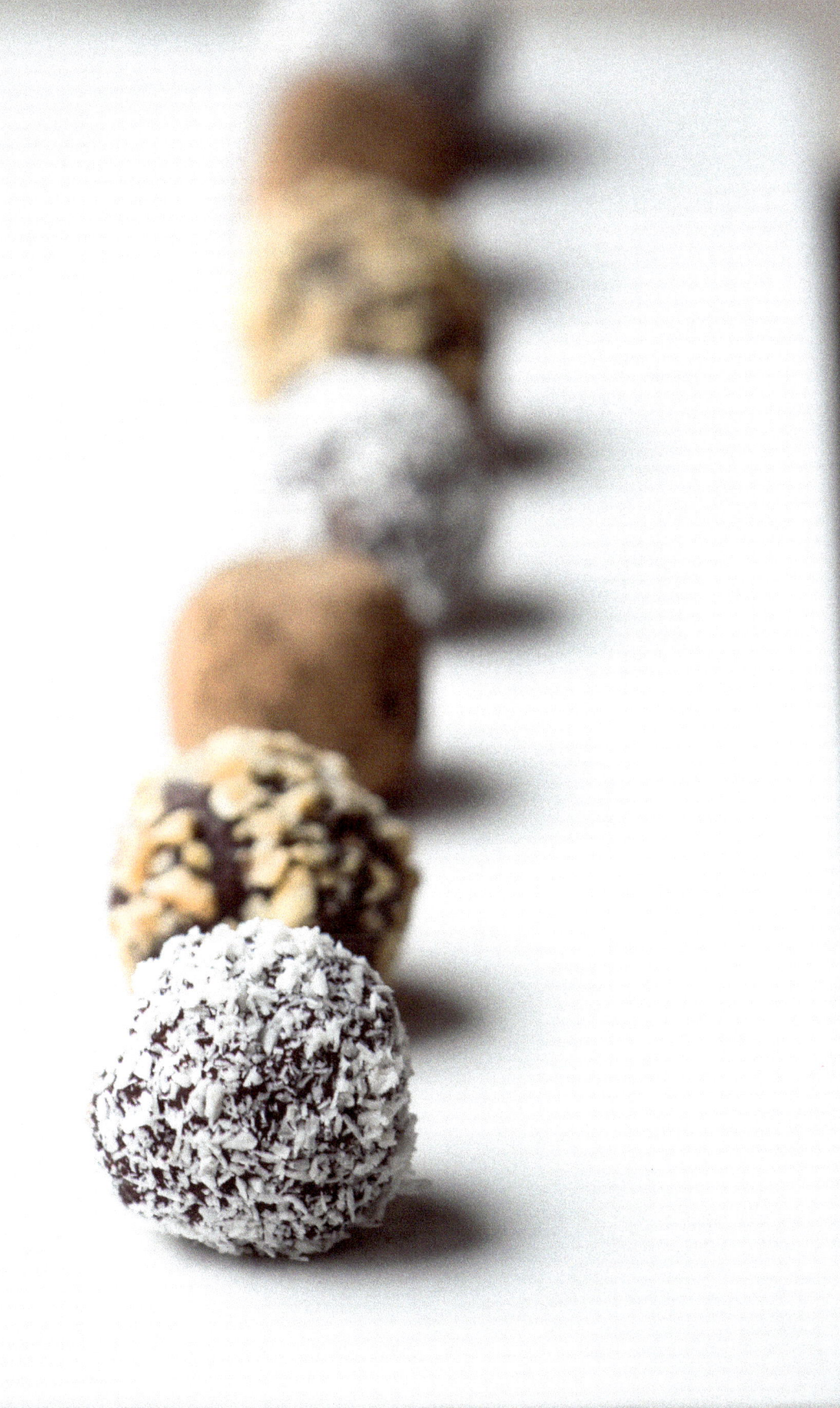

DECADENT CHOCOLATE TRUFFLES

Forget diamonds, I think chocolate is truly a girl's best friend. Looking for a healthier version of the original? Try these date-based truffles and don't be afraid to have them with a small glass of red wine. You deserve it!

 Prep time: about 20 minutes   **Servings:** makes about 20-25 truffles

Ingredients

- 2 cups Medjool dates (pits removed)
- ½ cup peanuts or hazelnuts
- ½ cup almond unbleached flour/meal
- ⅓ cup extra dark chocolate morsels
- 3 tbsp. cocoa powder
- 1 tsp. vanilla
- 1 tsp. raw honey
- ⅛ tsp. salt

Optional Garnish Rolling Toppings

- ½ cup shredded coconut
- ½ cup cocoa powder
- ½ cup crushed peanuts or hazelnuts

Directions

- Soak dates in warm water for about 10 minutes to soften them up a little.
- In a food processor, add peanuts or hazelnuts and almond flour and process until a fine powder.
- In a small saucepan, melt the chocolate morsels. Stir frequently so chocolate does not burn.
- Then add the medjool dates, melted chocolate, cocoa powder, vanilla, raw honey, and salt to flour mixture in the food processor. Process mixture until combined. It will form a sticky dough-like texture.
- Scoop a tablespoon of the mixture into your hands and form a small ball. Roll lightly in either coconut or cocoa powder and place on a tray. Repeat this process until all the mixture is gone. Place tray in freezer for about 15 minutes or until the truffles harden up and are not sticking together.
- Transfer to an airtight container and store in refrigerator until you are ready to eat.

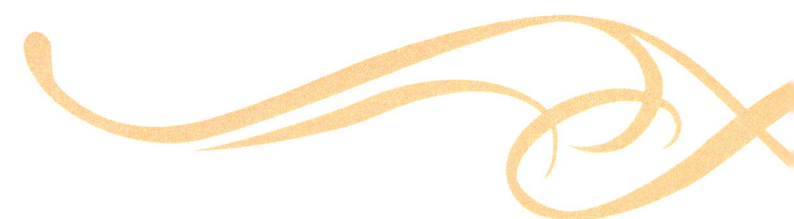

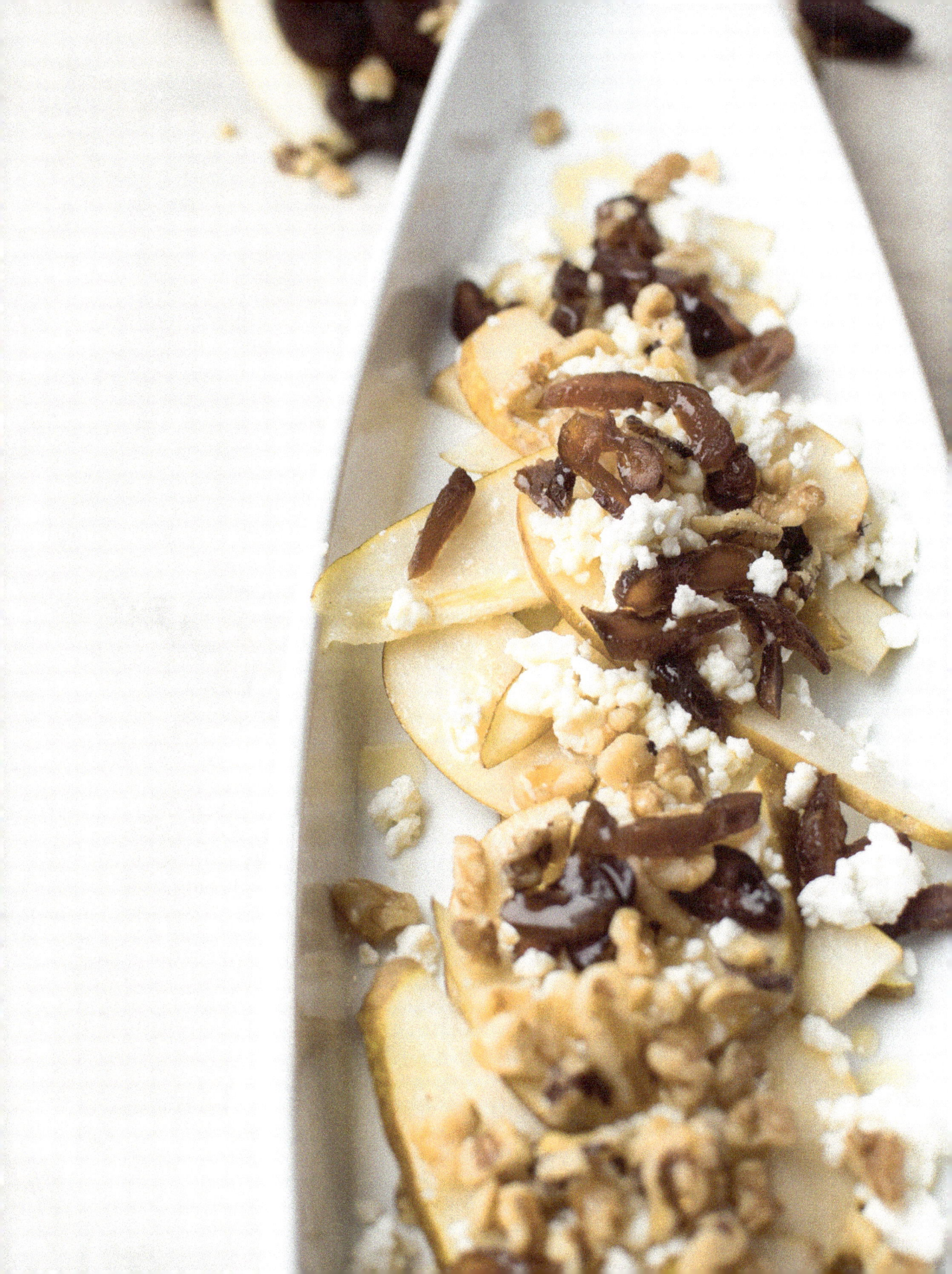

Danielle Formaro

PEAR WITH GOAT CHEESE, HONEY, TURKISH APRICOTS, AND PECANS

This is a dessert that you serve when you want to be a Miss Fancy Pants. I almost want to call this healthy dessert porn. The flavors marry each other so nicely and eating it is almost like an art. The sweetness of the pear with the creaminess of the goat cheese is just delightful. Top it off with the rest of the ingredients and the rest is history.

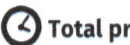 **Total prep time:** 10 minutes   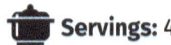 **Servings:** 4

Ingredients

- 2 pears (peeled, cored, and sliced)
- 3-4 oz. soft fresh crumbled goat cheese
- 6 Turkish apricots (finely chopped)
- 12 chopped pecans
- 2 tbsp. raw organic honey

Directions

- On a flat dish, align sliced pears across the plate.
- Layer with crumbled goat cheese.
- Layer with chopped Turkish apricots.
- Sprinkle the top with chopped pecans.
- Evenly drizzle honey over the entire dish.

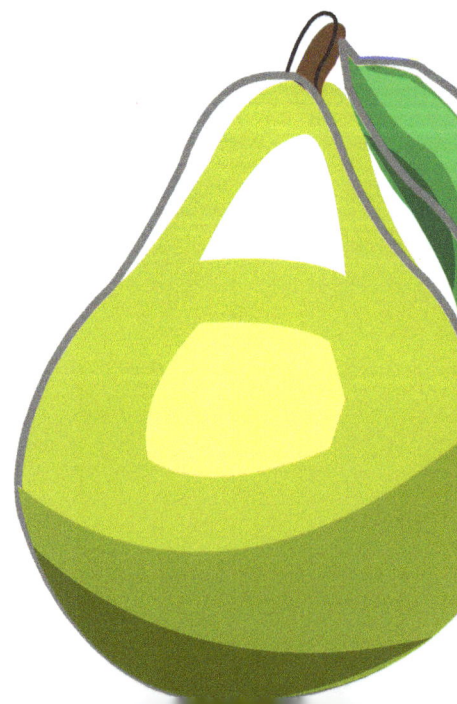

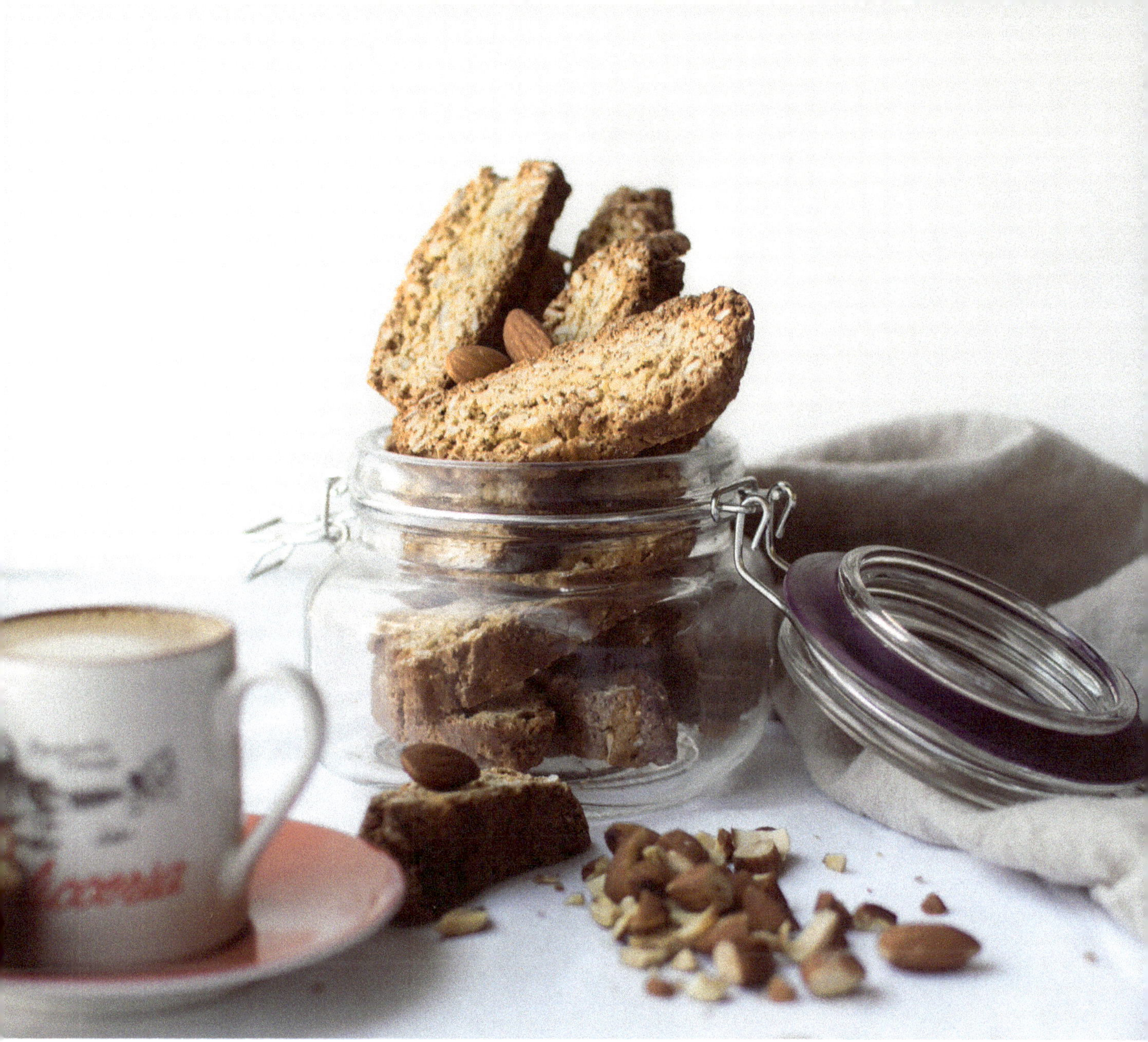

ALMOND BISCOTTI

I love having Italian cookies with my coffee but not necessarily all the sugar. Every time I go to the bakery I have to pick these up. The only problem is they are not necessarily the healthiest cookie. So I decided to create a lightened-up version that did the trick.

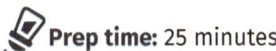 **Prep time:** 25 minutes   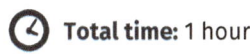 **Total time:** 1 hour   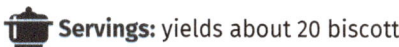 **Servings:** yields about 20 biscotti

Ingredients

- 3 cups roasted whole almonds
- 1 (16 oz.) package of almond flour/meal
- ¾ cup wheat flour
- ½ tsp. ground cinnamon
- 2 tsp. baking powder
- 3 jumbo eggs (beaten)
- 2 tsp. pure vanilla extract
- ¼ cup agave nectar
- ¼ cup raw organic honey
- zest of 1 large orange (about 1-2 teaspoons)
- one more egg, lightly beaten for brushing tops of loaves

Directions

- Pre-heat oven to 350°F.
- Line two large sheets with parchment paper.
- Place almonds in a single layer on a baking sheet and toast in the oven at 350°F for 10 minutes. Remove and set aside.
- In a large bowl, hand mix toasted almonds, almond flour, wheat flour, cinnamon, and baking powder.
- In a small bowl, whisk eggs. Add the vanilla, agave nectar, raw honey and orange zest, then whisk until well blended.
- Add wet mixture to the flour mixture. Work the batter together with lightly floured hands. The mixture will be sticky; you can also use an electric mixer if you have one. Keep squeezing the batter with your hands until a dough starts to form. Once the dough is firm, form a ball. Divide the ball into four equal pieces.
- On a lightly floured surface, take one of the 4 pieces of dough, and using your hands, roll into a log shape that is approximately 8 inches long, 2 inches wide, and ¾ of an inch high. Repeat with remaining three pieces of dough. Place two logs per baking sheet.
- Beat the remaining egg. Then Brush tops of each log with the egg mixture.
- Bake for 40 minutes, or until the tops of the loaves are shiny and deep golden.
- Cool on a rack for about 20 minutes before slicing.
- While the biscotti is cooling, reduce the oven temperature to 250°F.
- Place a loaf on a cutting board, and using a large serrated knife, slice cookies ¾ of an inch thick on the diagonal. If the cookie is crumbling, then let it cool a few more minutes. Don't let it rest too long, however, or they could become too hard to slice.
- Place slices back onto the baking sheets on their sides. Place in the oven and roast 5 minutes on each side. If you wish to have them even harder, you can turn off the heat in the oven and let rest in oven for an additional 25-30 minutes to the desired hardness.

APPLE CRUMBLE WITH VANILLA FROZEN YOGURT

I love this dessert in the fall. We all love apple pie and crumble, but may not like the calories that come along with it. So for you, I created a lightened-up version that is still just as pleasing. There's nothing better than a combo of creaminess and a crunch.

Ingredients

For the Apples
- 4 tbsp. butter
- 2 red apples (such as Gala) (peeled, cored, and sliced)
- ¼ tsp. cinnamon

Vanilla Frozen Yogurt:
See recipe on page 218

Crunchy Granola:
See recipe on page 110-111

Directions

- Prepare frozen yogurt.
- Prepare granola and put aside.
- In a medium-sized frying pan on medium, melt the butter.
- Add diced apple and cook and stir occasionally on medium-high until they become soft (about 6 minutes), then add cinnamon. Once cooked and soft, remove and turn off flame.
- In a small bowl, prepare the apple crumble. Take one scoop of vanilla frozen yogurt and place in bowl. Top with a few spoonfuls of your cooked apples, then sprinkle the top with your homemade granola.

Danielle Formaro

NECTARINE, HEIRLOOM TOMATO, AND MINT SALAD

This was my mom's creation, and it is fabulous. Something about the acidity of the tomato and the sweetness of the nectarine just works. This is a unique blend that is refreshing and will add some convo at the table.

Prep time: 10 minutes   **Servings:** 4

Ingredients

- 2 white nectarines (peeled and sliced)
- 2 heirloom tomatoes (cored, sliced)
- 1 tbsp. white balsamic vinegar
- 2 tbsp. light olive oil
- salt and pepper

Directions

- Combine all ingredients in a bowl, toss, and refrigerate for one hour to marinate. Serve chilled.

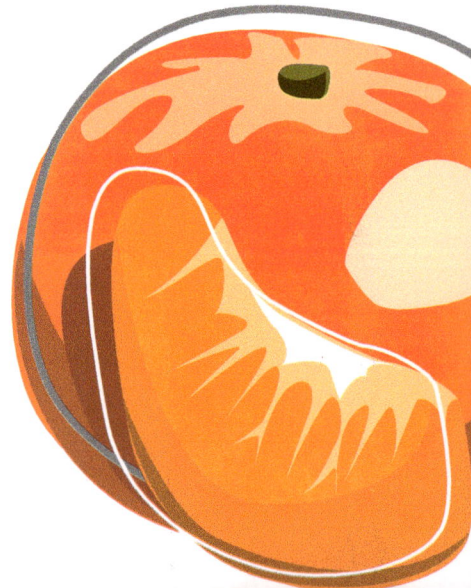

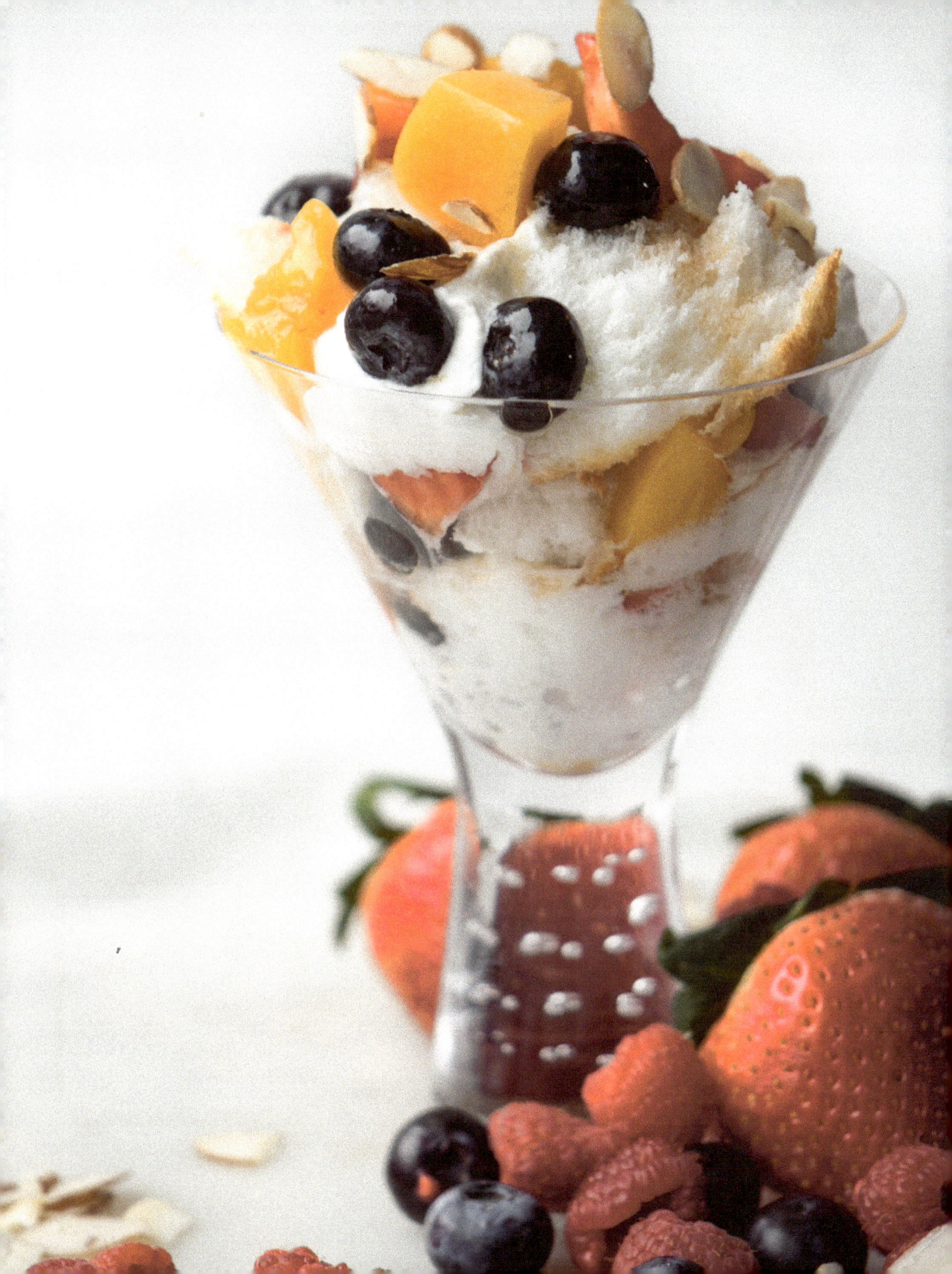

ANGEL FRUIT TRIFLE

For decades, angel food cake has been known as the diet-friendly cake. It gets its lift from beaten egg whites. No egg yolks and no butter mean the cake contains no fat. Without the fat, the cake is also lower in calories than say pound cakes, cupcakes, or ice cream. Although it does contain sugar, it is still a lighter option than your chocolate cake and buttery chocolate chip cookies, although I know those are delicious! I do love angel food cake simply because it is a neutral tasting cake that can be paired with any type of fruit. So by all means, mix and match your fruits of choice and enjoy.

 Prep time: 25 minutes 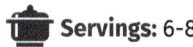 **Servings:** 6-8

Ingredients

- 3 cups strawberries (halved, stems removed)
- 3 cups raspberries
- 1 cup blueberries
- 1 cup jarred organic sliced peaches (drained and diced)
- 2 tbsp. agave nectar
- 1 tsp. vanilla
- 1 (10 oz.) angel food cake cut into chunks
- 2 (16 oz.) containers of soy whipped cream or low-fat whipped cream
- 1 cup sliced almonds, toasted

Directions

◎ In a bowl, combine strawberries, raspberries, blueberries, peaches, agave nectar, and vanilla. Let stand for 10 minutes. So fruit becomes glossy.

◎ Line bottom of a 12-cup trifle dish with one-third of angel cake chunks. Layer with 2 cups fruit mixture and then 2 cups soy whipped cream. Repeat layering process until all product is finished (about 2 more times).

◎ Cover with plastic wrap. Refrigerate until all juices have absorbed into cake, about 2-3 hours. Sprinkle with almonds before serving.

PRESENTATION TIP:

You can also layer in small Mason jars or other glass cup of choice for a little extra-cute presentation!

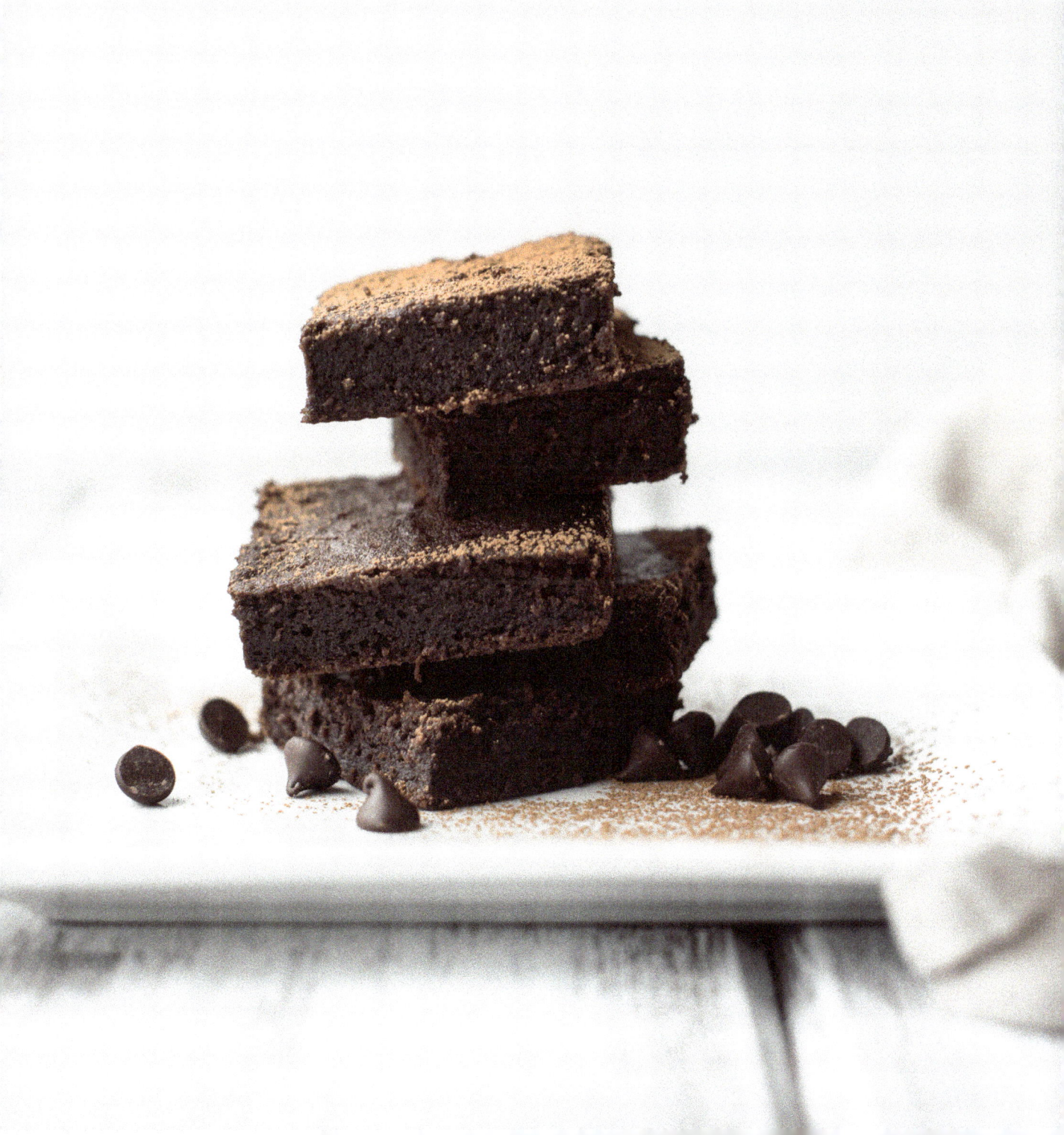

DECADENT FLOURLESS CHOCOLATE PEANUT BUTTER BROWNIES

Chocolate and peanut butter will never go out of style. It is just a match made in heaven. The great thing about these lightened-up brownies is that they are rich enough that a small serving will do. Most of the time we just need a nibble to satisfy a sweet craving. The richer in taste or the darker the chocolate is, I personally find I need less of it as well which is always wonderful for portion control.

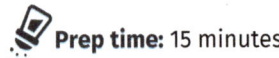 **Prep time:** 15 minutes   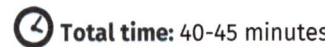 **Total time:** 40-45 minutes   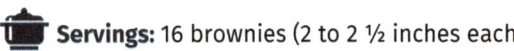 **Servings:** 16 brownies (2 to 2 ½ inches each)

Ingredients

- 6 tbsp. coconut oil
- 1 cup dark chocolate morsels
- ¼ cup unsweetened cocoa powder
- 3 tbsp. cornstarch
- ¼ tsp. salt
- 1 tsp. baking powder
- 2 eggs (beaten)
- ¼ cup raw organic honey
- 2 tsp. vanilla
- 4 oz. organic applesauce
- ½ cup natural peanut butter

Directions

- Preheat oven to 350°F.
- In a small saucepan, on low heat, add coconut oil and chocolate morsels, and mix together until fully melted. Turn off heat.
- In a small bowl, combine unsweetened cocoa powder, cornstarch, salt, and baking powder.
- In a medium-sized bowl, whisk together eggs, honey, vanilla, and applesauce. Add the dry mixture to the wet mixture, and whisk until blended.
- Then add the peanut butter and melted dark chocolate to the bowl, and whisk until fully combined and the mixture is smooth.
- In an 8 x 8-inch pan, line with parchment paper so that the brownies do not stick to the bottom and can be easily be removed, once baked.
- Pour brownie mixture into the pan, spreading evenly.
- Bake at 350°F for 18 minutes. Let rest for 15 minutes.
- Remove brownies by lifting parchment paper up from pan, and then resting them on cutting board.
- Cut into 4 even lines across and up and down.

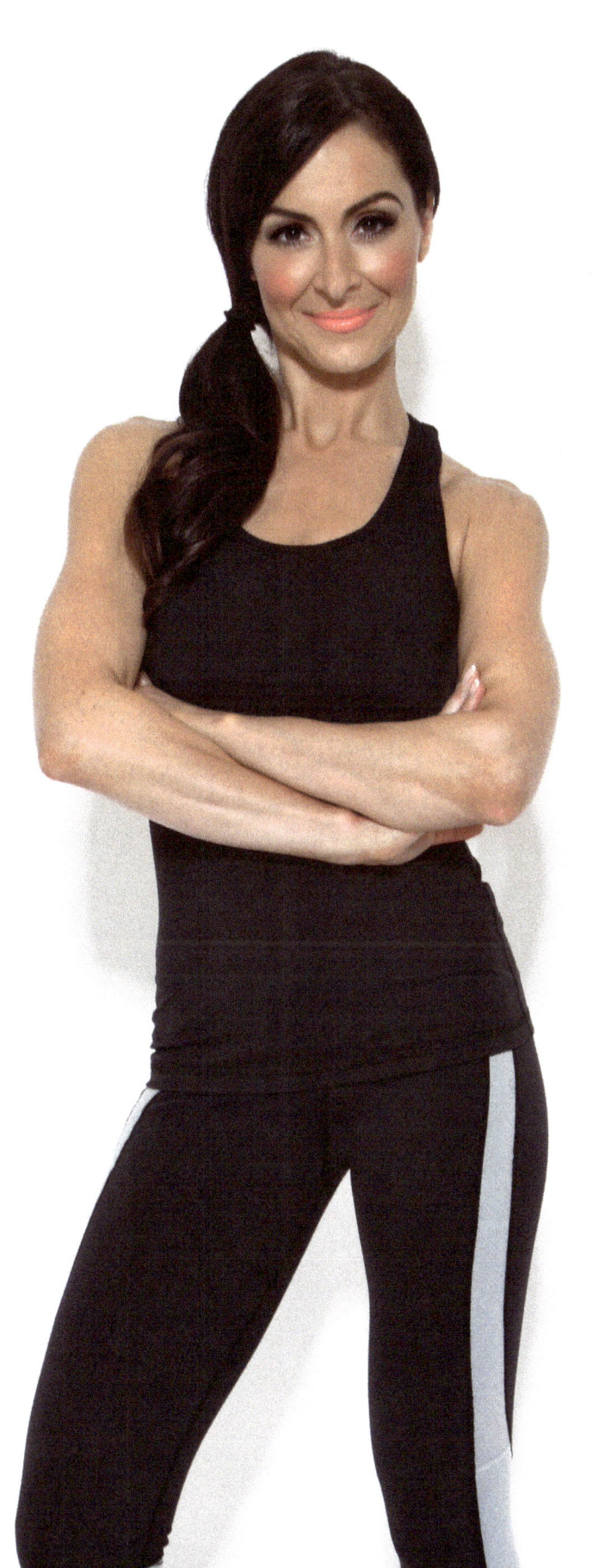

Add THIS to Your Plate!

Getting Back in the Saddle

#momproblems

In my opinion, nothing in the world is more amazing than being a mom. It is by far the hardest and most important job in the world. In fact, when I started going back to work again, my day job felt like a break, almost a short vacation. Motherhood takes a toll on us physically and mentally. Mentally, we are exhausted, and physically, we are left with a jiggly tush, possibly a belly button hernia, diastasis recti, and a weak bladder that gives you a wet surprise every time a sneeze occurs. The struggle is real! You feel as though you will never have a moment alone ever again. The thought of sleep seems like a distant memory. Going to the grocery store alone now feels like a treat! In fact, I vividly remember the first time I went to the grocery store alone a few months after my son was born. *"Praise the Lord!"* I felt like I had died and gone to Aisle 9 heaven. It was amazing to say the least.

Once we get the physical clearance from the doctor, the first mission we all seem to want to tackle is to reclaim that pre-baby body. We just want to feel sexy again rather than a giant, wet burp cloth. The challenge comes into play with this simple question: "When will I find the time and energy?"

Let's be honest for a minute. If someone said to you, "I will give you a million dollars if you lose twenty pounds in three months," would you do it? I bet you would haul some major ass and kick those pounds to the curb. So my point is, we can all figure it out if we really want to, but we have to believe that we can do it. We can't make excuses. Excuses are lies we tell ourselves so that it doesn't have to be our fault. Don't make excuses about why you can't find the time to take care of yourself; just get the ball rolling and don't look back.

We discussed effective time management previously in this book, so you have the tools to create an effective schedule. Now it's time to put it to use. I will tell you that it will not be easy, but with the right mindset and support, it can be done.

The biggest challenge you have in life is changing your thinking. The first part of the body I train with my clients is their mind—their ways of thinking. If we can train our mind that we can do anything, the sky is the limit. Believe that YOU DESERVE IT and that YOU ARE WORTH IT. When Mom feels good, Mom is happy. When Mom is happy, your positivity will be infectious. You are the main energy source in your home. You have mighty powers. You are a mighty mamma! Believe it or not, without you, nothing else will function. Your family needs you, so it is important that you take care of yourself. You will be faced with an array of new mom problems, but it will be ok, you just have to take things one step at a time. Remember, you are only human after all and this emotional roller coaster is all part of the ride.

Training the Mind Through Personal Development

As a lifestyle and fitness coach, one of the vital behaviors of my business is personal development. Personal development (PD) is food for the brain. You may be thinking to yourself, "Are you crazy? I don't have the time or energy to read." You are right, but I bet you have time to listen to some audio in the car, while you shower, while you cook the amazing recipes in this book, or perhaps while you do your makeup? I have always found traffic hour is a great time to listen to my PD resources. See how many opportunities you have? You can finish one book a week by doing this. Imagine how many you can read in a year.

According to Darren Hardy, author of *The Compound Effect,* 88% of very wealthy people spend 30 minutes or more reading to learn every day. Only a small percentage of those with lower incomes do this. Interesting, right? Still think you don't have time to listen to some audio? You bet your ass you can!

So what should you be listening to? Well, this is up to you! When it comes to training your mind, you have to figure out what your challenge is. What do you wish to be better at? If your challenge is motivation, then you will need to get some PD on how to be self-motivated. If you want to learn how to resist temptation, then buy some audio on that. Perhaps you have low confidence? Then you had better buy some audio on how to build confidence. One of my favorites is Jen Sincero's *You are a Bad Ass*. That will get your mindset back in the saddle! I am also a huge Chalene Johnson fan; I just love her.

You must be relentless about your goals. Establish a strong "why" or reason you want to conquer these goals, and write it down on sticky notes. Post them all over the house. I love the phrase, "Your why should make you cry." If your why is this strong, you will never give up. I have said this many times: it will be hard. I, too, understand it is hard to find the time and energy to work out, but it is even harder to not like who you see in the mirror each day. You will need to choose your *hard* and choose it wisely. Remember to strive for progress, and not perfection, as there is no such thing. Perfection is a reality that we create as individuals, something to always remember. Be proud of who you are and strive to be your personal best. You can do it!

Once and for All, the Truth about Weight Loss and Carbs

I bet your eyes immediately ran to this section. I don't blame you! Our changed bodies are probably one of the hardest things to accept postpartum. The good news is, you can get your old body back! Repeat after me: YES. I. CAN.

The most common way to lose weight is a simple calculation: you must put out more calories than you are taking in. There, of course, are many other contributing factors as well such as how often we eat, our hormones, and the way we combine our foods. In fact in my weight-loss program called "FROM SCRATCH," you actually are REQUIRED to eat carbs with every meal! Amazing right? But it is all about choosing the right types of carbs and of course portion control. But for the sake of keeping it real simple, let's start with the basics. For example, if you were to download an app on your phone that can track the calories you are currently taking in, then for the next two months, create a 500-calorie deficit each day while implementing a daily exercise regimen, you could lose about one to two pounds per week. Pretty nice, right? Now hang on ... pounds are not everything; inches are even more important, as I will get into in a bit. The bottom line is, with this behavior repeated consistently, you will see results. It's your inconsistency that will hold you back, plain and simple. The other BIG mistake people make is they take this rule to the extreme and go in starvation mode, this is not good either, not eating enough (which I also teach in my weight loss program "FROM SCRATCH") can slow your metabolism causing weight loss as well. This is why a 500 decrease in calories is plenty for a healthy realistic maintainable weight loss.

Forget about all the fad diets telling you to not eat carbs and load up on high-saturated-fat proteins instead. You know what I am talking about. I'll bet you know people who are binge eating bacon because they were told they couldn't eat carbs. Let's get something straight: YOU NEED CARBS. This drives me nuts! They are your body's main source of energy. People get confused and think all carbs are bad, but know there are many types of carbs. Bagels, chips, soda, and white bread are not the only ones that exist. So let's clear the air, shall we?

We have complex carbs (from vegetables, whole grains, pasta, beans, rice, and cereals) and simple carbs (sugar, including glucose from fruit and vegetables, lactose from milk, and sucrose from cane and beet sugars). In recent years, low-carbohydrate diets have been widely advocated by bestselling authors. Unfortunately, studies show that in the average American diet, carbohydrates contribute about half of those the calories, but most of these calories come from just eight sources: sodas, sweets, pizza, potato chips, white rice, white bread (and bagels, English muffins, buns, and rolls), beer, and French fries.

This type of diet is clearly not healthy and has low nutritional content. This can also lead to insulin resistance, which, in time, can lead to diabetes. Even if your body does not develop this resistance, the repeated rising and falling of insulin and blood sugar levels can set the stage for overeating as the brain sends out hunger signals in response to a sudden drop in blood sugar. This is why we have something called the glycemic index. It is a chart that ranks which carbohydrate foods may or may not cause an insulin surge and, eventually, pose a resistance problem.

But let's not give all carbohydrates a bad rap! Vegetables are amazing for us and, yes, they are carbs! White bread in large quantities may not be our best friend, but whole grains are wonderful. Not only do whole grains provide us with lots of nutrients, but they also aid in weight loss by keeping us full longer to slow the digestion factor, and by helping us cleanse out weight via the fiber. This is why you will see small changes in my recipes that, over time, can make a big impact on your weight management. I tend to swap white flour for whole-wheat flour, and I often replace white sugars with natural sweeteners, like honey or agave nectar, due to the rank on the glycemic index. Yes, they are still sugars, but our body responds better to natural sweeteners versus the processed ones. Now it's not to say you can't enjoy white pasta, now and again, but if you are trying to lose weight, limit your intake. Understand? Or as us Italians say ... *capisce*?

The other big problem with no-carb and high-protein diets is since protein is the last fuel source to burn in the body, consuming too much will create an excess, which usually turns into fat, not muscle. An athlete is the only person who may need to have additional protein due to the amount of energy they exert. Plus, protein excretes calcium, and too much-lost calcium can compromise bone health and cause stress on the kidneys. The average person needs to stay within reason and have a balanced diet in order to have the energy to get through their regular workouts. The more energy we have, the better we can perform, depending on what our goals are.

Ok, I will stop ranting on that. I hope you get the point of what I am saying, which is that too much of anything is no good, and extreme dieting is one of them. At the end of the day, you need to listen to your body more. I like to call this "Intuitive Eating." If something makes you feel good, do more of it. If something makes you feel lousy, then stop doing it! While some people may do well with limited carbs, some of us do better with more of them. While some people are vegetarians, this will not be a good option for all.

A lot of what your body needs also depends on your biological makeup and your genes! We are all created differently; therefore, we all have different needs. So stop listening to what people tell you and start listening to your gut (no pun intended). You will have to try a few things to see where you excel. Sometimes, you will need to remove certain things from your diet, but do this because of how it makes YOU feel, not because someone told you that you MUST do it. Does this make sense? My diet may not work for someone else, but it works for me. The general rule of thumb, however, is the simple science of caloric intake and watching this. Overall, if you can start to take action on what I mentioned above, you will see results.

The reality of the situation is that if you truly want to look and feel good forever, there is no magic pill. You must learn to lead a healthy lifestyle with balance and moderation for the rest of your life. I can tell you the longer you do it, the easier it will get. It will become second nature. This does not mean eating plain lettuce either. You have a book in your hands with pages of healthy family recipes, so hopefully, you have gained trust that eating healthy can be delicious! Even the dessert recipes have been lightened up, so things are already looking up! The key is portion *control*, which we will get into in just a bit.

No one said you should have to do this alone. As I mentioned above, I have actually developed a program just for us women called "FROM SCRATCH." In my program, I will teach you an easy method for losing weight and keeping it off, and guess what? We eat lots of carbs! The method teaches you how to create a positive mindset for motivation and provides a nutrition course on how to create fat-burning meals, with an array of fat-burning workouts to have you melting off the pounds. I also offer private coaching and a wonderful online community to give you all the support a woman needs. So if you feel you need some help to get you started, you have a great solution! Check out the first pages of this book for more info!

If you are looking to go the "do-it-yourself route," another great resource is https://www.choosemyplate.gov or http://www.foodpyramid.com/mypyramid/. These sites will go over caloric-intake needs based on your specific body type and lifestyle. It is a fantastic resource to really see what your plate should look like. To keep things even simpler, I can give you some easy tips on portion control in the next section as well.

Portion Control

Can you guess how many people were obese in America as of 2017? According to the National Institute of Diabetes, Digestive, and Kidney Diseases, more than two-thirds (**68.8 percent**) of adults are considered to be overweight or obese. The main reason is simply portion control. Below is a simple chart to help you practice portion control anytime and anywhere. If you are a working mom who eats out a lot, you can still stay in control. Here are the basic rules I teach in my weight loss program "FROM SCRATCH."

PROTEIN: Size of your palm and the thickness of a deck of cards.

FATS: Size of your thumb.

CARBS: The size of one fist!

VEGGIES: The size of your hands together open-palmed.

FRUITS: The size of one fist.

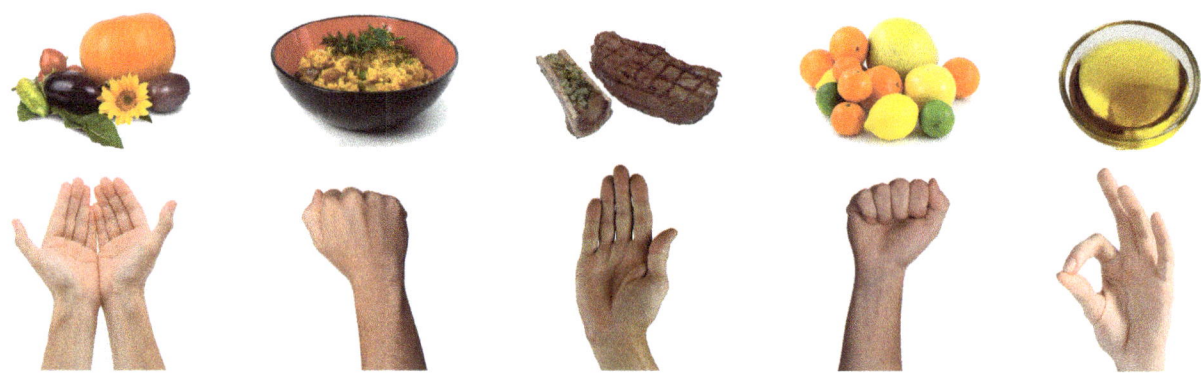

So now you are probably thinking, Ok, well how do I know how many of these portions I am supposed to have each day? Well, that all depends! Here is a sample guideline of what I do for my clients. Although individuals may need tweaking by a professional, this is just a basic outline that you can use that I find works for most. Also, I should preface it by stating that before you begin any new regimen your body is not used to, especially after pregnancy, you should always consult a physician.

BMI	19	20	21	22	23	24	25	26	27	28	29	30	31	32	33	34	35
Height							Weight in Pounds										
4'10"	91	96	100	105	110	115	119	124	129	134	138	143	148	153	158	162	167
4'11"	94	99	104	109	114	119	124	128	133	138	143	148	153	158	163	168	173
5'	97	102	107	112	118	123	128	133	138	143	148	153	158	163	158	174	179
5'1"	100	106	111	116	122	127	132	137	143	148	153	158	164	169	174	180	185
5'2"	104	109	115	120	126	131	136	142	147	153	158	164	169	175	180	186	191
5'3"	107	113	118	124	130	135	141	146	152	158	163	169	175	180	186	191	197
5'4"	110	116	122	128	134	140	145	151	157	163	169	174	180	186	192	197	204
5'5"	114	120	126	132	138	144	150	156	162	168	174	180	186	192	198	204	210
5'6"	118	124	130	136	142	148	155	161	167	173	179	186	192	198	204	210	216
5'7"	121	127	134	140	146	153	159	166	172	178	185	191	198	204	211	217	223
5'8"	125	131	138	144	151	158	164	171	177	184	190	197	203	210	216	223	230
5'9"	128	135	142	149	155	162	169	176	182	189	196	203	209	216	223	230	236
5'10"	132	139	146	153	160	167	174	181	188	195	202	209	216	222	229	236	243
5'11"	136	143	150	157	165	172	179	186	193	200	208	215	222	229	236	243	250
6'	140	147	154	162	169	177	184	191	199	206	213	221	228	235	242	250	258
6'1"	144	151	159	166	174	182	189	197	204	212	219	227	235	242	250	257	265
6'2'	148	155	163	171	179	186	194	202	210	218	225	233	241	249	256	264	272
6'3'	152	160	168	176	184	192	200	208	216	224	232	240	248	256	264	272	279
	Healthy Weight						Overweight					Obese					

1. First, I like to find out what my client's BMI is. BMI stands for Body Mass Index. Although it is not a perfect method and has some flaws, overall it is a good indicator of where you fall in your weight category. Again, there is always an exception to the rule where it may not be accurate (such as someone's height and body composition), but overall, it's a good tool. BMI is a person's weight in kilograms divided by the square of height in meters. The chart to the left was taken from health.gov is a basic guideline for where one would fall based on the calculation.

2. Now that you know where you fall, we can assess your goal. So depending on your goal, we can then take it to the next step, which would be to figure out how many calories you should be consuming per day. I take care of this part for all my online clients, but if you are doing this on your own, the easiest way to find this calculation is to go to https://www.supertracker.usda.gov which is the USDA guideline for weight loss depending on your age, sex, weight, and activity level. You can go on this free online source, create a profile and then get the information needed.

3. Lastly, you will need to now know how to break up those calories by food group. Again, this is where my clients and I figure out a meal plan that is the most efficient, by trial and error, in terms of what makes them feel the best and what is working. In my weight loss program "FROM SCRATCH" I took the guesswork out by creating an easy do-able system that anyone can follow. But should you want the do it yourself option, a great free tool you can use to figure out how many servings of each food group you should eat is available at https://www.choosemyplate.gov. These are the USDA's official guidelines. The guidelines are always changing, and each person's needs are different, therefore you can get an idea from this site to help you along.

Meal Prepping and Planning Ahead

Meal planning can really be a busy mom's best friend. Why? Because most likely, and if you are a working mom, *especially*, cooking every night may not be an option. For example, when I was working at the office all day (before I changed careers), I would take Sundays and Wednesdays as my cooking days. This way, I always had food in the fridge without having to cook from scratch every night. Let's face it, some nights, we are just too tired to do anything else. It's nice to have a grab-and-go dinner right at your fingertips.

Basically, the concept is to cook in bulk, enough for three to four days. Whether you are broiling a fillet or roasting an entire tenderloin, it shouldn't involve that much extra work or time. What it will do is open up a few evenings where you can put your feet up a little. Soups are also a really great option. They even taste better the next day as leftovers! You can also freeze them for a later time. I always have a chicken soup frozen for sickie emergencies.

The great news is the recipes in this book are, for the most part, four to six servings, and with soup recipes, even more. There should always be leftovers unless you have a Brady-Bunch-sized family. My suggestion is to pick a few entrees, a few sides, and a soup, and take a day to prepare them for the week. If you feel you need more than six servings to last a few days, you can always double the recipe. If cooking three days in advance is too much for you, rest assured that you should be able to get away with cooking every other night, since each meal should (unless you have a really large family) have leftovers. This is why the recipes in this book are meant to serve up to six portions. As I mentioned, I am Italian and Armenian, and we tend to supersize everything anyway.

Below is a sample of my weekly meal planners. (Yes, these simple recipes are in this book!) You will notice that a bunch of meals repeat themselves. It is because that week, I purchased only a few proteins, carbs, veggies, and fruit, and then prepared them all ahead of time, storing them in large Tupperware containers in my refrigerator. I only had to cook once that week. All everyone had to do was make a plate and reheat their food! I went food shopping on Saturday and prepped the Sunday before. I tend to eat out on the weekends, so this worked well for me. I was also eating on a specific calorie plan, so planning ahead was even more crucial. The reason we eat poorly, half the time, is because we wait until the last minute to eat and become so ravenous that the thought of cooking for an hour sounds like torture. So we resort to fast food or whatever snack is in the pantry. Sound familiar? If you have your good eats ready in a snap, it is more likely you will eat well, too!

Weekly Meal Plan
1,200 calories a day

SUNDAY	MONDAY	TUESDAY	WEDNESDAY	THURSDAY	FRIDAY	SATURDAY
	BREAKFAST	**BREAKFAST**	**BREAKFAST**	**BREAKFAST**	**BREAKFAST**	
Meal Prep Day	2 eggs with a serving of spinach and a half slice of dry wheat toast	1 cup steel cut oats with 1/2 banana and cinnamon	2 mini quiches with a cup of fruit	2 eggs with a serving of spinach and a half slice of dry wheat toast	Whole Wheat French Toast with serving of fresh fruit	Go Food Shopping
	SNACK	**SNACK**	**SNACK**	**SNACK**	**SNACK**	
Meal Prep Day	Apple with 1 tbsp. almond butter	Snack: Apple with 1 tbsp. peanut butter	Serving of raw unsalted nuts and a 0% fat free yogurt	Apple with almond butter	Apple with almond butter	Go Food Shopping
	LUNCH	**LUNCH**	**LUNCH**	**LUNCH**	**LUNCH**	
Meal Prep Day	Broiled salmon with broccoli & lemon and a serving of brown rice	Grilled chicken over garden salad with garlic/lemon dressing	Grilled flank steak with brussels sprouts and mediterranean quinoa salad	Baked Cod over Armenian bulgar wheat pilaf with broccoli	Broiled salmon with broccoli & lemon and a serving of brown rice	Go Food Shopping
	SNACK	**SNACK**	**SNACK**	**SNACK**	**SNACK**	
Meal Prep Day	Serving of nuts and a 0% fat greek yogurt	Serving of strawberry, mango & mint salad	Apple with almond butter	Serving of strawberry, mango & mint salad	Serving of nuts and a 0% fat greek yogurt	Go Food Shopping
	DINNER	**DINNER**	**DINNER**	**DINNER**	**DINNER**	
Meal Prep Day	Grilled flank steak with brussels sprouts and mediterranean quinoa salad	Broiled salmon with broccoli & lemon and a serving of brown rice	Baked Cod over Armenian bulgar wheat pilaf with broccoli	Grilled chicken over garden salad with garlic/lemon dressing	Grilled flank steak with brussels sprouts and mediterranean quinoa salad	Go Food Shopping

Danielle Formaro

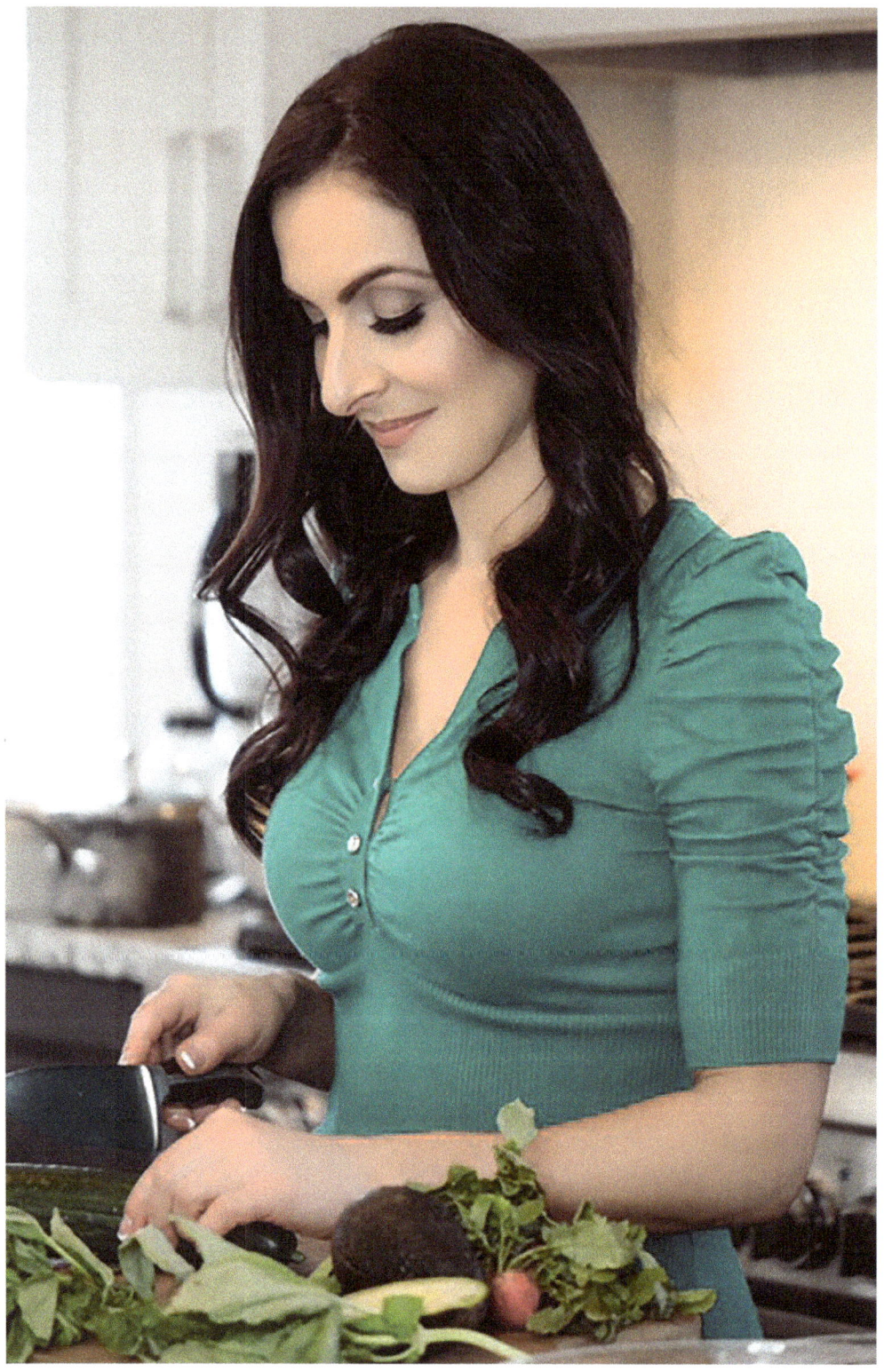

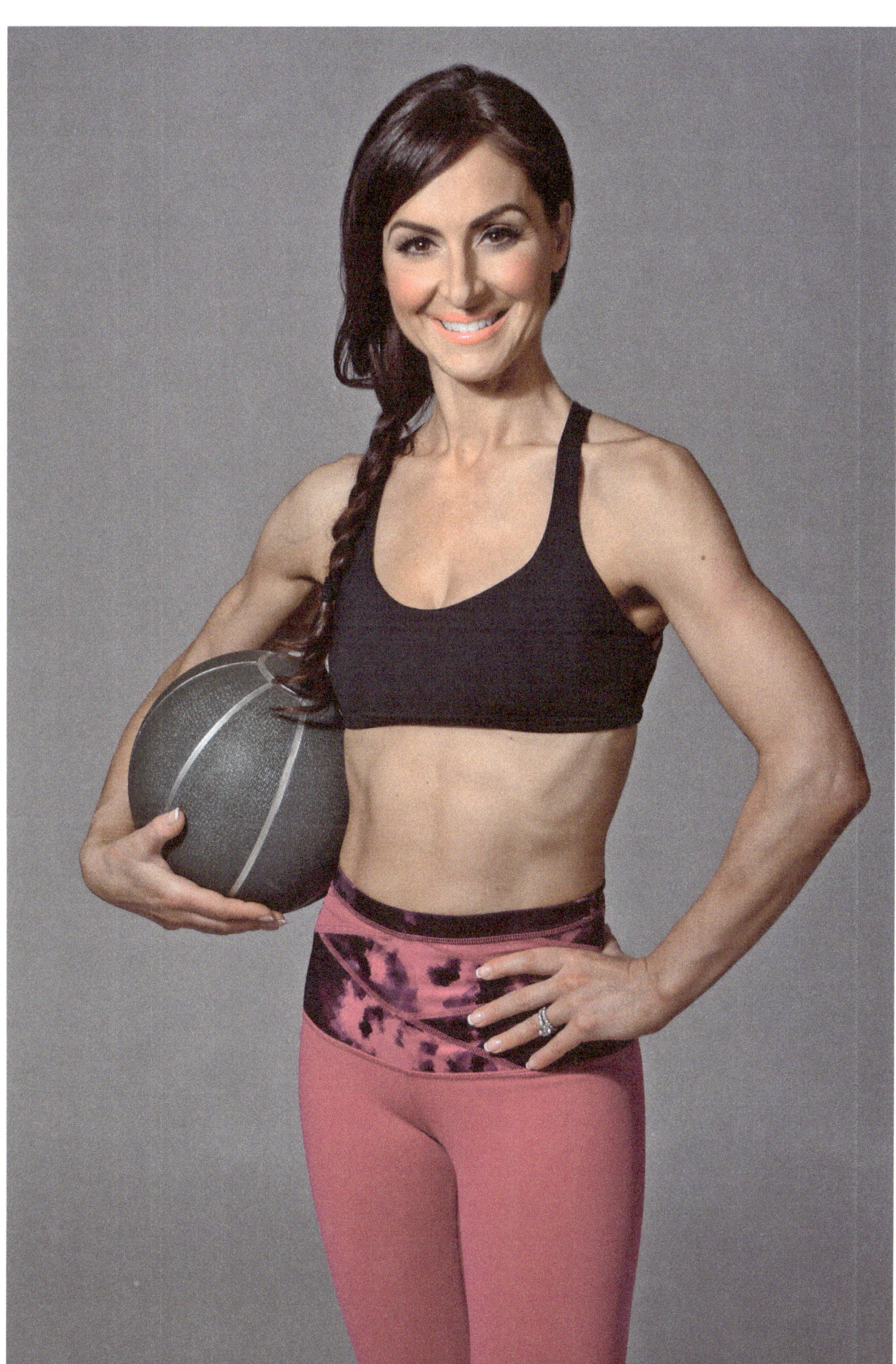

Finding a Fitness Program That Works for You

When it comes down to exercising, people either love it or hate it. Even the crazy people like myself who love super high-intensity workouts have days when motivation is a struggle. There are a few things you need to ask yourself when figuring out your plan.

1. What do you enjoy doing? With so many types of workouts these days, there truly is something for everyone. You can shake your tail feather or line dance like no one's business. It doesn't have to all be weight training and push-ups. Chances are, if you like what you are doing, you will continue to do it. It does not seem like rocket science, but I see it every day: people forcing themselves to do something they don't enjoy. It is no wonder they quit a week, or even days, later. No one likes to be tortured unless you are into that sort of thing. I'd rather save that for *Fifty Shades of Grey.* Right ladies? Wink, wink.

2. Figure out how much time you have to work out. If you only have twenty-five minutes a day, then don't pick a program or class that is sixty minutes. Find something that fits into your time schedule. Overall, we need either five days a week of moderate exercise or three days a week of something more high-intensity, if you are going to cut down the number of days a week you work out. I always give my clients an array of options from weights, martial arts, dance, interval training, circuit training, and more! Enjoying what you are doing is KEY.

3. Decide whether going to a gym or perhaps a home workout program will work best for you. For me, home-programming changed my life. I used to spend three hours a day going to the gym. Between packing a bag, driving, working out, and driving back, it was three hours. I then discovered home-programming, which took a fraction of the time (sometimes as little as twenty-five minutes a day), and believe it or not, my results were BETTER! Although I am a group fitness instructor, we instructors need motivation and guidance too! After having my son Giorgio, I just never had the time or luxury to go to a gym. I did my workouts at home while my son was asleep because that was, and still is, my only option. Home workouts have come a long way since the days of leg warmers and leotards and grapevines. But you need to decide what works best for you. Some people need the energy of a live-class, and that is ok too! In my newly released weight-loss program, "FROM SCRATCH," it is gym- or home-friendly; that is what is so great about it.

After you figure out the above, you will then need to schedule this into your calendar just like your baby's doctor appointments. Make it non-negotiable. No excuses, remember? Not only will you feel better, but you will release stress and have more energy.

Stop Looking at the Scale!

One of the first things I tell my clients is to forget about looking at the scale. Just forget it exists. In fact, throw your scale away. Ok well, you don't have to take it that far...but seriously, hide it away for a while. Why? Because no one likes a liar. OK, maybe I am being a bit harsh, but you will see why.

Do you know how many people tell me that they stopped working out because they gained weight, or that they were getting "bulky?" I could scream and then roll myself downhill. It makes for a funny mental picture, but yes, that is how angry it makes me.

Let's get something straight, moms: working out is not going to make you gain weight. Overeating will! What happens when we start working out is that our body's metabolism will speed up. A faster metabolism is great; however, you will need to fuel your body a little bit more as well and seriously hydrate.

The hydration alone is the biggest element I need to address. Do you know how many people mistake dehydration for hunger? Millions! If you are drinking half your body weight in fluid oz., that alone will reduce your appetite to half and increase energy and weight loss tremendously. What happens sometimes is people start overeating due to the increase in metabolism, or starve themselves all day and then overeat at night. We all know what that does, right? That is a great way to gain weight, so just don't do that and you won't gain weight. I know I make it sound simpler than it is but remember, it's all the mindset! The actual equation is simple.

Ok, another reason your weight can go up on the scale if you are not truly gaining weight is because you are gaining muscle. I am sure you have already heard that muscle weighs more than fat, right? It is true. Every year, based on your athletic performance, you will gain new muscle or new fat. With this said, your body composition will change with time. Following me so far? To sum this up, we cannot compare a previous year's weight with the following year's weight since the distribution of fat and muscle will keep changing as we become more or less fit. Pounds are just not the most accurate way of judging your success with weight management.

Just remember that you may be heavier on the scale as you start a new program at first, and this is temporary. Let me explain why. As you start to build your muscles, you may gain a few pounds because like I said, muscle weighs more than fat. BUT, the more muscle mass you have, the more calories you burn. So if you increase a few pounds in muscle, number one you will look better, AND more importantly, the amount of calories you will now burn moving forward will be far more than before, thus making your future weight loss goals much faster and efficient to achieve. You have to be patient and trust the system. Does this make sense?

The best way to judge your success is by taking measurements or perhaps working on fitting into a particular clothing size. The first thing my clients say to me, for example, is "Do you think I can lose 20 pounds in two months?" My answer is, "What size clothing would you be happy fitting into? If we get you into that size, will you be happy?" They always reply, "Yes." After all, if you are fitting into a pair of pants several sizes smaller than when you started, that would put a smile on your face, right?

Check out the picture below that shows you muscle vs. fat. Although the muscle will weigh more, you will have a more lean and toned look, yay! The best time to take your measurements is at the very beginning, and then every 30 days after that. Be sure to also take before and after pictures of yourself. Although the scale lies, pictures typically do not. Wear the same outfit for your before and after, and try to wear something that shows your body, such as a bathing suit or sports bra and shorts. Don't be camera shy! This is for your eyes only.

Example of Fat Vs. Muscle

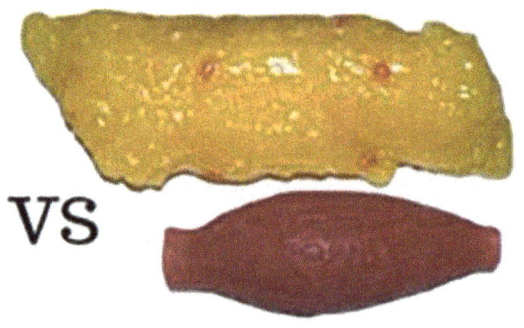

How to Take Your Measurements

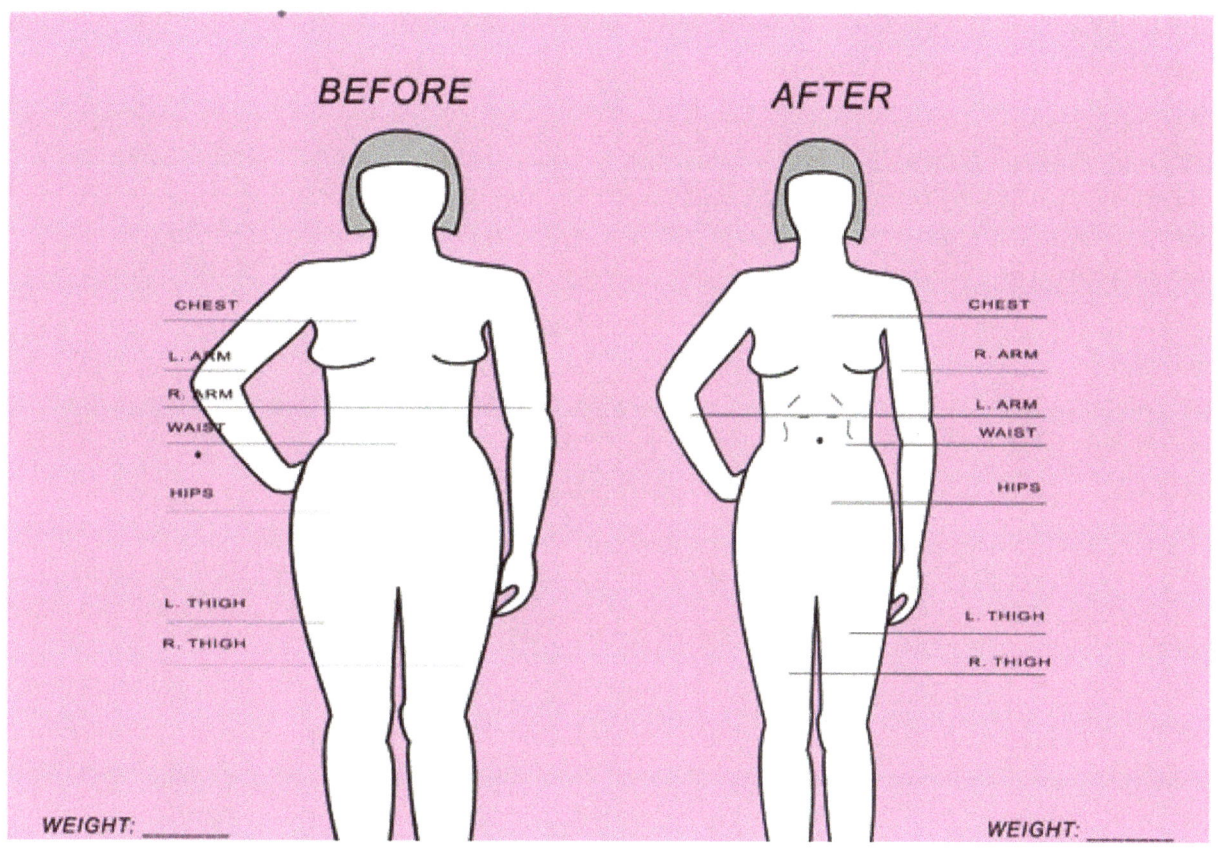

Finding a Success Partner

At the end of the day, the only person who is going to get you to do something is yourself. However, it never hurts to set up a support system for when the going gets tough. As people, we love to have partners. We have many other essential needs, including the need to be appreciated, respected, and accepted. We also all love when we get recognition on a job well done. Whether you ask a friend, a spouse, or perhaps join a group, this support system will be like your core: it will help hold everything together and keep you feeling strong.

Although I do love to work one-on-one with my clients, I also offer online coaching for those who may not live nearby. One of my favorite offerings to my clients is my online motivation and accountability groups. While I offer daily motivation and tips, members are encouraged to also post and share their journey with the rest of the group. It not only motivates the others to do the same, but it becomes a family of ongoing support.

My groups are mainly mothers who do not have time to go to the gym or cannot afford a personal trainer. Instead, I will put them on a home program and they have the responsibility of checking into our online accountability group each day. They get rewarded for participating and everyone has somewhere they can go to vent about their struggles or just to have some bragging rights.

Support systems are amazing because *they work*, it is just that simple. So before you begin your journey, ask a friend, your partner, or perhaps join a group where you can both keep each other accountable. Be sure the person is on the same mission as you so you can both be on the same page. You can set monthly goals for each other and then celebrate at the end of the month when you have accomplished these goals together. Setting incentives for each other is always fun. You can even have a one-on-one competition with each other. Who can shed more inches by the end of the month? Just don't overdo it; be healthy about it, make it fun!

Be aware: there will be haters. You know, the people who will want to deter you from doing well due to their own incompetencies. They may even mock you. Just remember, haters are only hating because they are mad at themselves for not doing what you are doing. So when you get a hater asking you why you are doing this or that, take it as a compliment that you are moving in the right direction. Your efforts are being noticed. Then guess what? That same person will probably reach out to you after you have success to ask you to help them! The irony always cracks me up, but that's a fact of life.

Saving the Best Recipe for Last

Ingredients

Self-Love

Directions

Create and practice every day.

Remember at the end of the day, your baby does not care about the extra pounds on your tush, and your family will love you unconditionally because you are a beautiful person inside and out. You just created the miracle of life. You are a superhero, a mighty mamma! Remember to not be too hard on yourself. Give yourself a break and start your goals when you are ready. Have fun with it; try not to make goals a punishment. Train your mind to see it as a fun adventure.

Giving yourself the gift of health is a blessing and should be a beautiful journey. Remember what we discussed at the beginning, which was training your mind, and with this, the body will follow. Remember to appreciate who you are and love every inch about yourself. You are special and unique. There is no one like you in the world, remember that. There is no such thing as perfect, so don't try to be.

Remember, we create our own realities. You will have times of destruction when life seems to be falling apart, and then you will have times of victory, where the world is all yours for the taking. You will cry your eyes out one day, and the next day you will feel like a rock star. That is life! Just remember love is the ultimate, most important ingredient to add to every one of your plates. You will have many plates to fill! So fill each plate with love. Whether you are feeding your baby her first teaspoon of vegetable puree, cooking a beautiful beef tenderloin for your family, or enjoying that chocolate truffle with a glass of wine, do it with LOVE, and I promise, you will be able to add ANYTHING to your plate.

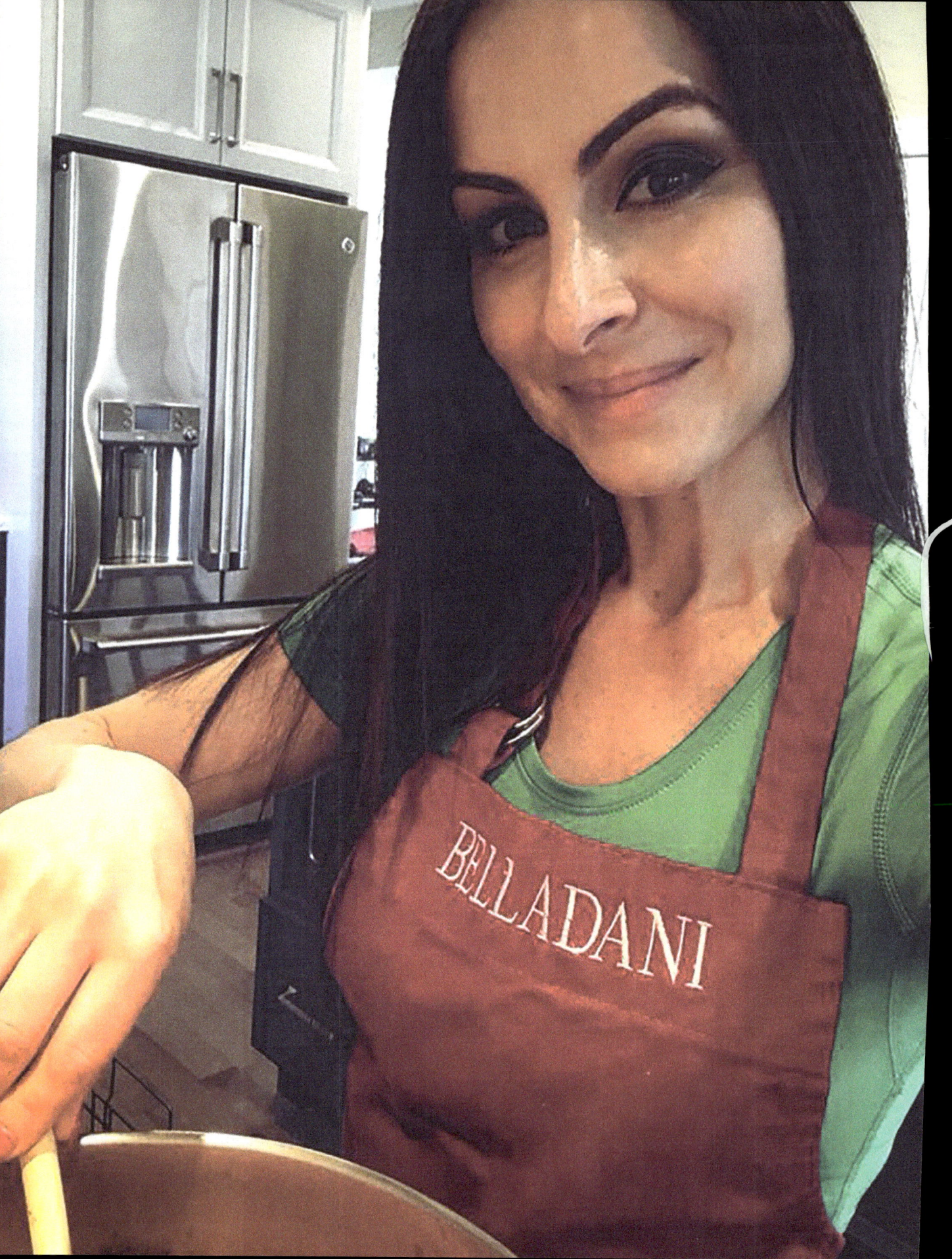

ACKNOWLEDGEMENTS

As we all know it takes many ingredients to make a recipe just right!

Thanks to everyone that helped season this book:

To my food testing team of moms, Rachel DiGiorgio, Sara Garcia, Gina Amato-Souza, Diana Muccio, Nadia Barsamian, and Jaclyn Davin. I could not have done this without you guys! Thank you for all your honest, constructive criticism and feedback to perfect these recipes!

To my good friend and talented chef, Eric Bogardus, for helping me make the dishes in this book photo ready! You are a food styling machine! Thank you for all the hours you spent with me in my kitchen perfecting each dish, making the camera drool with envy.

To my food photographer, Lauren Pariseau, for making my vision come to life. The photos in this book totally exceeded my expectations, thank you for all your hard work.

To my fitness photographer and friend, Stewart Smith. Thank you for always making me feel so comfortable in front of the camera. You have such great talent. Thank you for always capturing the perfect moment.

To Janet Choup, my hair and makeup hero! Thank you for always making me photo ready! You always know how to glam me up just right!

To my bestie, Candice Talbot. Thank you for the unlimited and forever support of your friendship. I don't know how I could get by without you. Thank you for always helping me find humor in every situation, especially the challenges of motherhood. Having you in my life makes every day so much more fun.

To my family, without you, I would not have all the right ingredients to make me who I am today. Thank you for seasoning my life, adding in the perfect spice, and creating so many memories never to forget. I love you all so much.

www.ingramcontent.com/pod-product-compliance
Lightning Source LLC
Chambersburg PA
CBHW061752290426
44108CB00029B/2974